Serious Games and Mixed Reality Applications for Healthcare

Serious Games and Mixed Reality Applications for Healthcare

Editors

Marco Gesi
Sara Condino
Giuseppe Turini
Rosanna Maria Viglialoro
Marina Carbone

MDPI • Basel • Beijing • Wuhan • Barcelona • Belgrade • Manchester • Tokyo • Cluj • Tianjin

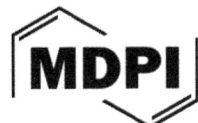

Editors
Marco Gesi
University of Pisa
Italy

Sara Condino
University of Pisa
Italy

Giuseppe Turini
Kettering University
USA

Rosanna Maria Viglialoro
University of Pisa
Italy

Marina Carbone
University of Pisa
Italy

Editorial Office
MDPI
St. Alban-Anlage 66
4052 Basel, Switzerland

This is a reprint of articles from the Special Issue published online in the open access journal *Applied Sciences* (ISSN 2076-3417) (available at: https://www.mdpi.com/journal/applsci/special_issues/Serious_Games_Mixed_Reality_Applications_Healthcare).

For citation purposes, cite each article independently as indicated on the article page online and as indicated below:

LastName, A.A.; LastName, B.B.; LastName, C.C. Article Title. *Journal Name* **Year**, *Volume Number*, Page Range.

ISBN 978-3-0365-4151-8 (Hbk)
ISBN 978-3-0365-4152-5 (PDF)

© 2022 by the authors. Articles in this book are Open Access and distributed under the Creative Commons Attribution (CC BY) license, which allows users to download, copy and build upon published articles, as long as the author and publisher are properly credited, which ensures maximum dissemination and a wider impact of our publications.

The book as a whole is distributed by MDPI under the terms and conditions of the Creative Commons license CC BY-NC-ND.

Contents

About the Editors vii

Sara Condino, Marco Gesi, Rosanna Maria Viglialoro, Marina Carbone and Giuseppe Turini
Serious Games and Mixed Reality Applications for Healthcare
Reprinted from: *Appl. Sci.* 2022, 12, 3644, doi:10.3390/app12073644 1

Christos Karapapas and Christos Goumopoulos
Mild Cognitive Impairment Detection Using Machine Learning Models Trained on Data Collected from Serious Games
Reprinted from: *Appl. Sci.* 2021, 11, 8184, doi:10.3390/app11178184 5

Vânia Guimarães, Elsa Oliveira, Alberto Carvalho, Nuno Cardoso, Johannes Emerich, Chantale Dumoulin, Nathalie Swinnen, Jacqueline De Jong and Eling D. de Bruin
An Exergame Solution for Personalized Multicomponent Training in Older Adults
Reprinted from: *Appl. Sci.* 2021, 11, 7986, doi:10.3390/app11177986 35

Serhii Shapoval, Begoña García Zapirain, Amaia Mendez Zorrilla and Iranzu Mugueta-Aguinaga
Biofeedback Applied to Interactive Serious Games to Monitor Frailty in an Elderly Population
Reprinted from: *Appl. Sci.* 2021, 11, 3502, doi:10.3390/app11083502 53

Alexandra Sipatchin, Miguel García García and Siegfried Wahl
Target Maintenance in Gaming via Saliency Augmentation: An Early-Stage Scotoma Simulation Study Using Virtual Reality (VR)
Reprinted from: *Appl. Sci.* 2021, 11, 7164, doi:10.3390/ app11157164 83

Yen-Ting Chen, Chun-Ju Hou, Natan Derek, Shuo-Bin Huang, Min-Wei Huang and You-Yu Wang
Evaluation of the Reaction Time and Accuracy Rate in Normal Subjects, MCI, and Dementia Using Serious Games
Reprinted from: *Appl. Sci.* 2021, 11, 628, doi:10.3390/app11020628 99

Nuno M. C. da Costa, Estela Bicho, Flora Ferreira, Estela Vilhena and Nuno S. Dias
A Multivariate Randomized Controlled Experiment about the Effects of Mindfulness Priming on EEG Neurofeedback Self- Regulation Serious Games
Reprinted from: *Appl. Sci.* 2021, 11, 7725, doi:10.3390/app11167725 113

Sara Condino, Giuseppe Turini, Virginia Mamone, Paolo Domenico Parchi and Vincenzo Ferrari
Hybrid Spine Simulator Prototype for X-ray Free Pedicle Screws Fixation Training
Reprinted from: *Appl. Sci.* 2021, 11, 1038, doi:10.3390/app11031038 137

Rosanna Maria Viglialoro, Sara Condino, Giuseppe Turini, Marina Carbone, Vincenzo Ferrari and Marco Gesi
Augmented Reality, Mixed Reality, and Hybrid Approach in Healthcare Simulation: A Systematic Review
Reprinted from: *Appl. Sci.* 2021, 11, 2338, doi:10.3390/app11052338 155

About the Editors

Marco Gesi

Marco Gesi (Full Professor) graduated from Pisa University (Italy) with a degree in Pharmacy in 1993, and subsequently gained his Ph.D. in 1997, the specialization in Pharmacology in 2000 and a degree in Physiotherapy in 2007. He is: Vice-Rector for Local Authority Relations, and the Delegate for Sport; Director of the departmental center of rehabilitation medicine "Sport and Anatomy"; President of the degree course in Physiotherapy at the University of Pisa; Director of the Joint Council for the post-graduate courses in Sports Physiotherapy, Hydrokinesis Therapy and the Theory and Techniques of Athletic Preparation for Football and Director of the proficiency course in Anatomy and Fascial Manipulation. Teaching Activity: Human Anatomy in Pharmacy, Pharmaceutical Chemistry and Technology and in Medicine and Surgery, and in the short cycle degree courses, specialization courses and in the Schools of Specialization of the departments in the Area of Health Science. Member of the Italian Society of Anatomy and Histology. Since 2012, he collaborates with the EndoCAS Research Center of University of Pisa for the development of applications of virtual/mixed/augmented reality; medical and surgical simulators; navigation surgical simulation. He published 2 books, 3 Teaching Manuals and over 300 papers or chapters.

Sara Condino

Sara Condino (Post Doc Researcher) received the master degree in Biomedical engineering from the University of Pisa, Italy, in 2008. She received the PhD degree from the University of Pisa, Italy, in 2012, with a thesis regarding the development of an electromagnetic navigation system for endovascular surgery and new strategies for innovative medical devices testing. At the present time her research is carried out in the context of computer-assisted surgery and in the development of innovative technologies based on virtual reality, physical and hybrid simulation for rehabilitation specialists. She is author of scientific papers on ISI journals and patents. In march 2012 she also founded a spin-off company: e-SPres3D s.r.l. The company offers high profile technological services to plan and simulate surgical interventions deploying the information contained inside the volumetric radiological images.

Giuseppe Turini

Giuseppe Turini (Associate Professor) received his M.Sc. in Computer Science from the University of Pisa (Italy) in 2004, specializing in computer graphics. In the same year he joined the Visual Computing Lab of the CNR-ISTI in Pisa (Italy), where he started working in computational geometry, and in particular on the processing of volumetric tetrahedral meshes for interactive physics simulation.

In 2005, he started working as a research fellow at the EndoCAS Research Center: the research center for computer-assisted surgery of the University of Pisa (Italy). During this period, he worked on the design and development of research grade software applications for minimally-invasive and robotic surgery as well as medical imaging. Then in 2011, he received his Ph.D. in Health Technologies (Computer Engineering) from the University of Pisa (Italy).

One year later, in 2012, he started working at Kettering University (Flint, Michigan, USA), where he is now an Associate Professor of Computer Science. Nevertheless, he still continues the collaboration with the EndoCAS Research Center as a visiting research associate.

His main research interests are in the fields of: computer graphics visualization, interactive physics simulation, computer-assisted surgery, medical imaging, human-computer interactions, virtual and augmented reality, and serious game development.

Rosanna Maria Viglialoro

Rosanna Maria Viglialoro (Post Doc Researcher) received the master degree in Biomedical engineering from the University of Pisa, Italy, in 2012. She received her Ph.D. inTranslational research and of new surgical and medical technologies", at University of Pisa, in 2018. Her main research interests are related to: mixed/augmented reality; surgical simulation; innovative technologies based on AR for rehabilitation specialists. She is author of scientific papers on ISI journals and of a patent.

Marina Carbone

Marina Carbone (Post Doc Researcher) received the master degree in Biomedical engineering from the University of Pisa, Italy, in 2009. She received her Ph.D. in Innovative Technologies at Scuola Superiore sant'Anna, Pisa, in 2013. Since 2009 she works in the EndoCAS center for computer assisted surgery joining in 2014 the Department of Information Engineering. Her main research interests are related to: medical Image segmentation and registration, surgical navigators, Augmented Reality based solutions for simulation and navigation, development and validation of surgical simulators also for medical/surgical training purposes. In march 2012 she also founded a spin-off company: e-SPres3D s.r.l. The company offers high profile technological services to plan and simulate surgical interventions deploying the information contained inside the volumetric radiological images.

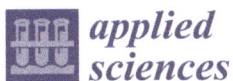

Editorial

Serious Games and Mixed Reality Applications for Healthcare

Sara Condino [1,*], Marco Gesi [2,3], Rosanna Maria Viglialoro [2], Marina Carbone [1] and Giuseppe Turini [4]

[1] Department of Information Engineering, University of Pisa, 56126 Pisa, Italy; marina.carbone@endocas.unipi.it
[2] Department of Translational Research and of New Surgical and Medical Technologies, University of Pisa, 56126 Pisa, Italy; marco.gesi@unipi.it (M.G.); rosanna.viglialoro@endocas.unipi.it (R.M.V.)
[3] Center for Rehabilitative Medicine "Sport and Anatomy", University of Pisa, 56121 Pisa, Italy
[4] Department of Computer Science, Kettering University, Flint, MI 48504, USA; gturini@kettering.edu
* Correspondence: sara.condino@unipi.it; Tel.: +39-050-995689

1. Introduction

Serious games are games in which the main goal is not entertainment, but a serious purpose ranging from the acquisition of knowledge to interactive training, to name just a few. These games are emerging as a promising educational technique across various domains (such as the military, education, politics, management, and engineering) and are attracting growing attention in healthcare thanks to the possibility of: increasing the level of interactivity of the application and the motivation of the user, allowing adaptation to the user's level of competence, flexibility over time, repeatability, and continuous feedback.

In recent years, there has been a growing interest in applying virtual reality (VR) techniques to the development of serious games for creating immersive experiences. VR and augmented reality (AR) have a long history in the healthcare sector, offering the opportunity to develop a wide range of tools and applications aiming at improving the quality of care and efficiency of services for professionals and patients alike.

The best-known examples of VR/AR applications in the healthcare domain include surgical planning and medical training by means of simulation technologies. The techniques used in surgical simulation have also been applied to cognitive and motor rehabilitation, pain management, and patient and professional education.

Recently, healthcare has also become one of the biggest adopters of mixed reality (MR), which merges real and VR content to generate new environments where physical and digital objects not only co-exist but are also capable of interacting with each other in real time. MR encompasses both VR and AR applications.

These novel applications are attracting growing attention from users and researchers, but many cognitive and perceptual issues still need to be completely understood and resolved to fully take advantage of the disruptive potential of these emerging technologies in healthcare, and to minimize side effects of VR/AR technologies such as "cybersickness". Moreover, efforts should be made to strengthen the experience of "presence", the level of acceptance, and the compatibility of MR technology with the general population (including the elderly and sick people).

In light of the above, this Special Issue was introduced to gather and publish original scientific contributions that explore opportunities and address the challenges of serious games, VR/AR, and MR applications in healthcare. There were 11 papers submitted to this Special Issue, and 8 papers were accepted.

2. Serious Games in Healthcare

Various topics have been addressed in this Special Issue, mainly focused on the description of innovative serious games with applications in the field of rehabilitation/training of elderly people or patients with degenerative diseases [1–5], and training for self-regulation of mental states [6].

The collected papers cover some of the key points in the development of serious games, namely: development of interactive and engaging tasks to increase user motivation, acquisition and analysis of quantitative data, and adaptation to the user's conditions.

In Sipatchin et al. [4], VR is proposed as a new assisting tool for patients suffering from macular degeneration. More specifically, a VR game that involves tracking and detecting changes in a moving object is proposed to re-define traditional tasks used for preferred retinal locus development studies and therapy, which can be repetitive, exhaustive, and tedious, ending in a decrease in the subject's motivation. Gamification, in this context, was intended to develop more entertaining tasks, resulting in greater participant engagement and rapid adaptation.

One of the possibilities offered by serious games for rehabilitation/training is the collection and analysis of quantitative data for different purposes, such as: to assess the initial disease state and/or exercise performance, and to monitor the patient's progress during therapy, just to name a few.

Three papers of this collection [1,3,5] focus on collecting and analyzing quantitative data, and two of them [1,3] employ artificial intelligence (AI) techniques. AI is becoming an important major asset for serious games to provide more facilities for the learner, but also more knowledge for the supervisor (educator, medical specialist, etc.) [7].

Shapoval et al. [3] describe the integration of biofeedback into a serious game to monitor frailty in an elderly population. The system is suitable for everyday use at home, but also for more in-depth observation of various biological parameters, such as the heart rate and temperature. It features a real-time tracking system of the body position, relying on the use of a webcam and a built-in motion recognition algorithm based on a neural network, for controlling the game and for analyzing the patient's activity. Acquired data may be subject to medical secrecy rules and will not be available to anyone other than the treating physician and the patient to monitor the outcome and progress of the rehabilitation process for different degrees and types of musculoskeletal disorders. All the data obtained can be visualized and examined at any time, thanks to a cloud interface where all the information is duplicated.

Karapapas et al. [1] propose the use of a serious game for early detection of mild cognitive impairment (MCI), which is an indicative precursor of Alzheimer's disease. More specifically, their work intends to test whether performance data collected during sessions of a serious game, specifically conceived for cognitive assessment and training of elderly people, can be used to create machine learning (ML) models to classify the patient's cognitive status.

Investigating the deterioration of cognitive functions is also the goal of the research work by Chen et al. [5]. Their serious game was designed in collaboration with psychologists and clinicians to be as simple as possible, given that the target patients are elderly and that most of them have no experience in playing video games. The aim of the game is to measure the subjects' performance, in terms of the reaction time and accuracy rate in reaching a target, to classify their cognitive abilities and distinguish normal subjects from MCI subjects and subjects with dementia.

Traditional sensing devices employed for serious games in rehabilitation include optical and inertial sensors. According to [2], the Microsoft Kinect (a 3D sensor based on time-of-flight technology and the intensity modulation technique [8]) is usually the preferred choice to track full-body movements, although accuracy drops when complex movements are executed. In Shapoval et al. [3], the main sensor required is a simple USB webcam: this makes the platform more affordable from the financial standpoint, and easy to install and use.

One work in this Special Issue by Guimarães et al. [2] employs two inertial sensors (one for each user foot) to simplify the setup and reduce costs. This serious game is designed to support personalized and multicomponent clinical interventions for older adults, and, more specifically, the goal is to train strength, balance, cognition, and the pelvic floor muscle, in one single session. In this work, reducing the system complexity was preferred over the use of additional sensors for full-body movement evaluation.

Recent studies have also integrated biosensors into games designed for physical rehabilitation and for the treatment of cognitive and neurological disorders. Biosensors indeed can be integrated into games to study the biological data of the participants during play as well as making games adaptive based on information extracted from the patient's bio-signals [9].

In this Special Issue, da Costa et al. [6] hypothesized the possibility of developing a "Neurofeedback assisted self-regulation machine" combining the technical, behavioral, psychological, emotional, and electrophysiological components of brain–computer interfaces (BCIs) based on electroencephalography (EEG), neurofeedback training (NFT), mindfulness meditation, and self-regulation of mental states in a single framework. The work investigates "how" a priming intervention right before NFT affects NFT performance and the emotional state, acquired using qualitative emotional state self-reports and quantitative emotional state biomarkers (i.e., galvanic skin response and heart rate variability). The proposed framework could potentially improve the efficacy of self-regulation serious games for therapeutic, performance, or entertainment purposes.

3. Extended Reality Applications and Hybrid Simulation in Healthcare

Among all the papers accepted in this Special Issue, three focused on extended reality (XR) applications and hybrid simulation for the healthcare sector [4,10,11].

Each one of these papers investigated a different aspect of the application of these technologies (VR, AR, MR, and hybrid simulation) in medicine, in particular: introducing VR and gamification in traditional patient treatment [4], using AR and hybrid simulation in medical training [10], and reviewing the current state of the art of AR/MR applications in healthcare simulation [11].

In [4], Sipatchin et al. presented a VR serious game for patients suffering from macular degeneration. This VR application includes both eye tracking of the user and motion tracking of a moving object, and its goal is to modernize conventional therapies for preferred retinal locus development. This novel VR game, by using gamification techniques, can improve patient engagement, motivation, and adaptation.

A hybrid simulator for the training of pedicle screw fixation in the spine was proposed in [10]. In this paper, Condino et al. describe a system for the preoperative planning and rehearsal of spine surgery, with the goal of improving both surgical workflows and postoperative patient outcomes. This hybrid simulation platform combines a 3D printed patient-specific spine model with AR functionalities and virtual X-ray visualization, obviating the need for any harmful radiation during the medical simulation.

Viglialoro et al. [11], in their review paper, summarized and discussed different medical simulators based on AR, MR, and hybrid approaches, analyzing their evaluation and validation as well. This work, by highlighting the drawbacks and advantages of each application, provides some guidelines for developing novel healthcare simulators and also outlines promising research trends in this field for the coming years.

Author Contributions: Conceptualization, S.C., M.G., R.M.V., M.C. and G.T.; methodology, S.C., M.G. and G.T.; validation, S.C., M.G., R.M.V., M.C. and G.T.; formal analysis, S.C. and G.T.; investigation, S.C. and G.T.; data curation, S.C., M.G. and G.T.; writing—original draft preparation, S.C., M.G. and G.T.; writing—review and editing, R.M.V. and M.C.; visualization, S.C., M.G., R.M.V., M.C. and G.T.; supervision, S.C. and G.T.; project administration, S.C., M.G., R.M.V. and G.T.; funding acquisition, S.C. and M.C. All authors have read and agreed to the published version of the manuscript.

Funding: This work was funded by the CRIO2AR project, Fas Salute 2018—Regione Toscana, Linea 3.6. This work was also supported by the Italian Ministry of Education and Research (MIUR) in the framework of the CrossLab project (Departments of Excellence) of the University of Pisa, Laboratory of Augmented Reality.

Acknowledgments: Thanks are due to all the authors, professional reviewers, and the dedicated editorial team of *Applied Sciences* for their valuable contributions to this Special Issue. We would like to take this opportunity to congratulate the authors and express our sincere gratitude to the editorial team of *Applied Sciences*. Special thanks to the Managing Editor for Computing and Artificial Intelligence, for the fruitful support offered that was essential for the success of this Special Issue.

Conflicts of Interest: The authors declare no conflict of interest.

References

1. Karapapas, C.; Goumopoulos, C. Mild Cognitive Impairment Detection Using Machine Learning Models Trained on Data Collected from Serious Games. *Appl. Sci.* **2021**, *11*, 8184. [CrossRef]
2. Guimarães, V.; Oliveira, E.; Carvalho, A.; Cardoso, N.; Emerich, J.; Dumoulin, C.; Swinnen, N.; De Jong, J.; De Bruin, E.D. An Exergame Solution for Personalized Multicomponent Training in Older Adults. *Appl. Sci.* **2021**, *11*, 7986. [CrossRef]
3. Shapoval, S.; García Zapirain, B.; Mendez Zorrilla, A.; Mugueta-Aguinaga, I. Biofeedback Applied to Interactive Serious Games to Monitor Frailty in an Elderly Population. *Appl. Sci.* **2021**, *11*, 3502. [CrossRef]
4. Sipatchin, A.; García García, M.; Wahl, S. Target Maintenance in Gaming via Saliency Augmentation: An Early-Stage Scotoma Simulation Study Using Virtual Reality (VR). *Appl. Sci.* **2021**, *11*, 7164. [CrossRef]
5. Chen, Y.-T.; Hou, C.-J.; Derek, N.; Huang, S.-B.; Huang, M.-W.; Wang, Y.-Y. Evaluation of the Reaction Time and Accuracy Rate in Normal Subjects, MCI, and Dementia Using Serious Games. *Appl. Sci.* **2021**, *11*, 628. [CrossRef]
6. Da Costa, N.M.C.; Bicho, E.; Ferreira, F.; Vilhena, E.; Dias, N.S. A Multivariate Randomized Controlled Experiment about the Effects of Mindfulness Priming on EEG Neurofeedback Self-Regulation Serious Games. *Appl. Sci.* **2021**, *11*, 7725. [CrossRef]
7. Frutos-Pascual, M.; Zapirain, B.G. Review of the Use of AI Techniques in Serious Games: Decision Making and Machine Learning. *IEEE Trans. Comput. Intell. AI Games* **2017**, *9*, 133–152. [CrossRef]
8. Caruso, L.; Russo, R.; Savino, S. Microsoft Kinect V2 vision system in a manufacturing application. *Robot. Comput.-Integr. Manuf.* **2017**, *48*, 174–181. [CrossRef]
9. Hughes, A.; Jorda, S. Applications of Biological and Physiological Signals in Commercial Video Gaming and Game Research: A Review. *Front. Comput. Sci.* **2021**, *3*, 37. [CrossRef]
10. Condino, S.; Turini, G.; Mamone, V.; Parchi, P.D.; Ferrari, V. Hybrid Spine Simulator Prototype for X-ray Free Pedicle Screws Fixation Training. *Appl. Sci.* **2021**, *11*, 1038. [CrossRef]
11. Viglialoro, R.M.; Condino, S.; Turini, G.; Carbone, M.; Ferrari, V.; Gesi, M. Augmented Reality, Mixed Reality, and Hybrid Approach in Healthcare Simulation: A Systematic Review. *Appl. Sci.* **2021**, *11*, 2338. [CrossRef]

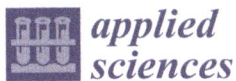

Article

Mild Cognitive Impairment Detection Using Machine Learning Models Trained on Data Collected from Serious Games

Christos Karapapas and Christos Goumopoulos *

Information & Communication Systems Engineering Department, University of the Aegean, 83200 Samos, Greece; icsdm117025@icsd.aegean.gr
* Correspondence: goumop@aegean.gr; Tel.: +30-22-730-82220

Abstract: Mild cognitive impairment (MCI) is an indicative precursor of Alzheimer's disease and its early detection is critical to restrain further cognitive deterioration through preventive measures. In this context, the capacity of serious games combined with machine learning for MCI detection is examined. In particular, a custom methodology is proposed, which consists of a series of steps to train and evaluate classification models that could discriminate healthy from cognitive impaired individuals on the basis of game performance and other subjective data. Such data were collected during a pilot evaluation study of a gaming platform, called COGNIPLAT, with 10 seniors. An exploratory analysis of the data is performed to assess feature selection, model overfitting, optimization techniques and classification performance using several machine learning algorithms and standard evaluation metrics. A production level model is also trained to deal with the issue of data leakage while delivering a high detection performance (92.14% accuracy, 93.4% sensitivity and 90% specificity) based on the Gaussian Naive Bayes classifier. This preliminary study provides initial evidence that serious games combined with machine learning methods could potentially serve as a complementary or an alternative tool to the traditional cognitive screening processes.

Keywords: mild cognitive impairment; serious games; machine learning; feature selection; data transformations; classification; elderly

Citation: Karapapas, C.; Goumopoulos, C. Mild Cognitive Impairment Detection Using Machine Learning Models Trained on Data Collected from Serious Games. *Appl. Sci.* **2021**, *11*, 8184. https://doi.org/10.3390/app11178184

Academic Editor: Marco Gesi

Received: 27 July 2021
Accepted: 30 August 2021
Published: 3 September 2021

Publisher's Note: MDPI stays neutral with regard to jurisdictional claims in published maps and institutional affiliations.

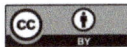

Copyright: © 2021 by the authors. Licensee MDPI, Basel, Switzerland. This article is an open access article distributed under the terms and conditions of the Creative Commons Attribution (CC BY) license (https://creativecommons.org/licenses/by/4.0/).

1. Introduction

Studies have shown that the cognitive functions of the elderly are negatively affected by a number of factors, such as heredity, lifestyle (e.g., diet, smoking, alcohol), and age-related pathological conditions [1]. With regard to normal aging, it appears that many cognitive functions remain stable throughout life with mild attenuation beginning gradually in the sixth or seventh decade of life [2]. Mild cognitive impairment (MCI) is often labeled as a precursor of dementia and especially of Alzheimer's disease (AD) [3] or just as an intermediate level of cognitive function that is lower compared to what is considered normal for a certain age and an educational level [4].

The current approach of MCI diagnosis is through a clinical check-up, performed by a specialist, that includes an interview with the subject, the collection of the subject's medical history, a series of neurological examinations to test the mobility, the balance, the functionality of the nervous system and finally a cognitive assessment, such as the Mini Mental State Examination (MMSE) [5] or the Montreal Cognitive Assessment (MoCA) [6]. Although this approach provides the specialist with a wealth of information, beyond an assessment score, which is assistive in drawing safe conclusions about the cognitive level of the subject, it also presents some disadvantages. Given that the assessment is part of a clinical check-up, the potential anxiety of the subject along with other convoluted factors might result in a decreased performance. This situation combined with the low repeatability of the clinical check-ups may lead to distorted assessments [7].

An aspect of the MCI detection is the stage at which it is performed. According to a research that was conducted with a cohort of 139 subjects and included two MoCA assessments with a difference of 3.5 years, subjects with normal cognition during their first assessment maintained their cognitive levels until the second assessment, whereas subjects with MCI during the first assessment presented an average decline of 1.7 units on the MoCA scale [8]. This suggests that the cognitive level of people with MCI has the tendency to decline faster, something that makes the early detection of MCI an important factor in cognitive intervention programs.

On the other hand, the evolution of technology now provides the possibility of MCI detection through computer programs, electronic games and mobile devices [9]. These innovations seem to be gaining ground in the field of cognitive screening compared to traditional methods, as they are less costly, more flexible, provide better administration conditions and more people have now access to these tools. In the same context, the development of serious games as a cognitive assessment and screening tool is an innovative practice that uses computer software to combine randomized visual, auditory and tactile stimuli, as a simulation of various everyday situations of the individual [10]. Such tools can provide the user with the sense of an engaging three-dimensional reality which encourages the implementation of the method in research and clinical practice.

Serious games are games that have an explicit and carefully designed educational purpose and are not intended to be used primarily for entertainment even though this does not prohibit the inclusion of enjoyment and fun aspects [11]. They have been used in several application domains, such as education, business, finance, cultural heritage, health and military training. In particular, in the healthcare domain the aim is to introduce innovative methods in the care, general health and rehabilitation processes, where the patient is less dependent on professionals. Serious games can be designed to bring about some behavior change in the patient, whether it is for prevention, treatment or for information about the disease.

The general goal of this work is to contribute to the research in the field of early MCI detection. Since MCI is a characteristic precursor of AD and other neurodegenerative conditions, early diagnosis is critical to restrain cognitive deterioration through preventive and rehabilitation measures. In the relevant literature, one can find numerous references to studies where serious games are utilized to support cognitive screening [12] or even rehabilitation [13] in a more engaging and fun way [14]. However, the specific objective of this work is to answer the research question of whether game performance data gathered during playing several sessions of serious games that were specifically designed for cognitive assessment and training of elderly people can be utilized to create machine learning (ML) models that could accurately classify users to the right cognitive state. The ultimate goal would then be, to make use of these models to classify new users to distinct cognitive levels judging by their in-game performance. The challenges that must be addressed in order to build such a model and to provide a service that would enable access of such a model for new data, were also investigated in this work.

2. Related Work

In the recent literature, a plethora of studies have been reported that demonstrate the advantages serious games are providing in order to improve the detection and evaluation of neurodegenerative diseases and precursor conditions of them, such as MCI. The research types of studies range from literature reviews [15], surveys [16] and methodological reviews [17], to more specialized research topics such as the use of special game-based metrics to detect MCI [18].

Although the perspective of using ML techniques to address cognitive screening in combination with serious games is mentioned in a few related works, eventually the problem is typically solved by employing statistical methods and correlations and the use of non-ML algorithms [12]. Furthermore, applying ML does not necessarily imply that a model is used directly to detect whether a subject has characteristics that are in the range of MCI. Instead there are plenty of cases that make use of ML for various other reasons. For example, in the work of Leduc-McNiven et al. [19], the use of reinforcement learning

(RL) techniques is demonstrated for the augmentation of the dataset with synthetic data so that when the data reach a sufficient volume, a classifier model could be trained to categorize new players based on their in-game performance. In a follow-up study by the same research group they leveraged bots simulating various degrees of impairment to produce synthetic data and on dense neural networks in order to explore the perspective to classify playing ranging from perfect to various degrees of impairment [20].

In the work of Solana et al. [21] the design and development of an algorithm is described that plays the role of a decision-making system which is built using data mining techniques. The system not only has the ability to classify the users by the level of cognitive impairment but it is also able to select the most appropriate tasks for each individual, in terms of game playing difficulty, thus aiming at cognitive improvement.

In the work of Banerjee et al. [22] a different approach regarding the ML methodology followed is given focusing on the datasets and the techniques applied on them. In particular, three different datasets were created composed of different feature subsets. Furthermore, the ML experiment is conducted four times, each time using a different technique for the model training process. Similar approaches can also be found in the methodology of our work, for example there are multiple datasets based on the selected features and there are multiple repetitions of the experiment that each employs a different training technique.

Another study that explores the potential of digital games in the detection of early symptoms of cognitive decline is reported by Sirály et al. [23]. A particular characteristic is the use of magnetic resonance imaging (MRI) to measure the volume of the cerebral structures as well as the use of several traditional cognitive screening tests including the neurophysiological test paired associates learning (PAL). A total of 34 subjects participated in the study playing the memory game 'Find the pair' and the main goal was to investigate the correlation between the MRI findings and the PAL results with the memory game results. The statistical analysis conducted based on Logistic Regression suggests that the number of trials a subject needs to complete the memory game could be used as an indicator to determine if the subject belongs to the healthy or the MCI group.

The work of Binaco et al. [24] presents a methodology that builds ML models trained on data from a digitized version of the well-known clock drawing test (CDT), which can be found also as part of the MoCA assessment. This specific work can be described as mostly a ML methods study since more focus is given to the methods needed to better prepare the dataset and the algorithms to train the classifiers, rather than to the evaluation of the models. For example, the SMOTE (synthetic minority oversampling technique) method is utilized to compensate for the minority class. Furthermore, three different neural networks are explored, multiple feature sets are selected, and the steps taken in the direction of optimization and more specifically to avoid overfitting are described. A detail that is interesting is the analysis of the challenges and the benefits that would arise in case a multi-class classification problem is targeted instead of a binary one. Both cases were examined with the binary classifiers resulting in a higher performance.

A work that lies in the same context to our research and includes the process of training classifier models based on in-game data is that of Valladares-Rodríguez et al. [25]. The scope of this study is much broader, since it also includes the process of creating the serious games, the selection of a suitable focus group, the inspection of collected data from a statistical point of view, the classifier training and finally the evaluation of the serious games based on participant's replies to the Game Experience Questionnaire. Regarding the classification models, three ML algorithms have been used, with a single dataset composed of features automatically selected based on their importance as calculated by a Random Forest based model. An evaluation study was performed with 16 seniors, including AD, MCI and healthy individuals as assessed by the MMSE scale. A dataset of 89 instances was assembled with several variables derived from the three games used. The binary classification model that was trained using logistic regression and support vector machine achieved an absolute prediction with no false negatives. Except for accuracy, the false positive and false negative ratios were measured, along with the metric of F-measure defined as the weighted harmonic mean of precision and recall.

To summarize there are only a few studies that are targeting MCI detection leveraging on ML models trained on data collected from serious games. Moreover, between the existing approaches there are significant differences in terms of the screening tools and the cutoff scores employed for assessing ground truth cognitive states, the game tasks involved, the cognitive functions targeted, the features engineered for model training, the ML methods applied, the measures taken to prevent high model bias/variance and the provision of an endpoint to access online classification services for new data. This entails that a simple comparison between existing methods may not be practical and that the discussion should take into consideration several characteristics. Table 1 provides an overview of such characteristics in order to associate our work to similar studies on MCI detection.

Table 1. Characteristics of related studies on MCI detection based on ML and game data.

Study	Game Suite	Subjects	Features	Classes	Dataset	ML Methods [a]	Accuracy	Bias [b]	CSAPI [c]
This work	COGNIPLAT platform	10	Game performance and demographic data	Healthy, MCI	119 game sessions	DT, GNB, kNN, LR, MLP, RF, SVM	92.14%	Addressed	Yes
[19,20]	War Cognitive Assessment Tool	Bots simulating various degrees of impairment to produce synthetic data	Game timing and hand tuned features	Random play, 75%/50%/25% impairment, perfect play	110,000 games played by bots	DNN	96.2%	Addressed	No
[23]	'Find the Pairs' memory game	34	Number of attempts and game completion time as predictor variables	Healthy, MCI	40 game sessions	LR for correlation analysis	Not applicable	Not applicable	No
[24]	Digital Clock Drawing Test	163	Dimensions and orientation of clock components, drawing time, drift from ideal placement	AD, MCI subtypes (binary classification combinations)	163 digital clock drawing tests	NN	83.44–91.49% depending on the binary classification problem	Addressed	No
[25]	Panoramix	16	Game performance data	Healthy, MCI/AD	89 instances	CART, LR, SVM	100%	Not discussed	Yes

[a] CART: Classification and regression trees, DNN: dense neural network, DT: decision tree, GNB: Gaussian Naive Bayes, kNN: k-nearest neighbors, LR: logistic regression, MLP: multi-layer perceptron, NN: neural network, RF: random forest, SVM: support vector machine. [b] Measures to prevent high model bias/variance, overfitting/underfitting avoidance. [c] Classification service application programming interface.

3. Methodology

CRISP-DM (cross-industry standard process for data mining) is one of the most established methodologies to apply data mining tasks [26]. In our approach existing methodologies were studied and adopted as guidelines, with CRISP-DM playing a major role in this procedure, to build a custom methodology consisting of a series of processes, each one focused on a particular task. According to recent studies CRISP-DM is the methodology of choice for several projects in health as well as other domains [27].

Overall, the methodology that was used as a guide for this research could be described as an extension of the CRISP-DM methodology, with the exception of the deployment step which was not applied. Examining the approach in a macroscopic level, the involved steps could be organized into the following four major processes which will be elaborated in the following sections:

- Extract-Transform-Load (ETL)
- Exploratory Data Analysis (EDA)
- Production Model Creation (PMC)
- Classification Service Application Programming Interface (CSAPI)

In Figure 1 an overview of the methodology is given as a general workflow of the processes involved. The association with the game platform employed is also given. The platform on the one hand provides the game data that are used to train the models, and on the other hand, classification results would be requested on demand by implementing a method to send game session's data to the CSAPI component through REST (REpresentational State Transfer) requests.

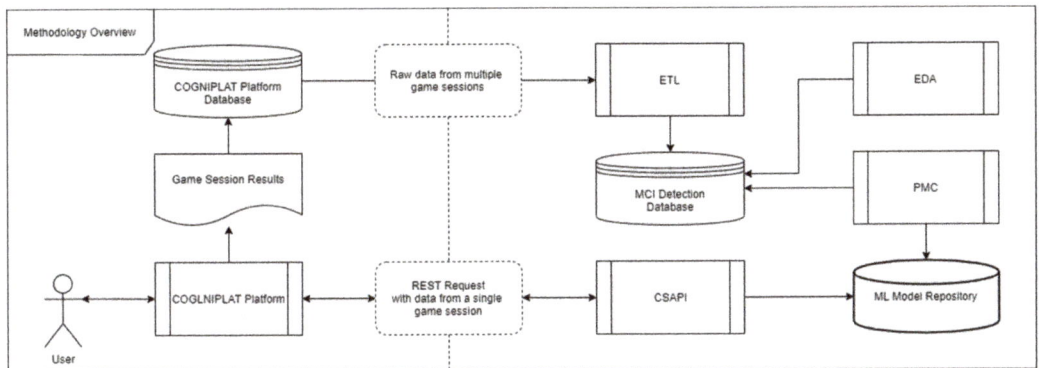

Figure 1. Methodology overview.

3.1. COGNIPLAT Platform and Data Collection

The data used in this work were collected in the context of COGNIPLAT project (A Gaming PLATform for Restoration of COGNItive Functions of the Elderly People) [28]. A basic aim of this project is to design and implement a serious gaming platform based on rehabilitation methods suggested by the scientific research, so that its employment as part of a therapeutic program, would alleviate MCI symptoms. The COGNIPLAT game platform was built based on a multi-disciplinary approach combining theories of neuropsychology, cognitive linguistics and speech therapy organized in six domains, one diagnostic and five training domains focused on enhancing cognitive functions through different game exercises. In addition, the platform has been designed to automatically adjust the complexity and type of exercises by adapting the cognitive requirements of the games to the characteristics of each patient through an ontology-based knowledge model [29]. In this work data from ten serious games used in the diagnostic mode were collected. Table 2 describes the game types and the associated cognitive functions.

Table 2. COGNIPLAT games used in this study and the corresponding cognitive function targeted.

Game Type	Description	Cognitive Function
Puzzle	Solving a photo puzzle	Attention
Maze	Finding the exit from a maze	Visual-motor perception
Recall (Anaklisi)	Recall a random sequence of numbers	Short-term memory
Calculations	Solving arithmetic crosswords	Working memory
Naming	Naming specific types of objects given a set of images shown on the screen	Episodic memory
Sound Matching	Listening to sounds and selecting the corresponding image	Acoustic memory
Orientation	Placing shuffled images in chronological order in order to create a brief story	Spatio-temporal orientation
Language	Finding word antonyms/synonyms	Semantic memory
Logical Order	Selecting the right pattern to reasonably complete the given sequence	Executive functions
Memory Cards	Revealing pairs of alike pictures	Visual memory

Every game played earns points. Different points are awarded for each successful game at a different difficulty level. The calculation of points is based on a formula that combines the level of difficulty and the difference between the completion time of the game and the total time available. The formula for calculating the total score is given below:

$$\textbf{Score} = Difficulty\_Level\_Points * \left(1 - \frac{game\ completion\ time}{available\ total\ time}\right) \qquad (1)$$

The design and development of the COGNIPLAT platform was based on the principles of user-centered design in terms of its technological dimension. In recent years there has been a shift in the creation of user-centered systems, especially in the field of health, which while providing care and support, this is done in a way that the patient is not mentally burdened, while entertainment is served. Each game screen was designed in such a way that useful conclusions can be drawn about the performance achieved, such as the speed of initial interaction with the game screen, the speed of successful completion of each task, the number of tasks successfully completed and other relevant statistics that can be collected. Figure 2 provides some examples of COGNIPLAT game screens.

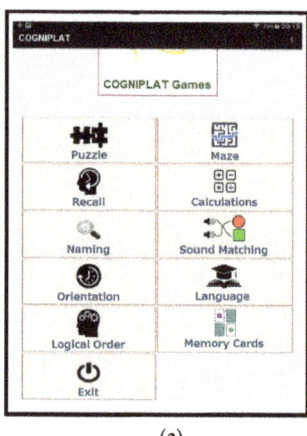 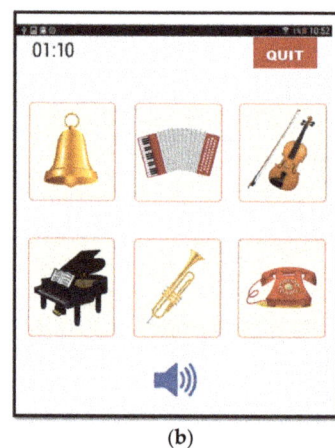 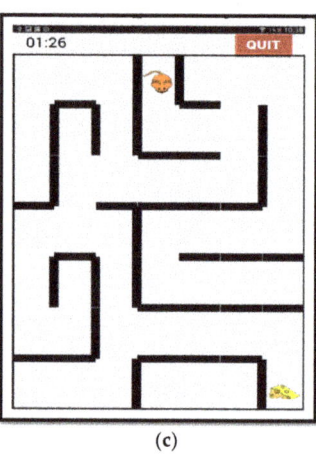

Figure 2. Examples of COGNIPLAT game screens: (**a**) the main menu; (**b**) the sound matching game; (**c**) the maze game.

The most important feature of the games is the ability to statistically analyze and draw useful conclusions from them. Taking into account the history of player performance and using game performance data, it is possible to observe performance over time and any changes can be noted and analyzed. In addition, the cognitive profile and cognitive status of each user can be monitored through game analysis. The adaptability or the ability of the system to dynamically adapt the difficulty of the game to the players is an additional important feature of the platform.

An experimental evaluation study of the COGNIPLAT platform took place with the participation of 10 elderly at a daily care center (7 male and 3 female, mean 76.1 ± 7.05 years of age, mean 9.60 ± 2.37 years of education). The games were accessible as an Android application on a tablet device. Each participant had the opportunity to complete twelve game sessions during the evaluation period, which lasted for about three months. During the study, the subjects had the freedom to play any of the games for an arbitrary number of rounds and in any order.

Although the main objective of the experimental study was to assess the feasibility, engagement and acceptance of serious games for the elderly people, leveraging on this evaluation our aim is to classify participants to cognitive levels by using data which were collected from the game platform and relevant questionnaires. The MoCA test was used to assess the ground truth cognitive level of the participants and their score ranged between 20 and 28 (mean 24.40 ± 2.88). MoCA has been validated for the Greek population by providing normative data [30]. Table 3 gives the distribution of the participants according to the MoCA diagnostic classification [30] and other basic characteristics of the sample.

Table 3. Distribution of participants according to their MoCA score and basic characteristics.

Characteristic	MCI	Normal
N	6	4
Age	76.67 ± 9.27	75.25 ± 2.06
Gender (Male/Female)	4/2	3/1
MoCA	22.50 ± 1.87	27.25 ± 0.96
Education Years	8.5 ± 2.26	11.25 ± 1.50
Technology Familiarity	1.83 ± 0.75	2.50 ± 0.58

MCI participants were distinguished from the "healthy group" with a cutoff score of 23 (2 cases) for low educational level (≤6 years) and a cutoff score of 26 (4 cases) for middle educational level (7–12 years). The mean MoCA score for the MCI group was 22.50 ± 1.87 and the corresponding score for the Normal group was 27.25 ± 0.96. The morphology of the sample for the two groups has similar characteristics in terms of age and gender. The mean age is comparable between the two groups although the variance is higher in the MCI group. The mean education years of the MCI group was 8.5 ± 2.26 and for the Normal group was 11.25 ± 1.50. The technology familiarity (e.g., frequency of computing devices and internet usage) was assessed with relevant questionnaire items in a scale of 0 to 4 and was found to be less than average for the MCI group (1.83 ± 0.75) and above average for the Normal group (2.50 ± 0.58).

The MoCA test can assess various cognitive domains of a subject, such as attention, concentration, executive functions, memory, language, visuospatial, as well as abstraction, delayed recall and orientation. The assessment is administered in approximately 10 min. The total points a subject can score is 30. The person who administers the assessment, sums the subtotals of each individual task that are recorded on the right-hand of the questionnaire during the MoCA process.

On top of that, an additional questionnaire was administered in order to collect demographic, medical and lifestyle information. A classification of the questionnaire data is performed according to standardized categories [31], as shown in Table 4.

Table 4. Grouping of questionnaire data according to the type of medical data source.

Medical Data Source	Questionnaire Field
Demographics (HL7)	age, gender, education level, marital status
Medical Profile (Diagnosis)	family medical history, depression, hypertension
Lifestyle	smoking, exercise, familiarity with technology (smartphones, Internet)

The data concerning the in-game performance of each subject is contained in two tables, the *game sessions* holding data such as which user is logged in and when, and the *game rounds* holding data such as game type, difficulty level, game outcome (success/fail), game completion time, earned points and other details regarding a single game round. During the evaluation period, in terms of recorded data entries, there were 10 subjects, 10 different game types, 119 game sessions and 2951 game rounds in total. These data are essential for this study in order to answer the main research question.

3.2. Extract-Transform-Load

The process of ETL plays a crucial part in our methodology. The main purpose that it serves is to merge all the data from the individual schemas, due to the fact that during the evaluation multiple tablet devices were used and each tablet had its own local database. The merging was done after a database migration to a new slightly improved schema.

3.2.1. Data Extraction and Partial Preprocessing

The schema migration was done in order to create *parameter* tables for each field with categorical values and use the key field from those parameter tables whenever these values are referenced in other tables such as game sessions and rounds. In turn, this practice helped to reduce the need for encoding functions until later in the EDA process. However, a drawback of this practice is that it can only be applied on ordinal features, since the non-ordinal features would still need to be treated with more appropriate techniques such as One-Hot-Encoding, as it was done for the feature of marital status.

3.2.2. Data Transformation and Feature Engineering

The next step, as part of the data transformation and before data loading at the scripting level, is feature engineering [32]. This process includes arithmetic and cumulative transformations to produce new features that were later inspected in the EDA process, for their importance and correlation to the target classification class.

In addition, apart from a couple of features with random values that were created to be used as reference points of the minimum importance a feature can have [33], the rest represent aggregated information about game rounds. The reason to customarily define how new features are calculated, instead of applying brute force or any other existing feature selection technique is the necessity for these features to be explainable and recreatable. The former is required to know exactly what a feature represents in a specific context, in other words to know how it relates to the target class. As for the latter, it denotes the ability to understand how the value of a feature is calculated, since this is essential to set up the process that recreates the feature from raw data of future datasets before feeding them to the model for the actual prediction.

The engineered features typically are aggregated data of individual game rounds found in a game session, as for example, total points earned in a session and average game completion time in a session. Other more composite aggregations can be also defined such as the importance of a game type which is measured as the ratio between total points won in successful game rounds of a game type in a session divided by the average points won in successful rounds for that particular game type in all sessions recorded. Table 5 gives an outline of the features that were defined and used in the MCI detection methodology.

Table 5. The entire feature set defined and explored in the developed models.

Feature	Data Type	Description
age	Categorical (Ordinal)	The age of the subject. 0: <60, 1: 60–69, 2: 70–79, 3: 80–89, 4: >89
gender	Categorical (Ordinal)	The gender of the subject. 0: Male, 1: Female
education	Categorical (Ordinal)	The education level of the subject. 0: Illiterate, 1: Primary incomplete, 2: Primary integrated, 3: Secondary incomplete, 4: Secondary integrated, 5: Tertiary, 6: Postgraduate, 7: PhD
laptop_usage	Categorical (Ordinal)	Frequency of laptop usage. 0: Never, 1: Seldom, 2: Sometimes, 3: Often, 4: Always
smartphone_usage	Categorical (Ordinal)	Frequency of smartphone usage. 0: Never, 1: Seldom, 2: Sometimes, 3: Often, 4: Always
smoking	Categorical (Ordinal)	Smoking level of the subject. 0: None, 1: Low, 2: Moderate, 3: Heavy
alcohol_use	Categorical (Ordinal)	Alcohol use by the subject. 0: None, 1: Low, 2: Moderate, 3: Heavy
family_med_history	Categorical (Ordinal)	History of memory loss or related illnesses of the subject. 0: None, 1: Low, 2: Moderate, 3: Heavy
exercising	Categorical (Ordinal)	Exercising level of the subject. 0: None, 1: Low, 2: Moderate, 3: Heavy
depression	Categorical (Ordinal)	Depression level of the subject. 0: None, 1: Low, 2: Moderate, 3: Heavy
hypertension	Categorical (Ordinal)	Hypertension level of the subject. 0: None, 1: Low, 2: Moderate, 3: Heavy
marital_status	Categorical (Non-Ordinal)	The marital status of the subject. 0: Single, 1: Married, 2: Divorced, 3: Widow. This feature is encoded with One-Hot-Encoder to derive separate Boolean features
marital_status_1	Boolean	One-Hot-Encoding of marital_status for 1: Married or 0: Not-Married
marital_status_3	Boolean	One-Hot-Encoding of marital_status for 1: Widow or 0: Not-Widow
total_gr_in_gs	Real number	The total number of game rounds in a game session
total_success_rounds_in_session	Real number	The total number of successful game rounds in a game session
total_win_gr_points_in_gs	Real number	The total points won in a game session
avg_gr_time_in_gs	Real number	The average completion time of a game round in a game session
avg_gr_time_win_gr_in_gs	Real number	The average completion time of a successful game round in a session
rf_integer_3	Integer	A feature with random integer value in the range between 1–3
rf_decimal_100	Real number	A feature with random decimal value in the range between 1–100

Table 5. *Cont.*

Feature	Data Type	Description
puzzleImp	Real number	
mazeImp	Real number	
anaklisiImp	Real number	
calcImp	Real number	The importance of a game, expressed as a ratio between the total points won in successful game rounds of a game session divided by the average points won in successful rounds for that particular game in all sessions.
namingImp	Real number	
soundImp	Real number	
orientImp	Real number	
langImp	Real number	
logicImp	Real number	
memoryImp	Real number	

3.2.3. Data Loading

The output of the ETL process is a data view that contains the information required to train the machine learning models. The dataset contains 119 instances with all the features derived from each game session. The last step, therefore, of the process is to load the data, at the scripting level for starting the EDA process.

3.3. Exploratory Data Analysis

The exploratory analysis could be described as the main process in the effort to create models, measure their performance and draw a conclusion regarding the research question of this work. The aim of this process is to explore all the important aspects that would provide a better understanding of the collected data and will support making decisions on the importance of each feature, testing various ML algorithms and observing the results to avoid overfitting and underfitting. Additionally, it is the most appropriate process to compare different standardization strategies, in other words secure the model from concept drift in future datasets. Python and the *Scikit-learn* library [34] were used as the development environment for the experimentation process.

The EDA process receives as input the data formulated at the end of the ETL process. The output of the EDA process takes the form of the information inferred by its sub-processes, which will enable the selection of the optimal feature set, the best performing algorithm and the most suitable optimizations. At this stage and before starting any data transformation, getting the quantile and the descriptive statistics of the engineered features, as shown in Tables 6 and 7 respectively, allows one to gain a better insight of the data.

Table 6. Quantile statistics of the game-based engineered features.

Feature	Quantile Statistics								
	Min	5th Perc.	Q1	Median	Q3	95th Perc.	Max	Range	IQR
total_gr_in_gs	1	4	16	24	31	48	60	59	15
total_success_rounds_in_session	1	1	2.5	7	11	12.1	14	13	8.5
total_win_gr_points_in_gs	5	11.6	43	97	167.5	323.3	361	356	124.5
avg_gr_time_in_gs	12.448	20.385	27.620	34.760	47.314	65.469	120.800	108.351	19.694
avg_gr_time_win_gr_in_gs	6	14.245	27.4	37	50.166	86	114.500	108.500	22.766
rf_decimal_100	1.140	6.093	24.322	51.228	74.437	93.357	97.827	96.687	50.114
puzzleImp	0.158	0.364	1.056	1.742	2.059	4.224	5.702	5.544	1.003
mazeImp	0.069	0.277	0.555	0.936	1.179	2.219	2.289	2.219	0.624
anaklisiImp	0.194	0.292	0.740	0.779	1.480	1.519	1.558	1.363	0.740
calcImp	0.090	0.090	0.428	1.037	1.465	2.286	2.976	2.885	1.037
namingImp	0.198	0.331	0.546	0.993	1.705	2.441	3.510	3.312	1.159
soundImp	0.106	0.156	0.424	0.848	1.590	2.932	6.734	6.628	1.166
orientImp	0.072	0.289	0.650	1.011	1.228	2.087	2.384	2.312	0.578
langImp	0.183	0.366	0.686	0.869	1.419	1.648	2.930	2.746	0.732
logicImp	0.382	0.473	0.812	0.908	1.290	1.725	1.768	1.385	0.477
memoryImp	0.213	0.355	0.711	0.995	1.422	1.991	2.204	1.991	0.711

Table 7. Descriptive statistics of the game-based engineered features.

Feature	Descriptive Statistics						
	STD	Coeff. of variation	Kurtosis	Mean	Median Abs. Dev.	Skewness	Variance
total_gr_in_gs	12.730	0.513	−0.044	24.798	8	0.347	162.060
total_success_rounds_in_session	4.082	0.610	−1.507	6.686	4	0.032	16.666
total_win_gr_points_in_gs	95.309	0.796	0.038	119.636	59	0.982	9083.866
avg_gr_time_in_gs	16.395	0.422	4.929	38.828	8.527	1.666	268.799
avg_gr_time_win_gr_in_gs	21.046	0.505	1.492	41.668	10.888	1.129	442.966
rf_decimal_100	28.731	0.579	−1.222	49.550	24.837	−0.066	825.518
puzzleImp	1.117	0.600	1.516	1.860	0.475	1.098	147.000
mazeImp	0.633	0.623	−0.501	1.015	0.381	0.731	0.401
anaklisiImp	0.459	1.016	−1.434	0.596	0.389	0.426	0.368
calcImp	0.729	0.686	0.136	1.062	0.4961	0.726	0.532
namingImp	0.730	0.620	0.496	1.177	0.529	0.919	0.533
soundImp	1.037	0.888	13.422	1.166	0.583	2.907	1.075
orientImp	0.561	0.548	−0.075	1.023	0.361	0.587	0.315
langImp	0.528	0.507	1.691	1.040	0.412	0.833	0.278
logicImp	0.372	0.363	−0.327	1.025	0.143	0.620	0.138
memoryImp	0.531	0.483	−0.673	1.098	0.426	0.329	0.282

3.3.1. Target Class Selection

Given that the participants of the study were invited to complete both the MMSE and the MoCA cognitive assessments, before and after using the COGNIPLAT platform, there are more than one candidate variables that could be used as the target class. Aiming to select one of these two assessments, the criterion that was most influential had to do with the distribution of scores across the scale of cognitive performance for the MMSE (Figure 3a) and the MoCA (Figure 3b). Both assessments have a similar value range between 1 and 30, however, the cutoff scores of the different cognitive levels differ significantly for each assessment type. This is important as it affects the difficulty to distinguish a subject between the cognitive classes.

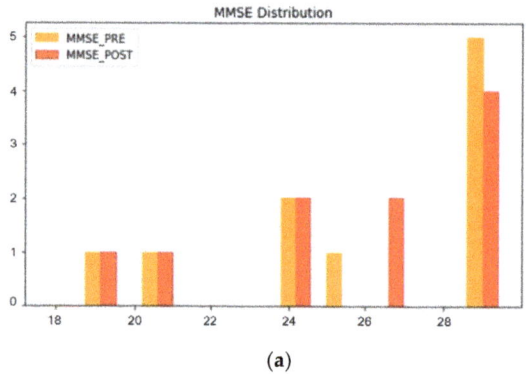 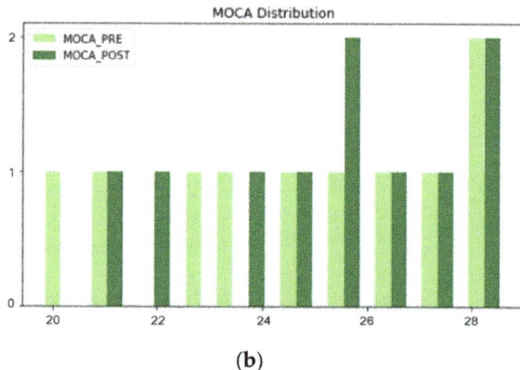

Figure 3. (a) Distribution of MMSE scores before (MMSE_PRE) and after (MMSE_POST) the intervention; (b) Distribution of MoCA scores before (MOCA_PRE) and after (MOCA_POST) the intervention.

As initially demonstrated by Nasreddine [6], the ranges between the cognitive levels are much less discrete in the MMSE assessment compared to the MoCA assessment. Other researchers confirmed also that the MoCA assessment presents a much better sensitivity in distinguishing subjects with MCI compared to the MMSE due to the fact that often subjects are achieving higher scores in the latter assessment [35]. Finally, normative data for the Greek population are available for the MoCA scale but not for the MMSE.

Therefore, in this study the MoCA assessment was selected. In particular, the test performed before using the COGNIPLAT platform was chosen due to the following reasons. Firstly, because the two tests were performed in a relatively short period of time it allowed subjects to score better in the latter one due to repetition. Secondly, even with a moderate usage of serious games designed to train cognitive abilities it was expected to have a positive impact on the follow up MoCA test. Thirdly, as shown in Figure 3b, the distribution of scores in the first MoCA assessment (MOCA_PRE) was slightly more homogeneous than the distribution in the second assessment (MOCA_POST).

3.3.2. Preprocessing

Missing Values Management

In the case of our dataset, the only entries with missing values were a few entries representing game rounds that terminated due to application exceptions. Since these rounds were only a few and they had most of their fields missing the decision was to discard and not include them in the schema migration following the tuple ignoring technique [36].

Management of Outliers

Outliers apply only to values of fields that represent in-game data and not to fields that are related to the demographics and other questionnaires that the subjects completed and cannot deviate from predefined values. Given that the size of the dataset is relatively limited, removing entries that contain outlier values in one or more fields is probably not the best option. On the other hand, leaving those values as-is could potentially affect the results in the process of scaling, depending on the algorithm that will be selected to apply.

Ideally, when a game session resembles an assessment, it provides a specific number of game rounds, in a specific order, with a specific difficulty progression. The COGNIPLAT platform which was used for data gathering serves a dual goal both for cognitive assessment and for exercising cognitive functions of the elderly. As a consequence, the level of difficulty was customizable allowing the application or the caregiver to adjust it in order to meet the capabilities of each subject. On the other hand, the game performance in terms of points won in a game round is directly related to the game difficulty level. Additionally, the subjects had the option to repeat a level for several times. These characteristics resulted in some game sessions with distinctly differentiated scores.

The way the issue of outliers was addressed was by value replacement and by applying the Winsorization technique [37]. The technique was implemented to calculate new values based on the following strategy. If the feature represented a total, for example the total points gathered in the successful game rounds of a session, and the value for this feature in an entry was too high, then it was replaced with the maximum value (Q3 + 1.5*IQR) of the distribution of the feature. Respectively the low-end outlier values of an entry for a feature representing a total value, were replaced by the minimum value (Q1 + 1.5*IQR) of the distribution. On the other hand, for features that represent an average value, for example the average completion time of a successful game round, the outlier values were replaced by the median value of their distribution.

Both discretization and scaling can be affected by outliers, therefore the process that manages the outliers was explicitly placed to precede both discretization and scaling to avoid any effect of outliers in the outcome of these processes [38].

Discretization

Although discretization by binning is a relatively simple data transformation, in our methodology binning of feature values to higher levels is an essential step and it has been applied for the target class and for features derived from in-game data with continuous values.

Firstly, discretization was applied to the target class, which represents the MoCA scores recorded before the game sessions. The implementation is affected by the type of the target class field because it defines what kind of ML algorithms, between regression and classification, can be used to train the model. Additionally, this affects the way a prediction is interpreted, since an answer in the MoCA range of results would give a specific estimate while the objective is to get a broader estimate of the cognitive level of the subject as a classification between two cognition levels: normal cognition (NC) and mild cognitive impairment (MCI).

Secondly, before moving to feature selection, some normalization method needs to be applied to avoid the outweighing of features with low value ranges. In the case of the target class, the exact range of each bin is known beforehand, which happens to be the MoCA cutoff scores of each cognitive level. However, in the case of the rest of the features several binning methods are available to be applied, since discretization can be achieved with various strategies, such as equal width levels, equal frequency levels or any other custom approach. What was used on the implementation level, was the *KBinsDiscretizer* method of the *Scikit-learn* library, with the quantile option, which is described as an equal frequency discretization strategy [34].

Low Variance Features Removal

The first step that was done towards feature selection was the removal of any low to zero variance features. Those features have no useful information to offer to the model, thus, a threshold was set and in case the values of a feature are the same in 80% or more of the total entries, that feature is removed. As a result of applying this method, the features of "smoking", "alcohol", "hypertension" and the importance of the Calculations game were removed from the dataset. Although most of the feature selection steps follow the preprocessing, on an implementation level, the step of low variance removal precedes the data standardization to avoid having the variance threshold method being affected by the transformation of the values.

Data Standardization

Standardization has been used to further ensure that values of our features will be on the same scale and thus avoid certain features being outweighed. By applying this technique, effects from a potential concept drift in future datasets is minimized [39]. Furthermore, standardization of individual features is considered a prerequisite for many of the classifiers to be able to perform as expected [34]. The standardization method that was applied is literally an implementation of the Z-score normalization technique, where the mean of each feature distribution is centered at 0 and the values are scaled to represent the result of the division by the feature standard deviation.

3.3.3. Feature Selection

Following the data curation that was described in the preprocessing section, the methodology continues with the process that most of the data mining and ML guides define as feature selection. The advantages of reducing the features to a subset of them are well described in the literature [40], and affects many aspects of a ML experiment, such as the speed of training, the accuracy and the explainability of a model.

Feature selection algorithms, based on their output, can be categorized into two different categories. The first category is feature weighting which returns the same number of input features along with their weights by employing wrapper feature selection algorithms. The second category is subset selection which returns a subset of the input features by employing either a filter or embedded model feature selection algorithms.

Our methodology involved the selection of two feature subsets based on two different strategies. The first strategy primarily aims at creating a subset of features in which at least some of the in-game related features will be included. The mandatory inclusion of some of these features is related to the research question of this work, since it would have been pointless to train a model based only on data from the questionnaires. The second strategy used the method of feature selection with the *chi2* statistic as the scorer function, a method that eliminates features with low correlation to the target class.

Feature Correlation Inspection

At first, the pairwise correlation between each feature is inspected. For this task, Pearson's correlation was calculated and projected on the heatmap shown in Figure 4. The purpose at this stage is to recognize the highly correlated features and eliminate the so-called redundant features, which are those that cannot append additional information to the model [41].

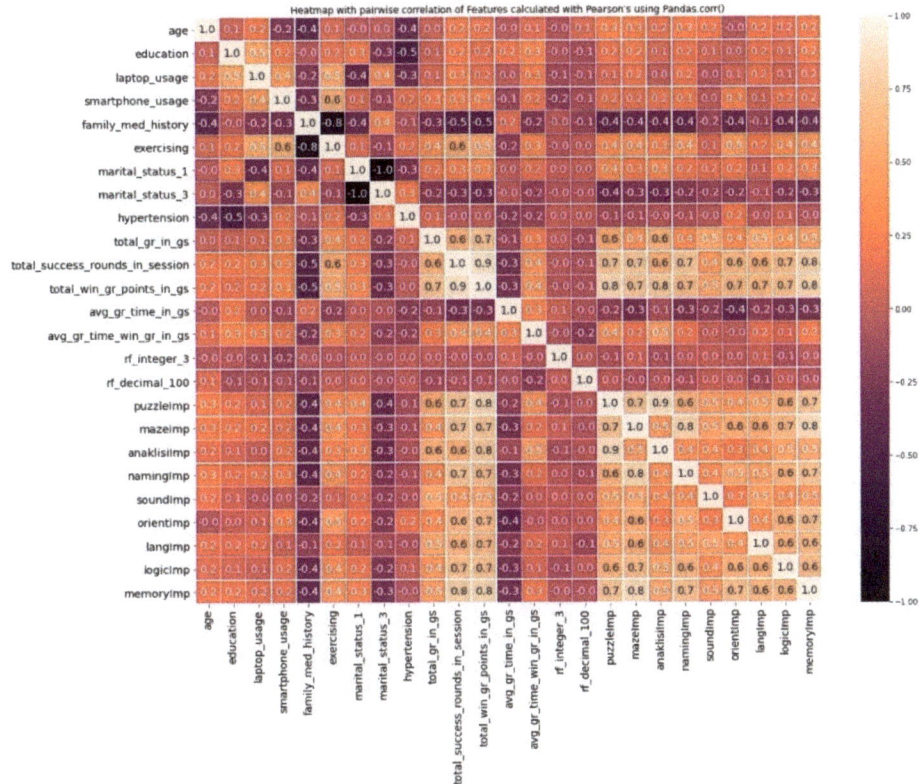

Figure 4. Heatmap of pairwise correlation of features calculated with Pearson's correlation.

To avoid the daunting task of manually using the heatmap to find the highly correlated features, a function that performs agglomerative clustering, was used, resulting in feature clusters separated based on the degree of their correlation which were previously calculated [42]. The dendrogram in Figure 5 projects the clusters that are formed based on a threshold value of 36% that was empirically selected and represents the maximum pairwise distance observed which in this case happens to be 4.68.

Feature Importance Inspection

Having every feature grouped into clusters of highly correlated features, the next step of the methodology is to inspect their significance against the target class, with the ultimate goal of keeping only the most important one of each cluster. To decide whether a feature is important or not two metrics were incorporated, the mean decrease in impurity (MDI) and the mean decrease in accuracy (MDA), also known as permutation importance. Essentially, this is a form of feature weighting, thus a wrapper method is needed in order to calculate these metrics. The wrapper method that was implemented incorporates a Random Forest classifier that is used as an estimator both for the MDI and the MDA metrics. The wrapper method was then called once for the complete set of features, excluding those already removed in the preprocessing, and then once for each cluster separately (Figure 6a,b).

To proceed with the custom selection process, judging by the MDA and MDI scores, the features that appear to perform worse than the two randomized features were excluded, followed by the exclusion of the less important features of each cluster. The features that remained after the low variance feature removal, were inspected for their pairwise correlation and for their importance against the target class in order to create an optimized feature subset. This subset is identified next as the manually selected features.

Apart from the custom wrapper method that was implemented to measure the MDA and MDI metrics, another wrapper method that measures the P-value and the F-score for each feature, was used for an automatic selection of the k-best features. Figure 7 projects the values of these metrics for each feature cluster.

Thus, a second subset was created using an automatic feature selection method which selects features according to the *k* highest scores by computing the *chi2* statistic. This subset is identified next as the automatically selected features. In Table 8, the feature subsets for each feature selection strategy is provided.

3.3.4. Classifier Selection

Having completed the preprocessing and the feature selection, the next major step of the EDA process for this methodology is the classifier selection. The outcome of this process is the performance evaluation of a series of ML algorithms. The criteria for whether an algorithm performs well or not, besides accuracy, is any indication about the bias and the variance of the model and also the statistics regarding the sensitivity and specificity metrics (Figure 8).

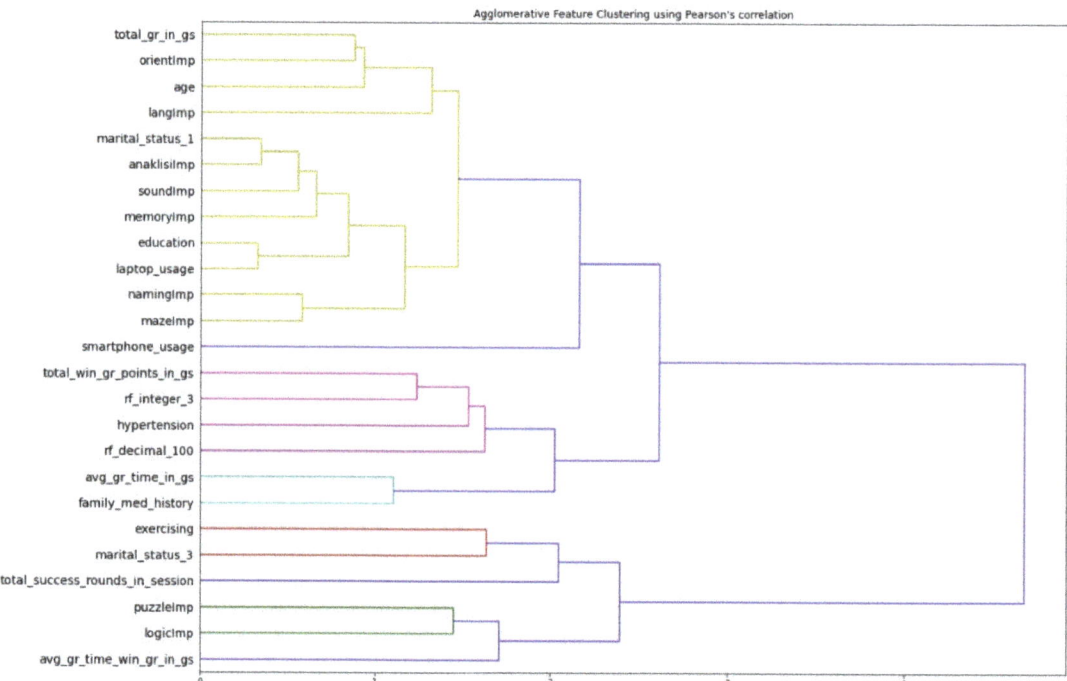

Figure 5. Dendrogram of the feature clusters created with Pearson's correlation values.

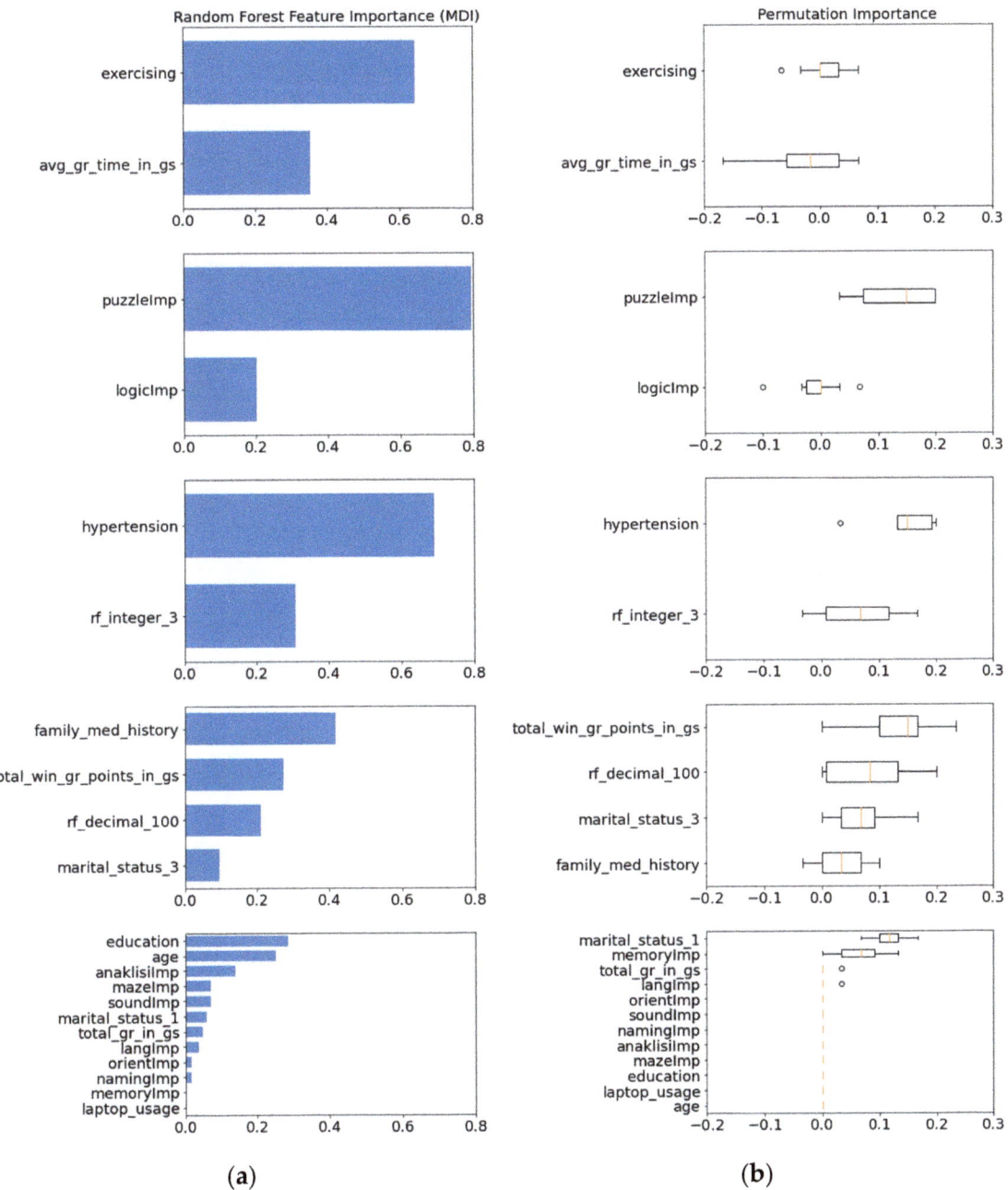

Figure 6. (**a**) Results of MDI metrics for every feature cluster; (**b**) Results of MDA metrics for every feature cluster.

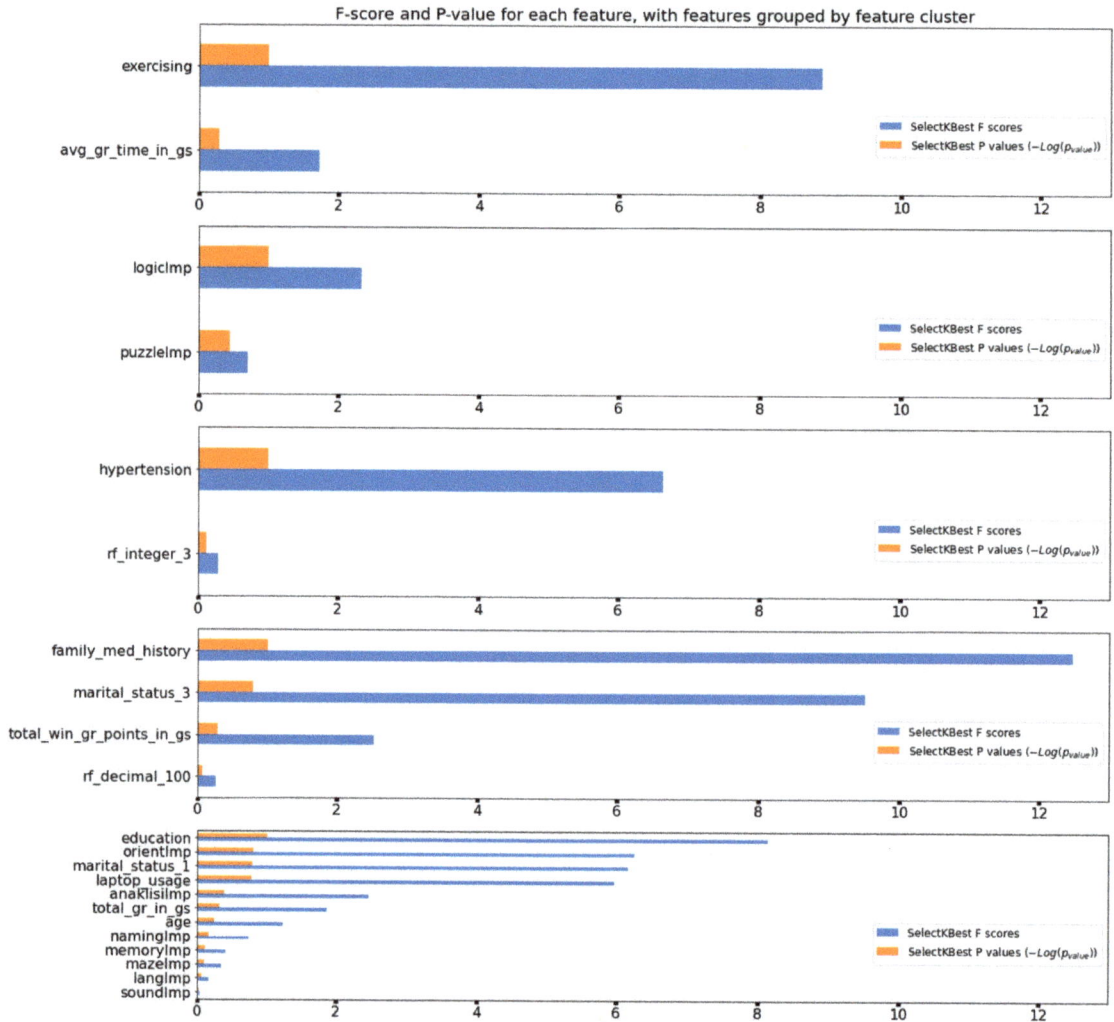

Figure 7. Results of F-score and P-value metrics for each feature cluster.

Table 8. Overview of feature subsets for each selection strategy.

Manually Selected Features	Automatically Selected Features
Age	Education
Family Medical History	Laptop Usage
Exercising	Smartphone Usage
Education	Family Medical History
Avg. Game Round Time in Game Session	Exercising
Orientation Game Importance	Marital Status 1 (Married)
Naming Game Importance	Marital Status 3 (Widow/er)
Memory Game Importance	Total Round Points for Rounds won
Recall (Anaklisi) Game Importance	Recall (Anaklisi) Game Importance
	Logic Game Importance
	Memory Game Importance

		Predicted Class		
		MCI	NC	
Actual Class	MCI	True Positive	False Negative	Sensitivity TP/(TP+FN)
	NC	False Positive	True Negative	Specificity TN/(FP+TN)
		Precision TP/(TP+FP)	NPV TN/(TN+FN)	Accuracy (TP+TN)/(TP+TN+FP+FN)

Figure 8. Primary model evaluation metrics definition based on the mapping of the positive-negative labels between the actual and the predicted class.

As already stated, the final model would have the role of complementing screening tests like the existing MoCA and MMSE assessments, which means that it aims to be a tool to provide the likelihood, and not a definitive answer, of someone having MCI or not, as per the definitions of diagnostic and screening tests presented in the work of Trevethan [43]. Therefore, given that the outcome of our work is a binary classification model that distinguishes subjects, between having or not MCI, the most appropriate metrics to take into account for model performance evaluation appear to be those of sensitivity and specificity. This is also backed up by the plethora of publications that examine the performance of the MoCA assessment where the sensitivity and specificity metrics have been the focus of the evaluation [30,44].

From a machine learning perspective, in order for a model to continue being accurate in future datasets, the bias/variance tradeoff needs to be taken into consideration. In other words, the model needs to be accurate enough, yet able to generalize effectively, disregarding any noise in data [45].

The following ML algorithms have been tested for the aforementioned evaluation metrics: logistic regression (LR), decision tree (DT), random forest (RF), support vector classifier (SVC), k-nearest neighbors (kNN), Gaussian Naive Bayes (GNB), multi-layer perceptron (MLP) and a custom ensemble that includes all the ML algorithms except from MLP and the output of the base models is combined considering a majority voting aggregation function. At this stage, two models were trained for each type of algorithm, one for each selected feature subset (Table 8). Those models serve as baseline models and their results as a reference point to evaluate the difference in performance after performing the optimization process.

To accomplish that kind of evaluation of the models, apart from the percentage of accuracy, which is a good starting point to recognize overfitting, the decision boundary for each model has been plotted, as shown in Figure 9. The way the decision boundary helps in the process of model evaluation is by allowing the inspection of the model complexity and how it would behave with noise such as outliers in data [46].

However, plotting the decision boundary on a two-dimensional plane presupposes a similar dimensionality of the dataset, otherwise we would have to repeat the plotting multiple times, each time for a features pair. The solution to that problem, on the implementation level, was given by plotting the decision boundary after applying the principal component analysis (PCA) method [47], where the dataset consists of two component features and the target class.

3.3.5. Optimization

At this stage, having trained and evaluated a series of baseline models, various optimization techniques are applied in order not only to improve the evaluation metric scores but also to improve the interpretability of these models. The optimization scenarios with the methods applied to the baseline models are outlined in Figure 10.

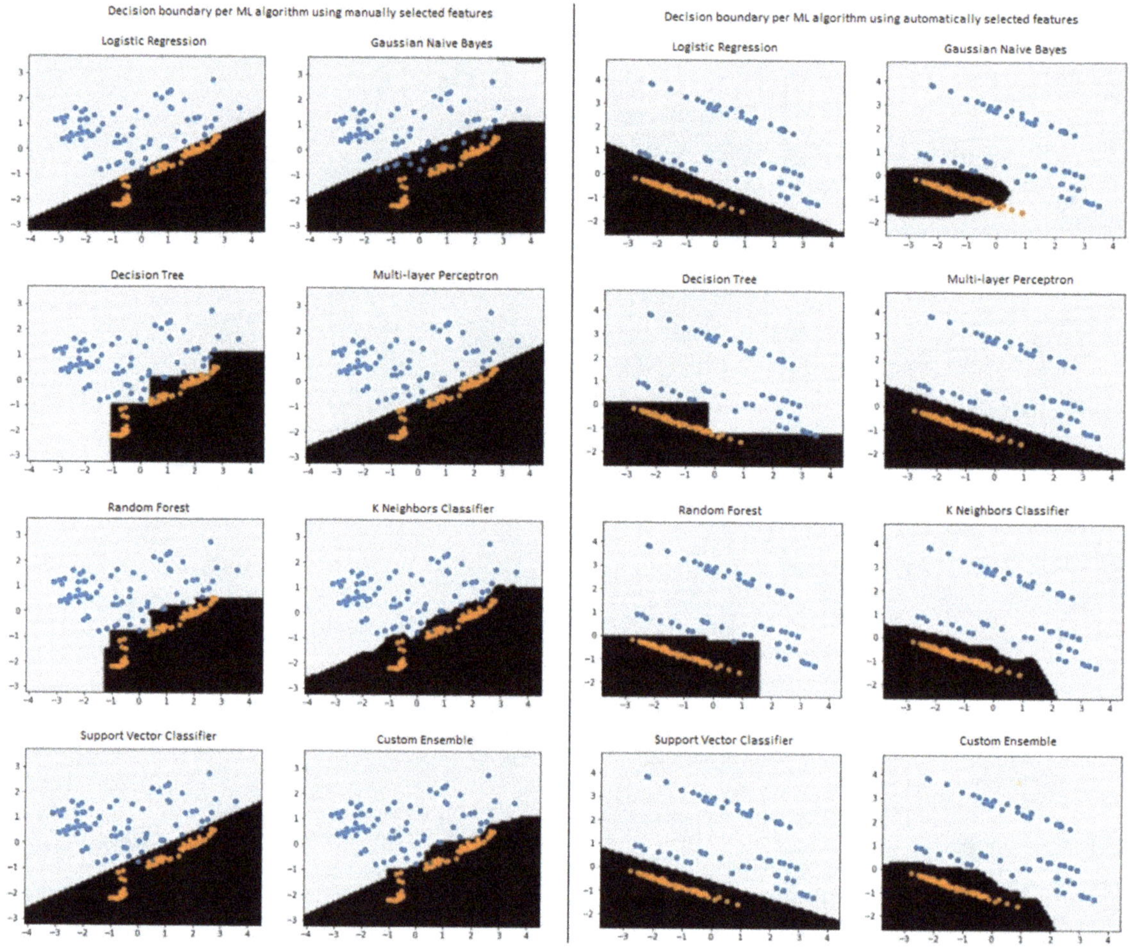

Figure 9. Decision boundaries for each ML model for the manually (on the left) and the automatically (on the right) selected features. Each dot represents a game session entry, where the blue dots in the light background represent game sessions of subjects within the MCI class and the orange dots in the dark background represent game sessions of subjects with the NC class.

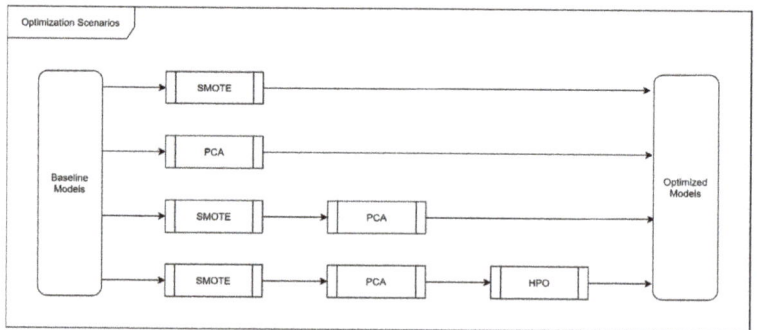

Figure 10. Optimization scenarios that describe which methods were applied and in what order.

Data Augmentation

A major issue that had to be addressed in order to avoid biased results in our model was the imbalanced number of game sessions between the two target classes, MCI and NC. Two of the widely used methods to solve that problem are undersampling and oversampling. Since the dataset is of relatively small dimensionality, especially after the process of feature selection, undersampling would probably be a good option. However, due to the fact that the dataset also has a rather small number of entries, the oversampling method was preferred, in order to avoid discarding useful information. At the implementation level the algorithm used was the synthetic minority oversampling technique (SMOTE) [48].

Interestingly, there seems to be a discussion on whether oversampling should be applied before or after feature selection. In this work, the approach which introduces oversampling after the feature selection was preferred, in order to avoid having artificially created data affecting the feature selection process, as similarly suggested by other studies [49].

Dimensionality Reduction

The PCA technique is one of the most well-known techniques for dimensionality reduction. Although PCA is fully capable of replacing the process of feature selection, especially if the dimensionality of a dataset is not too large [50], it is incorporated in our methodology for a different reason.

The first reason is to repeat the experiment having extracted a small number of components and see if there is any fluctuation in accuracy and the rest of the metrics used to evaluate the baseline models. The second reason is to reduce the dimensionality to a number of components that would allow the dataset to be visualized along with the decision boundary of each model. This means a reduction to either two components and plotting the dataset into a two-dimensional plane with the decision boundary being a line, or three components and plotting the dataset into a three-dimensional space with the decision boundary being a plane.

As illustrated in the optimization scenarios workflow (Figure 10), PCA has been applied in two different cases, right after the baseline models and after the oversampling. For the actual implementation, the first step in utilizing PCA is to decide the optimal number of principal components to extract. This was done using the *GridSearchCV* method of the *Scikit-learn* library, which allows to inspect the accuracy of a classifier having the number of components as a variable. The Gaussian Naive Bayes was the classifier selected for that process and the range of the components was set between 1 and the number of features minus one. In addition, cross-validation was used to get a standard deviation for the accuracy for each number of components. As seen in the grid search results on Figure 11, the case with two components presents the optimal performance between 0.95 and 0.99 accuracy. For further increase in the number of components, from 3 to 6, clear evidence of overfitting is shown since the model reaches an accuracy between 0.97 and 1.

The next step in applying PCA, is to observe the results by plotting the components against the total variance that they represent, as shown in Figure 12a and also the entire dataset, after the transformation, against the target class to inspect how easily the two classes could be distinguished as shown in Figure 12b.

Hyperparameter Optimization

One of the most applied methods for hyperparameter optimization (HPO) is grid search. From a computational perspective, it is a costly operation since it essentially is a brute force black-box task. However, it allows us to find the optimal values for the parameters of multiple algorithms without human interaction. According to the literature, one can find a few alternatives to grid search, such as the population-based methods of random search, genetic algorithms, particle swarm optimization, the Bayesian optimization methods and others that are less computationally expensive [51]. However, for this work, since the dataset is of relatively small size, the grid search method was preferred.

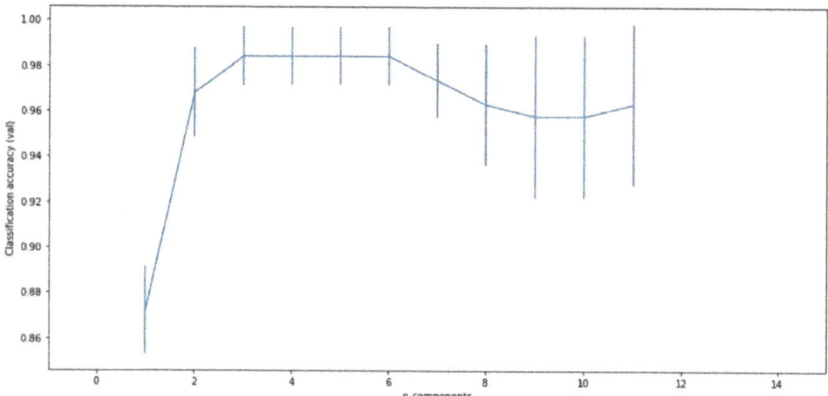

Figure 11. Classification accuracy with SD per number of principal components, created with grid search to find the optimal number of components.

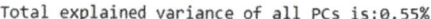

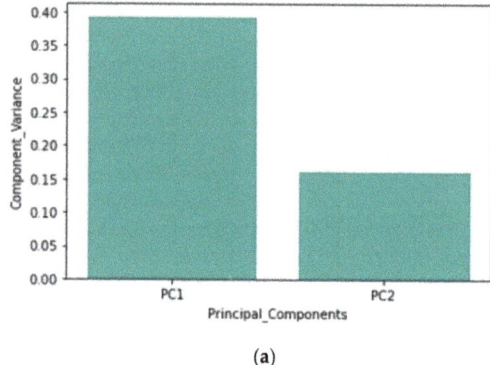

(**a**)

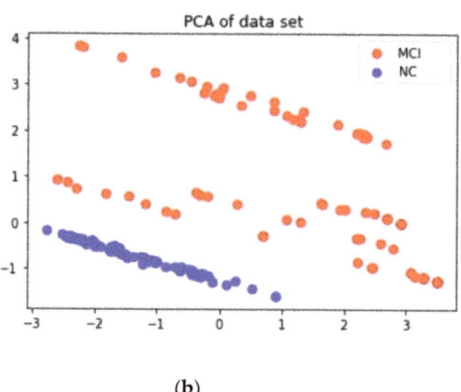

(**b**)

Figure 12. (**a**) Percentage of variance explained per principal component; (**b**) Two dimensional depiction of the principal components against the target classes.

3.4. Production Model Creation

To be able to claim that one of the trained models can be considered production ready, the aforementioned optimization processes are not sufficient. There is at least one important factor that could potentially introduce bias to the trained models and that is data leakage, as it is well described by Bussola et al. [52]. The final process of this methodology focuses on solving that issue.

Amongst all the possible forms data leakage can take, we focus on solving the leakage that could possibly occur during preprocessing from the training subset to the testing subset. The culprit, for this type of data leakage, is considered to be the transformations that the dataset goes through during the preprocessing and more specifically the transformations that precede the splitting of the dataset between training and testing subsets [53].

The challenge that arises here is the fact that we are already at a late stage regarding the methodology workflow, considering that even optimization has already been applied. Thus, to be able to implement a solution for data leakage, we incorporated a method to safely preprocess and train a model after splitting the dataset. On the other hand, a major advantage of this practice is that upon prediction there is no need to separately load any transformers to edit the future data, instead, preprocessing is now part of the model itself.

3.5. Classification Service API

For the final stage of the proposed methodology, we have experimented with building a classification service Application Programming Interface (API) to study and record any challenges that could come up from such a task. The structure of this service is rather simple, as it consists of a Flask server with a main method that loads the model and a controller to receive REST requests for prediction from the COGNIPLAT game suite application. In a production environment, these requests would contain the in-game data recorded throughout a game session. The response returned from the controller contains the label of the cognitive class predicted by the loaded model, i.e., MCI or NC and the confidence score for the specific prediction, given of course that the loaded model supports the export of that information.

4. Results

To evaluate the trained models, a wrapper function was created to efficiently get the metric scores, relevant confusion matrices and the receiver operating characteristic (ROC) with the area under curve (AUC) and the precision–recall diagrams. The evaluation of each classification model is performed by applying the k-fold (k = 5) cross validation technique on a stratified hold-out sub-dataset that was kept initially specifically for the purpose of model evaluation. A split of the initial dataset was performed yielding a training sub-dataset (70% of the dataset) and a test sub-dataset (30% of the dataset). The performance of models with different configurations is then evaluated on the hold-out set, for the purpose of selecting the best performing model. This approach is useful to measure the prediction performance of the final production model or compare predictions with reference to held-out samples [54].

The performance results of all the models trained are presented in two separate tables. Table 9 records the results that are related to the baseline models, the application of the SMOTE, PCA and HPO methods using the two feature subsets selected. Table 10 records the results of the models that were trained using pipelines. A pipeline in the context of ML can be described as a utility method that allows the design of a procedure from the data preprocessing to the training of the classifier offering some advantages over the manual execution of these steps. The purpose of the pipeline is to assemble the above methods that can be cross-validated together while setting different parameters in the context of using the *Scikit-learn* library [55]. The pipeline method eventually implements the solution for avoiding data leakage.

Table 9. Evaluation results, by ML algorithm, for the training and testing processes, for both feature selection strategies, from the stage of baseline models up to applying hyperparameter optimization.

Algorithm	Manually Selected Feature Set			Automatically Selected Feature Set		
	Accuracy (%)		SD	Accuracy (%)		SD
	Training	Testing		Training	Testing	
			Baseline Models			
Logistic Regression	100	100	0	93.33	93.33	13.33
Decision Tree	100	100	0	96.67	96.67	6.67
Random Forest	100	100	0	96.67	96.67	6.67
Support Vector Classifier	93.33	93.33	4.71	93.33	93.33	8.16
Gaussian Naive Bayes	100	100	0	100	100	0
Multi-layer Perceptron	90	90	8.16	90	93.33	8.16
k-Nearest neighbors	76.67	76.67	9.43	96.67	93.33	8.16
Custom Ensemble	100	100	0	96.67	96.67	6.67

Table 9. Cont.

Algorithm	Manually Selected Feature Set			Automatically Selected Feature Set		
	Accuracy (%)		SD	Accuracy (%)		SD
	Training	Testing		Training	Testing	
	Baseline Models					
	SMOTE					
Logistic Regression	97.78	97.78	3.14	97.92	98	4
Decision Tree	100	100	0	100	100	0
Random Forest	100	100	0	100	100	0
Support Vector Classifier	97.78	97.78	3.14	100	97.778	4.44
Gaussian Naive Bayes	100	100	0	100	100	0
Multi-layer Perceptron	97.78	97.78	3.14	97.92	98	4
k-Nearest neighbors	85.14	85.14	12.8	85.28	91.56	7.62
Custom Ensemble	100	100	0	100	100	0
	PCA					
Logistic Regression	70	70	14.14	76.67	73.33	13.33
Decision Tree	76.67	76.67	12.47	80	73.33	8.16
Random Forest	80	80	8.16	86.67	90	13.33
Support Vector Classifier	80	80	0	86.67	83.33	0
Gaussian Naive Bayes	70	70	8.16	96.67	96.67	6.67
Multi-layer Perceptron	73.33	73.33	9.43	86.67	86.67	19.44
k-Nearest neighbors	76.67	76.67	4.71	83.33	76.67	22.61
Custom Ensemble	73.33	73.33	17	86.67	86.67	12.47
	SMOTE + PCA					
Logistic Regression	95.56	95.56	6.29	95.83	95.78	5.18
Decision Tree	85.14	85.14	2.77	93.61	89.78	10.96
Random Forest	93.47	93.47	5.45	97.78	97.78	4.44
Support Vector Classifier	95.56	95.56	6.29	95.83	98	4
Gaussian Naive Bayes	93.47	93.47	5.45	95.69	95.78	5.18
Multi-layer Perceptron	95.56	95.56	6.29	95.83	95.78	5.18
k-Nearest neighbors	95.56	95.56	6.29	91.67	91.33	8.27
Custom Ensemble	95.56	95.56	6.29	97.92	93.78	5.1
	SMOTE + PCA + HPO					
Logistic Regression	95.56	93.33	8.89	95.83	95.78	5.18
Decision Tree	85.14	85.11	12.48	93.61	89.78	10.96
Random Forest	91.39	89.11	7.04	97.78	97.78	4.44
Support Vector Classifier	95.56	95.56	8.89	100	100	0
Gaussian Naive Bayes	93.47	93.56	8.79	95.69	95.78	5.18
Multi-layer Perceptron	91.39	89.11	7.04	100	100	0
k-Nearest neighbors	95.56	95.56	8.89	95.83	95.78	5.18
Custom Ensemble	95.56	95.56	8.89	90	86.67	12.47

Table 10. Evaluation results, by ML algorithm, for the training and testing processes, for both feature selection strategies using the pipeline method.

Algorithm	Accuracy (%)	Accuracy (%)	SD	Sensitivity (%)	SD	Specificity (%)	SD
Manually Selected Feature Set	Training			Testing			
Logistic Regression	100	91.79	6.74	96.6	6.8	70	20
Decision Tree	100	86.07	9.06	96.6	6.8	50	24.72
Random Forest	98.79	88.93	10.62	96.6	6.8	70	20
Support Vector Classifier	98.79	91.79	6.74	93.20	6.33	90	10
Gaussian Naive Bayes	84.33	83.57	10	93.20	6.33	60	17.42
Multi-layer Perceptron	100	94.64	6.59	96.60	6.8	90	10
k-Nearest neighbors	98.79	89.29	9.58	90	13.25	90	10
Automatically Selected Feature Set	Training			Testing			
Logistic Regression	96.38	89.64	8.66	89.4	6.62	90	10
Decision Tree	100	86.79	6.72	90	6.52	80	14.49
Random Forest	100	83.93	10.07	89.4	6.62	70	14.49
Support Vector Classifier	96.38	89.64	8.66	89.4	6.62	90	10
Gaussian Naive Bayes	98.79	92.14	8.2	93.4	6.2	90	10
Multi-layer Perceptron	100	89.64	8.66	89.4	6.62	90	10
k-Nearest neighbors	100	89.64	8.66	89.4	6.62	90	10

In Table 9, the accuracy of each model is provided both for the training and the testing dataset. In the latter case the cross-validation accuracy is shown. At this point, by inspecting the accuracy during training and testing it is possible to recognize which algorithms tend to create models that overfit or underfit. Therefore, first a set of baseline models are trained and tested, then SMOTE and PCA are applied separately, followed by the application of combined SMOTE and PCA on the same dataset and finally a set of models are created by combining SMOTE, PCA and hyperparameter optimization. By inspecting the results, it is observed that most of the baseline trained models for the manually selected features tend to either overfit or underfit, contrary to the dataset composed of the automatically selected features. Moving to the results of the datasets when the SMOTE technique is applied, a slight decrease of overfitting for the dataset of the manually selected features and a significant increase of overfitting for the dataset with the automatically selected features are observed. Inspecting the datasets when the PCA method is applied, a significant underfitting for both datasets can be observed. Examining the results after the sequential application of both SMOTE and PCA, a better consistency of the accuracy for both datasets is observed ranging between 85.14% and 95.56% for the dataset with the manually selected features and between 89.78% and 97.78% for the dataset with the automatically selected features. Finally, only marginal variations in performance are observed when comparing these results to those that are achieved from the sequential application of SMOTE, PCA and HPO for the dataset with the manually selected features and in some cases for the dataset with the automatically selected features where the models either present overfitting (SVC, MLP) or underfitting (custom ensemble).

Moving on to the results of the next stage of our methodology, the final models of this study are given which are built with the usage of pipelines to avoid any possible bias from data leakage. For these models, there is an interest to study their performance in terms of sensitivity and specificity as shown in Table 10. The first conclusion that can be drawn from this evaluation is that for both datasets there are models that score 100% on accuracy in training, so these models clearly overfit and they should be discarded. Hopefully, there are also models that do not overfit during the training, yet they do maintain relatively acceptable scores regarding the accuracy and the rest of the evaluation metrics. Taking into account the scores of sensitivity and specificity, we can distinguish as the best performing models those that are trained using the SVC and GNB algorithms. More specifically, the SVC based model yields an accuracy of 91.79% (6.74% SD), a sensitivity of 93.20% (6.33% SD) and a specificity of 90% (10% SD) for the dataset trained on the manually selected features, while the GNB based model yields an accuracy of 92.14% (8.2% SD), a sensitivity of 93.4% (6.2% SD) and a specificity of 90% (10% SD) for the dataset trained on the automatically selected features. Another remark about this batch of models is the relatively abrupt values of the specificity metric, which is related to the fact that the SMOTE is now part of the pipeline, thus the oversampling for the minority class happens much later than the dataset split, which consequently leads small numbers in false positives to have significant impact on specificity.

Figure 13 provides relevant confusion matrices to visualize the classification performance of the models using the testing dataset for a single prediction. Note that the testing dataset is a stratified hold-out sub-dataset, roughly 30% of the original dataset, yielding 38 instances.

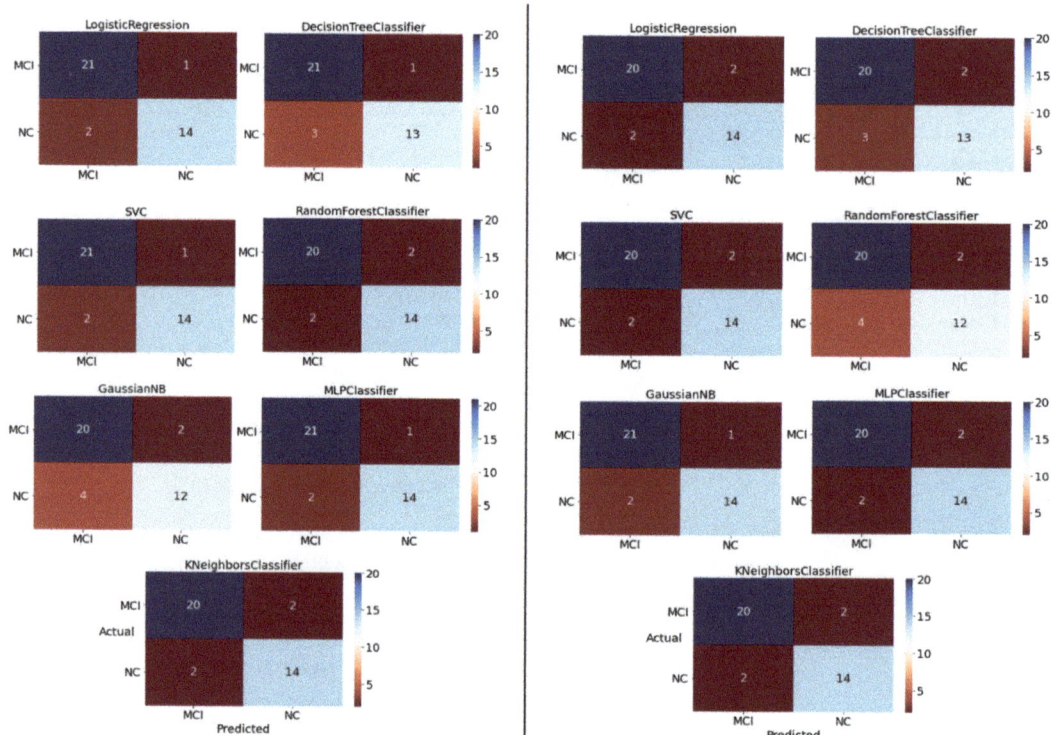

Figure 13. Confusion matrix per ML algorithm for the models trained using the pipeline method for the manually selected features (on the **left**) and the automatically selected features (on the **right**).

The custom wrapper method for model evaluation is also configured to plot the ROC-AUC and the precision–recall diagrams as shown in Figures 14 and 15, respectively. The AUC of SVC for the production level model and the manually selected features is 0.98 whereas the AUC of GNB for the automatically selected features is 0.97. These diagrams along with the precision–recall diagrams affirm the efficiency of the aforementioned ML models.

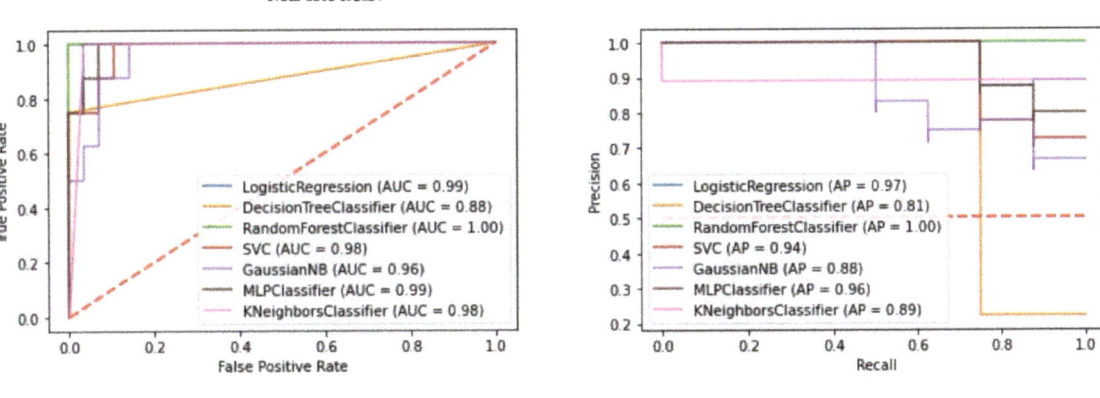

Figure 14. (**a**) ROC-AUC for the production level models and the manually selected features; (**b**) Precision–recall/sensitivity for the production level models and the manually selected features.

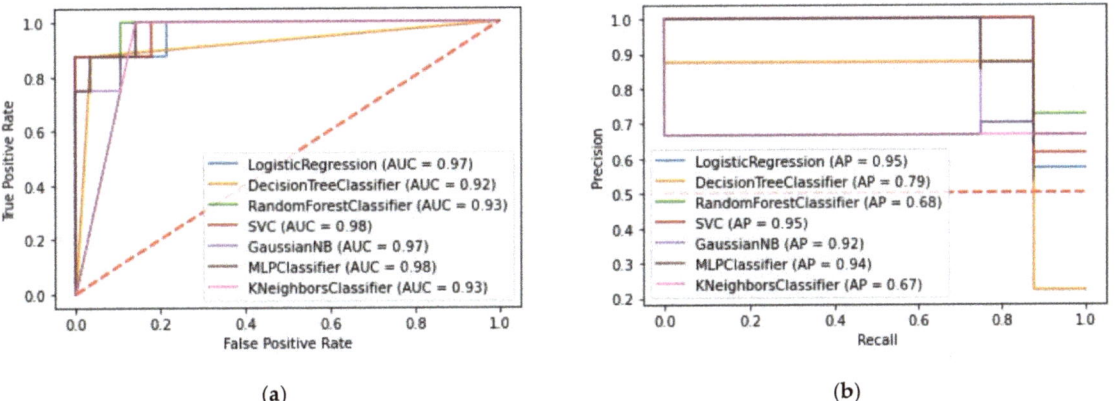

Figure 15. (**a**) ROC-AUC for the production level models and the automatically selected features; (**b**) Precision–recall/sensitivity for the production level models and the automatically selected features.

5. Discussion

This work has shown that it is possible to create ML models based on data collected from serious games and transformed to engineered features along with relevant subjective information. These models can be used then to accurately classify whether a subject belongs to the MCI or NC group as attested by the MoCA cognitive test. In this context, a focal point of the research performed was the development of a custom methodology to train such MCI detection models with low bias and variance and to validate the models using established and solid metrics and techniques, while being attentive to maintain high performance in terms of sensitivity and specificity.

There are 31 features that originally were defined to train the models from which 15 are related to the games, 14 are related to demographic and health data and 2 are artificial variables used as reference points to filter features with a lower importance than them during the feature selection process. Mixing technology-based and subjective data in order to improve the predictive performance of a cognitive impairment detection model is not unprecedented, as a similar approach has been demonstrated in other studies [56]. The inclusion of features that represent demographics, health and lifestyle cater for improving not only the performance but also the generality of the prediction. As a matter of fact, such factors are taken into account also when traditional assessments are used to evaluate cognitive impairment [57]. For example, in MoCA assessment, a score adjustment is allowed depending on the education level of the subjects [6,30].

For the production model trained with the manually selected features and the Support Vector Classifier integrating all the optimization techniques and in the context of the pipeline method an accuracy of 91.79%, a sensitivity of 93.20% and a specificity of 90% were achieved. On the other hand, for the production model trained with the more verbose set of automatically selected features using the Gaussian Naive Bayes algorithm under the pipeline context, the corresponding evaluation metrics were 92.14%, 93.4% and 90%. However, for the specificity metric a higher standard deviation is observed which is due to the fact that for the creation of the production model the testing dataset does not undergo the oversampling process which is now part of the pipeline and happens later in the workflow. Consequently, the true negative values are fewer and therefore small errors of the model lead to a large variation. Both feature selection strategies lead to models with roughly equal performance however the model with the manually selected features is 18% more compact. This model includes 9 features with 5 of them representing game data and 4 of them representing subjective data.

The COGNIPLAT game suite includes games which target cognitive functions that are linked to the assessment of MCI. From the features that have been selected in the machine learning models it is observed that the games that are associated with the cognitive areas of short-term memory, visual memory, episodic memory, spatio-temporal orientation and executive functions are the most important predictors of cognitive impairments. This is reasonable since the design of the corresponding games focused on several occasions on porting typical cognitive assessments in a gamified environment. For example, the *Orientation* game was inspired by Weschler's Picture Arrangement Subset [58] which is used to assess perception and problem-solving cognitive operations that are associated with spatio-temporal orientation. The *Logical Order* game is a digital emulation of the Wisconsin Card Sorting Test [59], frequently used to assess executive functions. The *Recall* game is a gamified version of the Digit Span Forward Test, a subsection also of the MoCA test, typically used to assess short-term memory. The *Naming* game is a gamified version of the Rey Auditory Verbal Learning Test [60] where the auditory stimuli are replaced by visual probes to assess the episodic memory. Consequently, this design approach ensures that each gameplay assesses the cognitive operation that was meant for.

The use of ML algorithms for cognitive impairment identification on the basis of game and subjective data goes beyond the classical approach of using statistical techniques. The MCI detection problem, as defined, calls for employing supervised ML algorithms for classification. Several such ML algorithms were evaluated in order to build the most effective models including probabilistic classifiers (i.e., LR and GNB), kNN, SVC, decision tree learning (i.e., DT, RF), neural networks (i.e., MLP) and ensemble learning. These algorithms were selected based on their suitability regarding the characteristics of the problem in hand and from a research perspective they provided the opportunity to test the created dataset on a broad spectrum of different methods for classification. The choice of ML algorithms is in accordance with other studies, especially in the area of disease prediction in the healthcare domain [61]. The best classification models for MCI detection that the proposed methodology delivered were based on SVC (an implementation of the support vector machine method in the Scikit-learn library) and GNB which are ranked amongst the top ML algorithms with superior accuracy in related problems [61]. The SVC algorithm proved capable of efficiently handling the mixed feature scope (in-game and subjective data) and showed endurance in the overfitting risk. On the other hand, GNB is a well-known classifier which is simple and able to handle both discrete and continuous data achieving a high performance even when the training dataset is limited.

There are several challenges that must be addressed in order to build an MCI detection model using data collected from serious games. Starting with the data available for model training an important issue had to do with their unequal distribution between the two categories of the target class. In particular, the game sessions that correspond to subjects in the MCI category were 71, in contrast to those in the NC category, which were 48. This issue could lead to the creation of biased models with respect to the majority class. To address this, the oversampling method was applied using the SMOTE algorithm, as described in the optimization task of the EDA process. Another data issue is related to features with very low variance which had almost the same values for all the subjects. These features were excluded from the model training (such as the alcohol and smoking variables) within the low variance feature removal procedure. Finally, due to the relatively small dataset, there is a limit to the application of more complex machine learning algorithms, such as deep learning algorithms.

Data leakage is another important issue to resolve. The effects of data leakage are essentially the possible alteration of performance results as the testing data are involved in the process of creating (fitting) the model. The solution to this problem was to use the pipeline utility method, where all transformations of the EDA stage are performed in a closed process that contains no elements of the testing dataset. The advantages of the pipeline include the encapsulation of the data transformations and the classifier, the ability to be used along with grid-search and the prevention of data leakage given that a dataset is split between training and testing sub-datasets beforehand. In our work, the usage of pipelines, apart from the data-leakage prevention and the overall simplicity in workflow design, offers the convenience of having the data preprocessing transformations included in the final model itself, which is very important for the deployment of the classification Service API. This allows new data to be loaded in a single entry point to get a prediction.

One of the optimization techniques applied was dimensionality reduction. In particular, the PCA technique was applied, thus managing to transform the independent variables of the dataset (i.e., the features) into two principal components, which contained a percentage of the original variance. There are other dimensionality reduction techniques that could be used. One alternative method is the linear discriminant analysis (LDA), which in contrast to the PCA method is a supervised learning technique, taking into account the target class for the creation of new components. The difficulty of the LDA method is that the number of new components that emerge is specific and is always the lowest value between the number of features and the number of categories of the target class. In our case this means that only one component could be used.

A limitation of the present study is that the number of participants is apparently small to draw safe conclusions even though the design of the study and the assembled sample were meticulously handled in terms of methodology (e.g., sample heterogeneity, informed consent, ethical approval). Undoubtedly, a larger sample would provide a sounder base regarding the effectiveness of the methodology. On the other hand, the dataset for training and testing the classification models consists of 119 instances, which correspond to the number of game sessions played by the participants. Each instance contains up to 32 variables, i.e., 31 features (as presented in Table 5) and 1 binary classification state. This configuration plausibly serves our preliminary study aiming to assess whether serious games combined with machine learning methods could potentially work as a tool for cognitive screening.

The research described in this paper could be enhanced in various directions. An extension of the research approach will be to explore a model that can classify multiple classes such as NC, MCI and Dementia given the diagnostic capability of the MoCA assessment. Since many subcategories of MCI have been identified such as amnestic MCI, single domain MCI, multiple domain MCI, dysnomic MCI, dysexecutive MCI and their combinations [62], it would be challenging to examine the association of low performance in specific games with specific MCI subcategories in order to create a model that would be able to classify multiple cognitive classes.

6. Conclusions

This work demonstrates that models trained on data gathered from serious games can distinguish, with sufficient accuracy, whether an individual belongs in the healthy or the MCI state in terms of cognitive competency. The research performed in this work is multifaceted and its scope ranges from the healthcare application domain in terms of exploring MCI characteristics, to the use of serious games in terms of collecting raw data and to the machine learning domain in terms of extracting features and building models that allow the early MCI detection. The contribution of this work is a methodology to train and evaluate models with ML algorithms, validate their results and reflect on the challenges addressed throughout the steps of this process. Eventually, the ultimate goal is to use the games and the machine learning models in services that could be used supplementary to the traditional cognitive assessment tools. Our preliminary results are promising and call for further research in the way to bring this methodology to the clinical practice of cognitive impairment diagnosis.

Author Contributions: C.G. planned and supervised the study, and C.K. designed the ML methodology. Analyses and writing of the manuscript were performed by both C.G. and C.K. Both authors have read and agreed to the published version of the manuscript.

Funding: This research has been co-financed by the European Regional Development Fund of the European Union and Greek national funds through the Operational Program Competitiveness, Entrepreneurship and Innovation, under the call ERA-NETS 2018 (ID:T8EPA2-00011, grant MIS:5041669).

Institutional Review Board Statement: The study was conducted according to the guidelines of the Declaration of Helsinki and approved by the Institutional Review Board (or Ethics Committee) of University of the Aegean.

Informed Consent Statement: Informed consent was obtained from all subjects involved in the study.

Data Availability Statement: The datasets generated during and/or analyzed during the current study are not publicly available due to ethical constraints in consideration of participants' privacy but are available from the corresponding author on reasonable request.

Acknowledgments: The authors would like to thank Georgios Koumanakos, Dimitrios Koumanakos and Maria Frounta from Frontida Zois for their support in implementing the evaluation study and the volunteers that took part in the study.

Conflicts of Interest: The authors declare no conflict of interest.

References

1. Plassman, B.L.; Williams, J.W., Jr.; Burke, J.R.; Holsinger, T.; Benjamin, S. Systematic review: Factors associated with risk for and possible prevention of cognitive decline in later life. *Ann. Intern. Med.* **2010**, *153*, 182–193. [CrossRef] [PubMed]
2. Langa, K.M.; Levine, D.A. The diagnosis and management of mild cognitive impairment: A clinical review. *JAMA* **2014**, *312*, 2551–2561. [CrossRef]
3. Albert, M.S.; DeKosky, S.T.; Dickson, D.; Dubois, B.; Feldman, H.H.; Fox, N.C.; Gamst, A.; Holtzman, D.M.; Jagust, W.J.; Petersen, R.C.; et al. The diagnosis of mild cognitive impairment due to Alzheimer's disease: Recommendations from the National Institute on Aging-Alzheimer's Association workgroups on diagnostic guidelines for Alzheimer's disease. *Alzheimer's Dement.* **2011**, *7*, 270–279. [CrossRef]
4. Petersen, R.C. Mild cognitive impairment as a diagnostic entity. *J. Intern. Med.* **2004**, *256*, 183–194. [CrossRef]
5. Folstein, M.F.; Robins, L.N.; Helzer, J.E. The mini-mental state examination. *Arch. Gen. Psychiatry* **1983**, *40*, 812. [CrossRef]
6. Nasreddine, Z.S.; Phillips, N.A.; Bédirian, V.; Charbonneau, S.; Whitehead, V.; Collin, I.; Cummings, J.L.; Chertkow, H. The Montreal Cognitive Assessment, MoCA: A brief screening tool for mild cognitive impairment. *J. Am. Geriatr. Soc.* **2005**, *53*, 695–699. [CrossRef] [PubMed]
7. Tong, T.; Chignell, M.; Tierney, M.C.; Lee, J. A serious game for clinical assessment of cognitive status: Validation study. *JMIR Serious Games* **2016**, *27*, e5006. [CrossRef] [PubMed]
8. Krishnan, K.; Rossetti, H.; Hynan, L.S.; Carter, K.; Falkowski, J.; Lacritz, L.; Cullum, C.M.; Weiner, M. Changes in Montreal Cognitive Assessment scores over time. *Assessment* **2017**, *24*, 772–777. [CrossRef] [PubMed]

9. Valladares-Rodriguez, S.; Fernández-Iglesias, M.J.; Anido-Rifón, L.; Facal, D.; Rivas-Costa, C.; Pérez-Rodríguez, R. Touchscreen games to detect cognitive impairment in senior adults. A user-interaction pilot study. *Int. J. Med. Inform.* **2019**, *127*, 52–62. [CrossRef]
10. Jin, R.; Pilozzi, A.; Huang, X. Current Cognition Tests, Potential Virtual Reality Applications, and Serious Games in Cognitive Assessment and Non-Pharmacological Therapy for Neurocognitive Disorders. *J. Clin. Med.* **2020**, *9*, 3287. [CrossRef]
11. Sawyer, B. *Serious Games: Improving Public Policy through Game-Based Learning and Simulation*; Woodrow Wilson International Center for Scholars: Washington, DC, USA, 2002.
12. Boletsis, C.; McCallum, S. Smartkuber: A serious game for cognitive health screening of elderly players. *Games Health J.* **2016**, *5*, 241–251. [CrossRef]
13. Ge, S.; Zhu, Z.; Wu, B.; McConnell, E.S. Technology-based cognitive training and rehabilitation interventions for individuals with mild cognitive impairment: A systematic review. *BMC Geriatr.* **2018**, *18*, 213. [CrossRef] [PubMed]
14. Lumsden, J.; Edwards, E.A.; Lawrence, N.S.; Coyle, D.; Munafò, M.R. Gamification of cognitive assessment and cognitive training: A systematic review of applications and efficacy. *JMIR Serious Games* **2016**, *4*, e5888. [CrossRef]
15. McCallum, S.; Boletsis, C. Dementia games: A literature review of dementia-related serious games. In *International Conference on Serious Games Development and Applications*; Springer: Berlin/Heidelberg, Germany, 2013; pp. 15–27.
16. Garcia-Ceja, E.; Riegler, M.; Nordgreen, T.; Jakobsen, P.; Oedegaard, K.J.; Tørresen, J. Mental health monitoring with multimodal sensing and machine learning: A survey. *Pervasive Mob. Comput.* **2018**, *51*, 1–26. [CrossRef]
17. Valladares-Rodríguez, S.; Pérez-Rodríguez, R.; Anido-Rifón, L.; Fernández-Iglesias, M. Trends on the application of serious games to neuropsychological evaluation: A scoping review. *J. Biomed. Inform.* **2016**, *64*, 296–319. [CrossRef]
18. Joshi, V.; Wallace, B.; Shaddy, A.; Knoefel, F.; Goubran, R.; Lord, C. Metrics to monitor performance of patients with mild cognitive impairment using computer based games. In Proceedings of the 2016 IEEE-EMBS International Conference on Biomedical and Health Informatics (BHI), Las Vegas, NV, USA, 24–27 February 2016; pp. 521–524.
19. Leduc-McNiven, K.; White, B.; Zheng, H.; McLeod, R.D.; Friesen, M.R. Serious games to assess mild cognitive impairment: 'The game is the assessment'. *Res. Rev. Insights* **2018**, *2*. [CrossRef]
20. Leduc-McNiven, K.; Dion, R.T.; Mukhi, S.N.; McLeod, R.D.; Friesen, M.R. Machine learning and serious games: Opportunities and requirements for detection of mild cognitive impairment. *J. Med. Artif. Intell.* **2018**, *2*. [CrossRef]
21. Solana, J.; Cáceres, C.; García-Molina, A.; Chausa, P.; Opisso, E.; Roig-Rovira, T.; Menasalvas, E.; Tormos-Muñoz, J.M.; Gómez, E.J. Intelligent Therapy Assistant (ITA) for cognitive rehabilitation in patients with acquired brain injury. *BMC Med. Inform. Decis. Mak.* **2014**, *14*, 58. [CrossRef]
22. Banerjee, S.; Chattopadhyay, T.; Biswas, S.; Banerjee, R.; Choudhury, A.D.; Pal, A.; Garain, U. Towards wide learning: Experiments in healthcare. *arXiv* **2016**, arXiv:1612.05730.
23. Sirály, E.; Szabó, Á.; Szita, B.; Kovács, V.; Fodor, Z.; Marosi, C.; Salacz, P.; Hidasi, Z.; Maros, V.; Hanák, P.; et al. Monitoring the early signs of cognitive decline in elderly by computer games: An MRI study. *PLoS ONE* **2015**, *10*, e0117918.
24. Binaco, R.; Calzaretto, N.; Epifano, J.; McGuire, S.; Umer, M.; Emrani, S.; Wasserman, V.; Libon, D.J.; Polikar, R. Machine learning analysis of digital clock drawing test performance for differential classification of mild cognitive impairment subtypes versus Alzheimer's disease. *J. Int. Neuropsychol. Soc.* **2020**, *26*, 690–700. [CrossRef]
25. Valladares-Rodriguez, S.; Pérez-Rodríguez, R.; Fernandez-Iglesias, J.M.; Anido-Rifón, L.E.; Facal, D.; Rivas-Costa, C. Learning to detect cognitive impairment through digital games and machine learning techniques. *Methods Inf. Med.* **2018**, *57*, 197–207. [CrossRef]
26. Schröer, C.; Kruse, F.; Gómez, J.M. A Systematic Literature Review on Applying CRISP-DM Process Model. *Procedia Comput. Sci.* **2021**, *181*, 526–534. [CrossRef]
27. Martínez-Plumed, F.; Contreras-Ochando, L.; Ferri, C.; Orallo, J.H.; Kull, M.; Lachiche, N.; Quintana, M.J.; Flach, P.A. CRISP-DM twenty years later: From data mining processes to data science trajectories. *IEEE Trans. Knowl. Data Eng.* **2019**, *33*, 3048–3061. [CrossRef]
28. COGNIPLAT Project. Available online: https://cogniplat.aegean.gr/ (accessed on 27 July 2021).
29. Goumopoulos, C.; Igoumenakis, I. An Ontology based Game Platform for Mild Cognitive Impairment Rehabilitation. In Proceedings of the ICT4AWE, Online Streaming, 21–27 June 2020; pp. 130–141.
30. Poptsi, E.; Moraitou, D.; Eleftheriou, M.; Kounti-Zafeiropoulou, F.; Papasozomenou, C.; Agogiatou, C.; Bakoglidou, E.; Batsila, G.; Liapi, D.; Markou, N.; et al. Normative data for the Montreal Cognitive Assessment in Greek older adults with subjective cognitive decline, mild cognitive impairment and dementia. *J. Geriatr. Psychiatry Neurol.* **2019**, *32*, 265–274. [CrossRef]
31. Weber, G.M.; Mandl, K.D.; Kohane, I.S. Finding the missing link for big biomedical data. *JAMA* **2014**, *311*, 2479–2480. [CrossRef] [PubMed]
32. Nargesian, F.; Samulowitz, H.; Khurana, U.; Khalil, E.B.; Turaga, D.S. Learning Feature Engineering for Classification. In Proceedings of the Twenty-Sixth International Joint Conference on Artificial Intelligence (IJCAI-17), Melbourne, Australia, 19–25 August 2017; pp. 2529–2535.
33. Stoppiglia, H.; Dreyfus, G.; Dubois, R.; Oussar, Y. Ranking a random feature for variable and feature selection. *J. Mach. Learn. Res.* **2003**, *3*, 1399–1414.
34. Pedregosa, F.; Varoquaux, G.; Gramfort, A.; Michel, V.; Thirion, B.; Grisel, O.; Blondel, M.; Prettenhofer, P.; Weiss, R.; Dubourg, V.; et al. Scikit-learn: Machine learning in Python. *J. Mach. Learn. Res.* **2011**, *12*, 2825–2830.

35. Aggarwal, A.; Kean, E. Comparison of the Folstein Mini Mental State Examination (MMSE) to the Montreal Cognitive Assessment (MoCA) as a cognitive screening tool in an inpatient rehabilitation setting. *Neurosci. Med.* **2010**, *1*, 39. [CrossRef]
36. Han, J.; Pei, J.; Kamber, M. *Data Mining: Concepts and Techniques*; Elsevier: Amsterdam, The Netherlands, 2011.
37. Ghosh, D.; Vogt, A. Outliers: An evaluation of methodologies. In Proceedings of the 2012 InJoint Statistical Meetings, San Diego, CA, USA, 28 July–2 August 2012; Volume 2012.
38. Brownlee, J. Data preparation for machine learning: Data cleaning, feature selection, and data transforms in Python. In *Machine Learning Mastery*; Machine Learning Mastery Pty. Ltd.: Vermont, VIC, Australia, 2020.
39. Sobolewski, P.; Wozniak, M. Concept Drift Detection and Model Selection with Simulated Recurrence and Ensembles of Statistical Detectors. *J. Univers. Comput. Sci.* **2013**, *19*, 462–483.
40. Liu, H.; Motoda, H.; Setiono, R.; Zhao, Z. Feature selection: An ever evolving frontier in data mining. In Proceedings of the Feature Selection in Data Mining, PMLR, Hyderabad, India, 21 June 2010; pp. 4–13.
41. Koller, D.; Sahami, M. *Toward Optimal Feature Selection*; Stanford InfoLab: Stanford, CA, USA, 1996.
42. Müllner, D. Modern hierarchical, agglomerative clustering algorithms. *arXiv* **2011**, arXiv:1109.2378.
43. Trevethan, R. Sensitivity, specificity, and predictive values: Foundations, pliabilities, and pitfalls in research and practice. *Front. Public Health* **2017**, *5*, 307. [CrossRef] [PubMed]
44. Goldstein, F.C.; Ashley, A.V.; Miller, E.; Alexeeva, O.; Zanders, L.; King, V. Validity of the montreal cognitive assessment as a screen for mild cognitive impairment and dementia in African Americans. *J. Geriatr. Psychiatry Neurol.* **2014**, *27*, 199–203. [CrossRef]
45. Briscoe, E.; Feldman, J. Conceptual complexity and the bias/variance tradeoff. *Cognition* **2011**, *118*, 2–16. [CrossRef] [PubMed]
46. Lever, J.; Krzywinski, M.; Altman, N. Points of significance: Model selection and overfitting. *Nat. Methods* **2016**, *13*, 703–705. [CrossRef]
47. Wall, M.E.; Rechtsteiner, A.; Rocha, L.M. Singular value decomposition and principal component analysis. In *A Practical Approach to Microarray Data Analysis*; Springer: Boston, MA, USA, 2003; pp. 91–109.
48. Blagus, R.; Lusa, L. SMOTE for high-dimensional class-imbalanced data. In *BMC Bioinform*; Rok, B., Lara, L., Eds.; BioMed Central: London, UK, 2013; Volume 14, p. 106.
49. Tang, L.; Liu, H. Bias analysis in text classification for highly skewed data. In Proceedings of the Fifth IEEE International Conference on Data Mining (ICDM'05), Houston, TX, USA, 27–30 November 2005; p. 4.
50. Kosmpoulos, A.; Paliouras, G.; Androutsopoulos, I. The effect of dimensionality reduction on large scale hierarchical classification. In *International Conference of the Cross-Language Evaluation Forum for European Languages*; Springer: Berlin/Heidelberg, Germany, 2014; pp. 160–171.
51. Feurer, M.; Hutter, F. Hyperparameter optimization. In *Automated Machine Learning*; Springer: Berlin/Heidelberg, Germany, 2019; pp. 3–33.
52. Bussola, N.; Marcolini, A.; Maggio, V.; Jurman, G.; Furlanello, C. AI Slipping on Tiles: Data Leakage in Digital Pathology. In *Pattern Recognition. ICPR International Workshops and Challenges*; Springer: Berlin/Heidelberg, Germany, 2021; pp. 167–182.
53. Saravanan, N.; Sathish, G.; Balajee, J.M. Data wrangling and data leakage in machine learning for healthcare. *Int. J. Emerg. Technol. Innov. Res.* **2018**, *5*, 553–557.
54. Chen, P.H.; Liu, Y.; Peng, L. How to develop machine learning models for healthcare. *Nat. Mater.* **2019**, *18*, 410–414. [CrossRef] [PubMed]
55. Assunção, F.; Lourenço, N.; Ribeiro, B.; Machado, P. Evolution of scikit-learn pipelines with dynamic structured grammatical evolution. *arXiv* **2020**, arXiv:2004.00307.
56. Alhanai, T.; Au, R.; Glass, J. Spoken language biomarkers for detecting cognitive impairment. In Proceedings of the 2017 IEEE Automatic Speech Recognition and Understanding Workshop (ASRU), Okinawa, Japan, 16–20 December 2017; pp. 409–416.
57. Milani, S.A.; Marsiske, M.; Cottler, L.B.; Chen, X.; Striley, C.W. Optimal cutoffs for the Montreal Cognitive Assessment vary by race and ethnicity. *Alzheimer's Dement. Diagn. Assess. Dis. Monit.* **2018**, *10*, 773–781. [CrossRef]
58. Wechsler, D. *Wechsler Adult Intelligence Scale*, 3rd ed.; Harcourt Assessment: San Antonio, TX, USA, 1997.
59. Heaton, R.K.; Chelune, G.J.; Talley, J.L.; Kay, G.G.; Curtiss, G. *Wisconsin Card Sorting Test (WCST): Manual: Revised and Expanded*; Psychological Assessment Resources: Lutz, FL, USA, 1993.
60. Schmidt, M. *Rey Auditory Verbal Learning Test: A Handbook*; Western Psychological Services: Los Angeles, CA, USA, 1996.
61. Uddin, S.; Khan, A.; Hossain, M.E.; Moni, M.A. Comparing different supervised machine learning algorithms for disease prediction. *BMC Med. Inform. Decis. Mak.* **2019**, *19*, 281. [CrossRef]
62. Díaz-Mardomingo, M.D.; García-Herranz, S.; Rodríguez-Fernández, R.; Venero, C.; Peraita, H. Problems in classifying mild cognitive impairment (MCI): One or multiple syndromes? *Brain Sci.* **2017**, *7*, 111. [CrossRef] [PubMed]

Article

An Exergame Solution for Personalized Multicomponent Training in Older Adults

Vânia Guimarães [1,*], Elsa Oliveira [1], Alberto Carvalho [1], Nuno Cardoso [1], Johannes Emerich [2], Chantale Dumoulin [3,4], Nathalie Swinnen [5], Jacqueline De Jong [6] and Eling D. de Bruin [7,8]

1. Fraunhofer Portugal AICOS, 4200-135 Porto, Portugal; elsa.oliveira@fraunhofer.pt (E.O.); alberto.carvalho@fraunhofer.pt (A.C.); nuno.cardoso@fraunhofer.pt (N.C.)
2. Dividat AG, 8834 Schindellegi, Switzerland; johannes@dividat.ch
3. School of Rehabilitation, Faculty of Medicine, Université de Montréal, Montréal, QC H3T 1J4, Canada; chantal.dumoulin@umontreal.ca
4. Research Center of Institut, Universitaire de Gériatrie de Montréal, Montréal, QC H3W 1W6, Canada
5. Faculty of Movement and Rehabilitation Sciences, KU Leuven, 3001 Leuven, Belgium; nathalie.swinnen@kuleuven.be
6. Physio SPArtos, 3800 Interlaken, Switzerland; j.dejong@artos.ch
7. Department of Health Sciences and Technology, Institute of Human Movement Sciences and Sport, ETH Zurich, 8093 Zurich, Switzerland; eling.debruin@hest.ethz.ch
8. Division of Physiotherapy, Department of Neurobiology, Care Sciences and Society, Karolinska Institute, 171 77 Stockholm, Sweden
* Correspondence: vania.guimaraes@fraunhofer.pt

Abstract: In addition to contributing to increased training motivation, exergames are a promising approach to counteract age-related impairments. Mobility limitations, cognitive impairment, and urinary incontinence are very common in older adults. To optimally address these conditions, exergames should include interventions for strength, balance, cognition, and pelvic floor muscle training. In this study, we develop a personalized multicomponent exergame solution for the geriatric rehabilitation of age-related impairments. The exergame can provide interventions for balance, strength, cognition, and urinary incontinence in one single session, accommodating the needs of older adults with multiple disabilities. For its development, we involved a multidisciplinary team that helped us to specify the structure and contents of the exergame considering training requirements, game design principles, and end-user characteristics. In addition to allowing the customization of the training components, the exergame includes automatic adaptation of difficulty/load, in line with player progress over time. The game mechanics ensures the fulfilment of training needs as defined by the therapist. The exergame is cross-platform compatible (web-based) and includes novel means of interaction with wearable sensors.

Keywords: exergames; personalized exergames; multicomponent training; wearable sensors; older adults; game design; interaction design

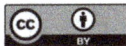

1. Introduction

Ageing is associated with a gradual decline in physical and cognitive abilities. Mobility limitations, cognitive impairment, and urinary incontinence are particularly common in older adults [1], having a negative impact on their lives. Moreover, these conditions are associated with gait impairments, increased risk of falling, and all-cause mortality [2–4].

Mobility and cognitive impairments share common underlying mechanics of decline, and often coexist in older adults [5]. Results from several studies also suggest that mobility decline and cognitive impairment are associated—and frequently coexist—with urinary incontinence [4,6–8]. According to [4] improving functional independence reduces urinary incontinence, and improves cognitive function in older adults.

Multicomponent exercises—including aerobic, strength, endurance, and balance training—were shown to improve physical performance and health [9], reduce falls, urinary incontinence, and risk of injuries [10–12], while improving cognitive functions [13–15], quality of life [16], and self-efficacy [17] in older adults. Cognitive training showed positive effects in specific cognitive functions and dual-task activities in older adults with or without cognitive impairment [18–21]. Additionally, pelvic floor muscle training is recommended for women with geriatric incontinence [22,23]. Still, lack of motivation and low adherence to physical activity constitute a barrier to the implementation of conventional training programs [24].

Exergames can be used to encourage physical activity in older adults [25,26]. Besides being widely available, leveraging autonomous use, and providing performance monitoring and individual adaptation capabilities [27,28], exergames can be used as an alternative to conventional training [29]. Exergames showed promising results to improve motor and cognitive functions in older adults [30–33], reduce the risk of falling [34], improve quality of life and enjoyment [30], improve balance and mobility [35], improve strength [36], and minimize urinary incontinence [37].

If, on one hand, we cannot deny the potential value of exergames in geriatric rehabilitation, on the other hand, practical implementation at clinics or at home is far from being ideal [28]: older adults may have difficulties following fast paced games; they may be afraid of falling or being injured; they may feel low confidence; and they may feel anxious or insecure working with technology [38]. These difficulties are aggravated by the fact that most exergames—especially those available commercially, such as Nintendo Wii^{TM} or Xbox Kinect^{TM}—were not developed specifically for older adults, neglecting their characteristics and preferences [39–41]. In contrast, very basic game design and game mechanics may end up compromising usability, enjoyment, and motivation [42].

Gamification refers to the use of game design elements (e.g., scores, feedback, and progression) to improve user experience and motivation [43]. Gamified concepts were applied to approach motor and cognitive training in older adults with or without cognitive impairment [31,44–47], and pelvic floor muscle training in older women [37,48]. To improve training variety, current solutions usually integrate several games that target different components of the training. However, individual training times (of each individual component) cannot be personalized, being training times usually controlled by the user according to the verbal or written guidelines provided by the clinician [48–50]. Current exergames also do not offer solutions for the multicomponent training of the three conditions—i.e., mobility limitations, cognitive impairment, and urinary incontinence—simultaneously, even though they are frequently associated and occur simultaneously in an older person.

In view of the above, the project VITAAL (funded by the European Commission through the Active Assisted Living Program) proposed the development of a personalized multicomponent exergame solution for mobility limitations, cognitive impairment, and/or urinary incontinence in older adults [51]. In this study, we propose an exergame design and mechanics targeting the three age-related disabilities, which allows the customization of the training components. The game mechanics ensures the implementation of training requirements, so that the training needs—as defined by the therapist—can be fulfilled in each training session. Gamification techniques and usability guidelines are incorporated for better user experience and motivation.

This study aims to describe the development and the theoretical foundations of the new exergame solution. We discuss how the proposed game mechanics adapts to the training needs of older adults with different age-related impairments and, simultaneously, how it answers to the needs of personalization and multicomponent progressive training in older adults. Finally, we discuss the challenges of the game design process and summarize a set of considerations for interaction design and implementation.

2. Related Work

Several exergames have been proposed to target mobility limitations, cognitive impairment, or urinary incontinence (Table 1). In 2015, the iStopFalls consortium proposed the development of an innovative home-based solution for fall prevention, comprising exergames for balance and cognition provided by a Kinect-based solution [46]. In more recent studies, Kinect continues to be the first choice when it comes to tracking and evaluating full-body movements [31,44,47]. However, according to [52], more than one Kinect sensor should be used to accurately track complex human movement sequences, which may compromise application in real scenarios.

Inertial sensors have been used by [45] in a previous project, Active@Home, to track the movements of the upper and lower limbs. To interact with the game, users had to point to the screen (like a cursor), or perform multidirectional steps (to interact with motor-cognitive games). Older adults had some difficulties alternating interaction with the cursor and the with the feet. The usability study also revealed some difficulties in visualizing movement feedback elements (while following an avatar), although these elements were placed as close as possible to the main action of the game [45]. The movements of the avatar were very clear and easy to understand. Due to the position of the sensor at the ankle, multidirectional steps could not always be correctly evaluated, which caused some frustration. The usability study recommended the inclusion of in-game design strategies to support interaction and autonomous use [45].

A freeware dance program, StepMania, was combined with pelvic floor muscle training, achieving some promising results [48,53]. The game required users to step in the direction of the arrows that reached the top of the screen; pelvic floor muscle contractions were represented by a red dot incorporated in the sequence of arrows [53]. The study did not include any gamification or game design concerns [48,53]. In [37], the pelvic floor muscle training was provided resorting to an adaptation of a Wii Fit Plus^{TM} exergame. Women would sit on the Wii Balance Board, and interact with the exergame resorting to pelvic movements. This intervention promoted a decrease in urinary symptoms; however, usability and game experience were not evaluated [37].

In [44] an augmented reality exergame was developed that combines a representation of the user body with a virtual environment. In [31], a virtual reality approach is employed, in which participants are required to wear virtual reality glasses. Although virtual and augmented reality promises many benefits for older adults, the use of these tools is still challenging due to lack of access and digital skills [54].

When designing exergames for older adults, the contents, mechanics, and interface of the exergames need to be tailored to the target group, considering their specific characteristics. Exergames designed specifically for older adults (as is the case of some of those presented in Table 1) incorporate some of the best practices for designing for older adults. Feedback, progression, time constraints and scores are considered particularly relevant for older persons' perceived performance while holding a training session [43]. Training principles such as feedback, optimal challenge and progression, and variety are also required for an effective training [23,38,49].

To improve training variety, studies usually integrate multiple exergames that target different components of the training. However, individual training times (of each training component) cannot be personalized, leaving it up the player to control training times as instructed by the clinician or researcher [48–50]. Current exergames offer no solutions for the simultaneous (multicomponent) training of mobility limitations, cognitive impairment, and urinary incontinence, even though these impairments frequently coexist in older adults.

Table 1. Exergames for motor-cognitive and pelvic floor muscle training in older adults.

Lead Author (Year)	Description	Technology	Limitations
Chen (2020) [44]	Three augmented reality exergames for simultaneous motor (strength and balance) and cognitive (attention, memory, and executive functions) training.	Kinect	Individual training times cannot be personalized. Training times are not ensured by the game.
Zhang (2021) [47]	The exergame combines cognitive and physical tasks to improve older adults' cognitive inhibition. The theme of the game (table tennis) is chosen considering the local popularity of this sport.	Kinect	Lack of progression mechanisms. Only cognitive inhibition and one type of physical exercise are targeted by the exergame.
Guimarães (2018) [45]	An exergame solution comprising dance (for balance), Tai Chi-inspired exercises (for strength) and motor-cognitive training. Dance and Tai Chi exercises are provided by a virtual instructor (3D Avatar).	Inertial sensors	Individual training times cannot be personalized. Training times are not ensured by the game.
Marston (2015) [46]	Three exergames for dynamic balance and stability based on weight shifting, knee bending and stepping. In addition, each exergame contains a cognitive component: memory, inhibition, and selective attention.	Kinect	Individual training times cannot be personalized. Training times are not ensured by the game.
Liao (2019) [31]	Two virtual reality-based physical training games and three virtual reality-based cognitive training games for people with mild cognitive impairment.	Kinect	Lack of progression mechanisms. Individual training times cannot be personalized.
Fraser (2014) [48]	A dancing (stepping) exergame combined with stimuli for pelvic floor muscle contractions.	Dance pad	Lack of progression mechanisms.
Botelho (2015) [37]	An exergame for the training of pelvic floor muscles. Women would sit on a pressure platform, and command the game through their pelvic movements.	Wii Balance Board	Not designed specifically for older adults.

3. Materials and Methods

The project VITAAL aimed at creating a technological solution—an exergame—to support personalized and multicomponent clinical interventions for older adults with mobility limitations, cognitive impairment, and/or urinary incontinence, while catering for individual capabilities and progress. Motivating the person through fun and entertainment was also an important goal of the project.

VITAAL was structured in three phases: investigation, development, and trials [51]. The investigation phase aimed at understanding user needs and expectations, for which partners in the project conducted a survey with end-users and a focus group with clinicians, whose results are reported elsewhere [51]. The development phase comprised the actual development of the solution using the methods thoroughly documented and discussed in this work. Following the development phase, the project foresees two evaluation loops that will assess (i) the acceptability and game experience of the users, and (ii) the feasibility of the intervention. In this study, we focus on the design and development of the VITAAL exergame solution.

The design and development of the VITAAL exergame considered inputs from older adults (resulting from the investigation phase of the project [51], and from the feedback obtained in a previous study [45]) and from a multidisciplinary team, including game designers, developers, user experience/user interface (UX/UI) designers, movement scientists, end-users, and clinicians. Through a set of meetings, and following an iterative design process, they helped us to specify the structure and contents of the exergame, ensuring its adequacy concerning training requirements, game design principles, and end-user characteristics.

In this section, we specify (i) the training requirements, (ii) the game mechanics, (iii) the game design, (iv) the minigames, (v) the evaluation and automatic progression adaptation, and (vi) the implementation details.

3.1. Training Requirements

Training requirements were identified with the help of clinicians—physiotherapists—and movement scientists with experience in geriatric rehabilitation. They all agreed that an exergame mostly based on the execution of multidirectional steps would fit the needs of the target population. Plus, multidirectional steps could be performed while answering to specific cognitive tasks, or contracting the pelvic floor muscles, which could largely improve the outcomes of the training [48,55]. Considering that most daily life activities require simultaneous performance of physical and cognitive functions, combining physical and cognitive exercises in a single exergame solution would potentially boost the benefits of both exercises [55].

According to the team, balance training should focus on the execution of multidirectional steps which have been previously recommended to prevent falls in older adults [56]. For optimal progression, the sequence and speed of steps should become increasingly challenging [57].

For strength training, exercises could be inspired by Tai Chi movements and focus on the hip, knee, ankle, and trunk muscles, as in a previous project Active@Home [45,49]. These exercises are mainly based on narrow and wide squats and should become increasingly challenging for optimal progression [49,58]. The team was responsible for defining the exercises, the number of repetitions and sets, and the progression within the exergame.

Cognitive training should focus on attention and executive functions (e.g., memory, reaction time, mental flexibility, and inhibition control) which are critical to control gait and walk safely [59]. For optimal load, the difficulty of the tasks must adapt to the person's abilities [38].

Exercises targeting urinary incontinence should involve strength (maximal contraction), endurance (repetitive or sustained contraction), and coordination (contraction prior to effort, e.g., prior to cough) training of the pelvic floor muscles [60]. For progression, pelvic floor muscle training should occur with multidirectional steps, following the challenges of the game [48]. The progressive training should increase the intensity and number of pelvic floor muscle contractions in line with patient performance [23,60]. The progression was defined by physiotherapists with experience on the treatment of urinary incontinence.

Studies recommend regular motor-cognitive training (targeting balance, strength, and cognition) in all three disabilities—mobility limitations, cognitive impairment, and urinary incontinence [48,61–63]. Additionally, women with geriatric incontinence should perform exercises for the training of the pelvic floor muscles [22]. The exergame should allow the training of the four training components, i.e., strength, balance, cognitive, and pelvic floor muscle training, in one single session. By personalizing the training times of each component, and adjusting its load, individual training needs should be optimally addressed [64].

3.2. Game Mechanics

To allow the integration of multiple training components within the game, we have structured it in a set of themes. The game mechanics was inspired on the SIMS (Electronic Arts Inc. (EA)) series of games, in which players take care of their virtual entities. In VITAAL exergame, the player should "take care" of each theme, ensuring that progress bars—associated with each theme—should be full by the end of the training session. Game mechanics was defined by game designers, together with a UX/UI designer, and considering the feedback from clinicians and movement scientists, to answer to the training requirements defined in Section 3.1.

Each training component (i.e., balance, strength, cognitive, and pelvic floor muscle training) was associated with one or more themes within the game. The themes were identified to target older adult preferences and interests—important to ensure adherence to the game [40]. The selected themes—nature, library, kitchen, farm, and supermarket—are related to the hobbies that were most commonly reported by older adults during the investigation phase [51]. Each theme includes two minigames targeting a single training component. Training components, themes, and minigames are depicted in Figure 1.

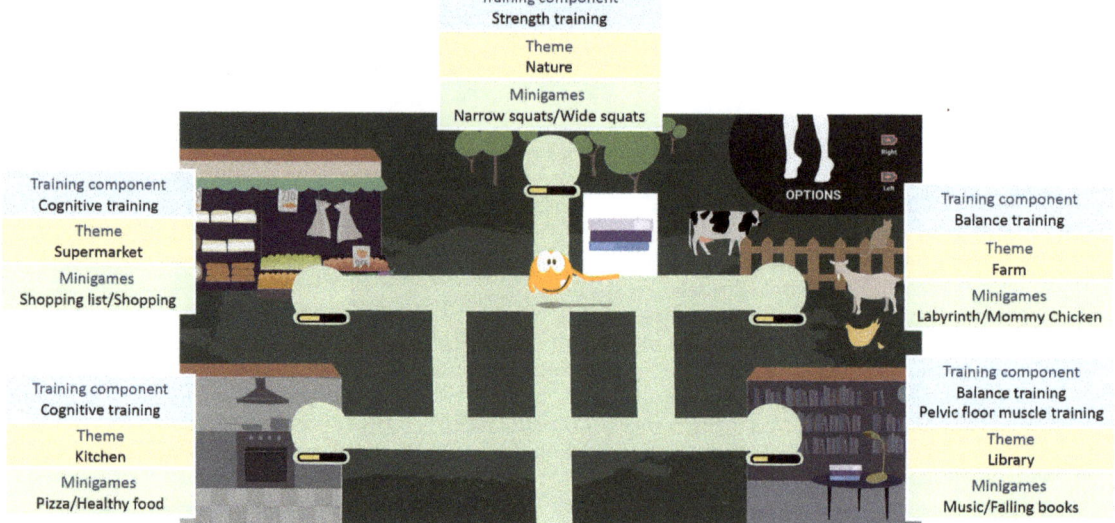

Figure 1. Main board: Training components, themes and minigames.

The game mechanics is illustrated in Figure 2 using a machinations diagram—a type of diagram used to describe game mechanics and its emerging gameplay dynamics [65]. Each progress bar has an initial state that is proportional to the prescribed training time (b)—defined by the therapist for a specific training component—within the total session time (a)—the total time of the session is the sum of the individual times prescribed for each training component. To update the status of the progress bar, the player should perform certain tasks (play minigames). The total time played (c) is used to update the status of the bar, which should increase proportionally to the percentage of time played (e). Progress bars provide information on training completion, and are used to guide the player through the themes and ensure the fulfilment of training needs—as defined by the therapist.

To ensure that recommended training times are not exceeded, the game engine also manipulates the duration of the minigames. This calculation is performed once when the player starts a new training session. The player is always able to repeat a minigame, even if the progress bars indicate 100% completion; when 100% is reached, the training times—as prescribed by the therapist—have been fulfilled.

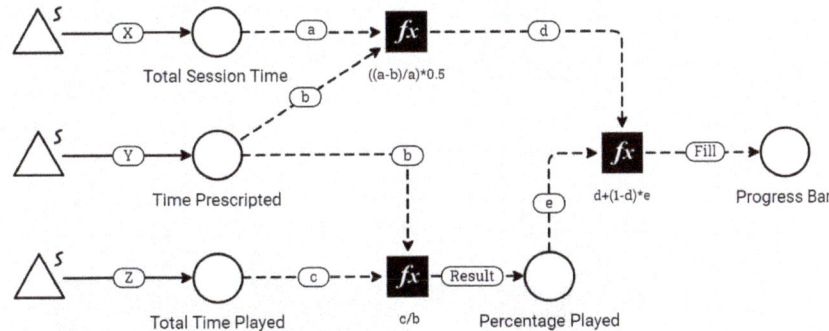

Figure 2. Game mechanics: initializing and updating the status of a progress bar.

3.3. Game Design

Previous literature pointed out several guidelines for designing for older adults [66–68]. Gamification strategies, within game mechanics and dynamics, had been implemented and experienced, in more serious contexts, as a means to enhance enjoyment and motivation towards the tasks [69]. Moreover, gamification techniques applied to elderly care have proven benefits, also challenges, for these group [43]. Our previous experience in designing exergames for older persons [45,70], have witnessed the impact of certain gamification techniques on older persons performance reflected in a positive engagement, despite some initial issues related to a first usage. VITAAL exergame makes use of several game design elements, namely feedback, progression, time constraints and scores—considered particularly relevant for older persons' perceived performance while holding a training session [43].

Game design, gamification strategies, and user experience were developed by a UX/UI designer with experience in designing exergames for older adults, considering feedback from clinicians—physiotherapists—movement scientists and game designers.

3.3.1. User Interface

VITAAL exergame user interface is based on grounded requirements for usability regarding older persons' experience with technological systems. The interface is designed to be displayed on a PC or TV monitor, placed at a suitable distance to ensure sufficient free space for the players' body movements, without compromising the proper visualization, and understanding, of what is being displayed. Realistic and unambiguous graphics should be considered for this purpose.

The user interface sought aimed to provide: (i) a good shape-understanding within a simple and unambiguous visual representation, e.g., characters' frontal view representation to be more easily recognized, contrasting colors, and proper dimensions, (ii) a clear distinction of actionable elements by its shape, color, size, and interactive state behavior, and (iii) auditory feedback to reinforce in-game actions and events.

3.3.2. Interaction

VITAAL exergame user interaction relies on specific movements, previously aligned with the training requirements that act as commands to play the game, i.e., multidirectional steps, to provide forward, backward, right, and left commands, and elevation of the heels (adapted from the calf rises from the Otago Exercise Program [71]) to pause the game and access the Options menu. The detection of these movements was performed using the data collected from inertial sensors placed on the feet, as described in [72]. Alternatively, people with severe physical limitations may use a computer keyboard as a game controller, which in this case may limit the interventions to the cognitive training component. Older adults may also play with the support of a walker, a cane, or alike.

To learn and experience the movements effectively, in a fun and contextualized setting, the design team proposed: (i) an in-game tutorial (as recommended by [45]) for the player to try the stepping, to learn how to open the Options menu and to be introduced to the progress bar, and (ii) a main character, named Vita (Figure 3) that represents the player within its position and action in-game. Vita floats from one place to another (instead of walking, to discourage players from moving in physical space), it gives feedback on the performance through its bold and animated expressions, while evoking an empathic and joyful atmosphere free of prejudice and discriminatory stereotypes.

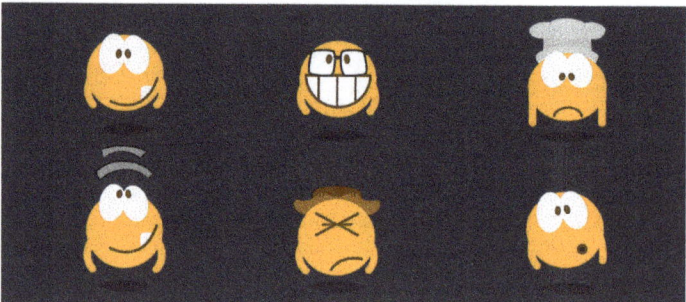

Figure 3. The main character, Vita.

3.3.3. Game Experience

VITAAL exergame experience (shown in Figure 4) is quite dependent on the training requirements, via specified body movements and cognitive exercises. In this regard the design team sought to keep the player motivated and engaged by balancing challenge and fun as follows: (i) distributing types and number of exercises by several minigames with different scenes and goals to promote variety and avoid monotony, (ii) adapting the difficulty level of each game according to the individual in-game progression to prevent frustration and foster learnability, and (iii) providing one single instruction and focus at a time to avoid an overwhelming experience. Through game mechanics progression and different difficult levels, we sought to answer to different user profiles.

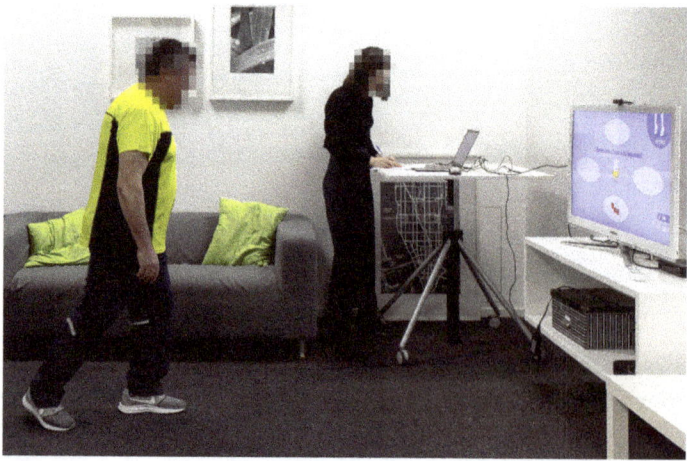

Figure 4. VITAAL exergame gameplay: interacting with the exergame by performing multidirectional steps.

3.4. Minigames

Six of the ten minigames developed for VITAAL are shown in Figure 5. Game designers, a UX/UI designer, clinicians and movement scientists were involved in the definition of the tasks and the specific objectives of each minigame. Additionally, the team relied on the feedback and developments performed under the scope of a previous project, Active@Home, which already included cognitive games based on multidirectional steps, and strength training based on Tai Chi-inspired exercises [45,49]. These games served as a basis for the development of minigames in VITAAL.

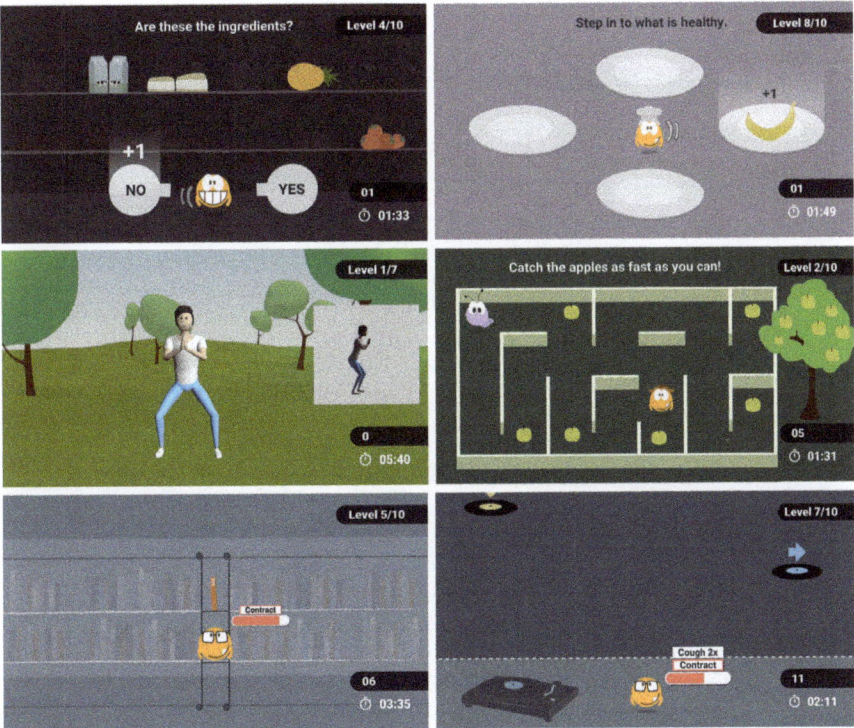

Figure 5. Six of the ten minigames. From left to right, top to bottom: Shopping list, Healthy food, Wide squats, Labyrinth, Falling books, and Music (the last two with the additional stimuli for pelvic floor muscle training in isolation or in coordination with a cough).

The tasks within minigames were defined according to the training components they represent: (i) *Cognitive training* focuses on cognitively challenging tasks that prompt the player to use multidirectional steps to provide 2- or 4-fold decisions; for instance, in the *Shopping list* minigame (Figure 5) users have a limited time to memorize a list of products and then confirm whether the products on the shelf correspond to those previously visualized or not; the *Healthy food* minigame (also shown in Figure 5) is an example of inhibition control that requires the patient to select healthy food as fast as possible, avoiding the selection of unhealthy food; (ii) *Strength training* tasks require the players to follow the movements of a virtual instructor who performs Tai Chi-inspired exercises based on narrow and wide squats; for better guidance, a frontal and lateral view of the avatar movement is provided (Figure 5); (iii) *Balance training* focuses mostly on steps that need to be performed to control Vita's movement towards an appropriate direction; for example, in the *Labyrinth* minigame (shown in Figure 5) users must avoid the worm and catch the maximum number of apples as fast as possible; (iv) *Pelvic floor muscle training* also focuses on quick and precise steps, where an additional stimulus to voluntarily contract the pelvic floor muscle (in isolation or in coordination with a cough) is included; these stimuli appear while playing the minigames *Falling books* and *Music*, as an additional task (Figure 5); when pelvic floor muscle training is not prescribed, these minigames will only target the balance training component.

A full description of all minigames developed for VITAAL is provided in Table 2.

Table 2. Minigames for motor-cognitive and pelvic floor muscle training.

Minigame	Training Component(s)	Description
Shopping list	Cognitive training (short-term memory)	Users have a limited time to memorize a list of products and then confirm whether the products on the shelf correspond to those previously visualized or not.
Shopping	Cognitive training (flexibility, divided attention)	In this game, the player needs to select whether two presented objects match in shape or in color. The correct answer evaluates the trueness or falseness of a sentence referring to the objects.
Healthy food	Cognitive training (inhibition)	The player must select healthy food as fast as possible, avoiding the selection of unhealthy food.
Pizza	Cognitive training (flexibility, selective attention)	The player must select the pizza slice that is pointing in the wrong direction while suppressing the impulse to select the most common direction.
Wide squats	Strength training	The player should follow the movements of a virtual instructor who performs Tai Chi-inspired exercises based on wide squats.
Narrow squats	Strength training	The player should follow the movements of a virtual instructor who performs Tai Chi-inspired exercises based on narrow squats.
Labyrinth	Balance training	The player must guide Vita inside the labyrinth to avoid the worm and catch the maximum number of apples as fast as possible.
Mommy chicken	Balance training	The player should catch as many eggs as possible, stealing them from the respective nests. Caution is required to avoid being caught by the chickens.
Falling books	Pelvic floor muscle training and/or balance training	The player should catch the maximum number of books, preventing them from falling off the bookshelves.
Music	Pelvic floor muscle training and/or balance training	In this game, the player must collect as many records as possible to score points. Special records will score additional points and switch to a different music style.

3.5. Evaluation and Automatic Progression Adaptation

Minigame scores reflect the performance of the player on a specific task, for instance, based on the number of right answers and average reaction time, the number of elements picked or, if applicable, the number of pelvic floor muscle contractions correctly performed.

The performance of strength training-related tasks is not evaluated within VITAAL, being maximum score achieved upon completion of the task. The team considered that by mirroring the movements of the avatar, older adults would challenge and strengthen their muscles—even without an objective evaluation and feedback for movement correctness. Reducing system complexity (using only two inertial sensors that evaluate the movements of the feet) was preferred over the use of additional sensors for full-body movement evaluation.

The exergame employs automatic progression adaptation that manipulates task difficulty and load. Each minigame includes a set of difficulty levels (a set of predefined game parameters that affect the difficulty of the game) and criteria (a set of predefined rules that describe when the player level should maintain, increase, or decrease). Difficulty levels were defined by game designers, with the support from clinicians and movement scientists, to ensure their adequacy concerning different training needs and end-user characteristics. Strength training exercises were arranged in a progressive order of difficulty, as defined by clinicians and movement scientists. The continuous adaptation of difficulty levels would ensure a progressively increasing training load and optimal challenge to prevent under- and overload [49].

The progression to the next (or previous) difficulty level is based on the scores achieved in previous training sessions. By default, all players start at the minimum difficulty level. If the last score of a task is excellent (above 90%), the difficulty level will automatically increase for the next play; otherwise, the average score of the last three plays—performed in the same level of difficulty—is used; the average score will decide whether the difficulty level should decrease (score below 50%), maintain (score between 50% and 75%), or increase (score above 75%). This set of rules apply to all tasks, except strength training-related tasks, where the fixed criteria of completing the task at least 5 times is enough to progress to the next level.

3.6. Implementation

The exergame was developed using the Unity Engine and compiled as a web-based tool to be readily accessible in any system without installation. Bluetooth® Low Energy-enabled inertial sensors—small size, portable, placed on the shoes, equipped with an accelerometer and a gyroscope—were used to monitor player movements (as described in [72]). Women with geriatric urinary incontinence may also use a vaginal dynamometer (tampon inserted into the vagina) [73] to monitor the pelvic floor muscle activation and strength while playing games for the treatment of urinary incontinence. Connection with Bluetooth devices was performed via browser using the Web Bluetooth API [74].

The VITAAL exergame was integrated with a backend (database) in connection with a clinician portal built on the Dividat Manager [75]. Among other functionalities, the backend allows recording session data, e.g., scores achieved, or training times. The clinician portal provides the clinician the ability to specify training times for a specific patient as well as perform and record standardized assessments, allowing further progress tracking and refinement of training plans [75]. Minigame parameters—e.g., scores, reaction time, difficulty level, time played—are displayed on the clinician portal through a set of graphs and tables that allow the clinician to follow the evolution of the parameters over time. System architecture is shown in Figure 6.

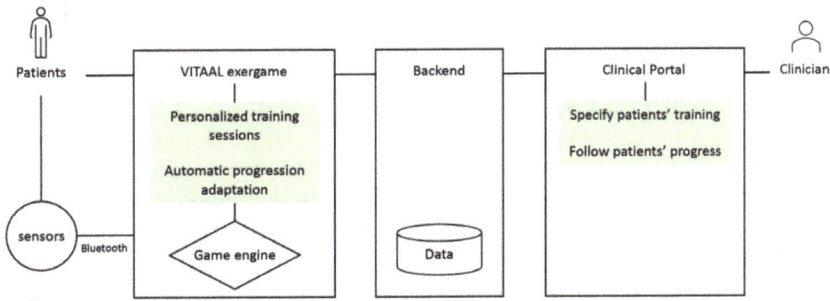

Figure 6. System architecture.

The system architecture was proposed to support exergame use by autonomously living older adults at their homes. Through the clinician portal, the clinician can remotely follow their patients' progress, as well as specify and refine training plans according to their individual progress. To play at home, patients need a laptop or PC, internet connection, and a set of sensors. Their data are recorded and stored on the backend, so that their progress can be followed over time. Alternatively, older adults (e.g., older adults living in residential care facilities) may play the exergame in a rehabilitation setting or long-term care facility, under the guidance of the clinician—as an alternative to conventional training. Under this scenario, the same equipment—laptop or PC and the set of sensors—can be shared, provided that each patient will use their credentials to sign into the game.

4. Results and Discussion

Studies recommend a multicomponent and personalized training approach for older adults with mobility limitations, cognitive impairment, and urinary incontinence [4,9,23,76]. Although exergames contribute to increased training motivation and can be used as an alternative to conventional training, current exergames fail to incorporate interventions for all required training components in one single session. To address this gap in the literature, we developed the VITAAL exergame, a personalized multicomponent approach for the geriatric rehabilitation of older adults with mobility limitations, cognitive impairment, and/or urinary incontinence.

Training requirements were evidence-based and adapted by the research team so that the training needs of the person should be optimally addressed and framed within the context of the exergame. The game design process sought to combine an effective intervention—within the specified clinical guidance—with concepts of gaming and enjoyment. The iterative design process, involving a multidisciplinary team, was crucial for the proper integration of all requirements and perspectives.

We developed an exergame solution comprising interventions for strength, balance, cognition, and pelvic floor muscle training. The clinician could specify the training times of each component, such that the intervention could adapt to the individual training needs of the patient. A set of progress bars provided information on training completion, guiding the player through the themes and ensuring the fulfilment of training needs as defined by the therapist. Other existing solutions relied on the player to control training times, assuming compliance with verbal or written instructions given by the therapist [48–50]. Our solution could manage training times automatically based on training requirements (obtained from the clinician portal) and player training times.

Ideal game experience and intervention requirements had to be balanced with the technical constraints on a take-home solution. For instance, the interaction—defined based on the movements that would suit an effective intervention—constrained the game narrative and user interface, as commands were limited to the four directions (plus the additional movement—calf rises—to access game menus). Moreover, driven by the requirement of providing an effective clinical intervention with a sustained and rich user experience, we avoided a game design based on linked stories and favored an implementation with unlimited replay value. On one side, we dropped all potential advantages of having linked stories—concerning engagement, motivation, etc. [77]; on the other side, we created a self-sustained concept: if it is sufficiently engaging and motivating, there is potential for continued play [78]. To improve game experience and user motivation, we have incorporated other gamification construction elements, such as feedback, progression, time constraints, and score [43]. According to [69], it is important to ensure an adequate level of gamification, as excessive elements may distract users from the main purpose of the activities. By design, the exergame allows the seamless integration of new contents, possibly contributing to sustain players engagement in the long-term [78], or even adapt the exergame to other disabilities.

Many exergame solutions use floor plates to support player interaction with respect to their movements [40]; others use handheld devices—e.g., the Wii Remote—that work as remote controls to interact with the game interface [40]. To evaluate full-body movements, Kinect is usually the preferred choice [31,44,47], although accuracy drops when more complex movements are executed [52]. In a previous work, four inertial sensors were used to track upper and lower limb movements, which added some complexity regarding interaction and system setup [45]. Yet, inertial sensors were considered a viable approach to monitor movements in the context of exergaming [45,79]. In this work we opted for using only two inertial sensors—placed on the feet—to simplify setup and reduce costs. However, complete movements (e.g., the strength training-related tasks) could not be evaluated. Reducing system complexity was preferred over the use of additional sensors for full-body movement evaluation. The use of the vaginal dynamometer was optional for women with urinary incontinence wanting to confirm pelvic floor muscle contraction.

We opted for a web implementation of the exergame to ensure cross-platform compatibility and easy access without installation. The complexity of the graphical game contents was adapted to meet the continuously increasing, but relatively limited performance of web browsers. Bluetooth-enabled devices could connect via web, allowing data processing in real time and interaction (and feedback) without any noticeable delay.

The VITAAL exergame was designed for use at clinics or at home—after an introductory session, the technical solution should promote independent use, with or without the support of a (remote) caregiver. Training at home is currently considered an alternative and/or complement to the training at clinics, allowing better access to services (e.g., in the context of a pandemic), promoting the continuity of treatments, and overcoming barriers related to the lack of resources at clinics [80]. The exergame operated in connection with a clinician portal that, besides allowing training specification, enabled the remote supervision of the training by the clinician. According to [81], exergames that fit older adults' characteristics and needs can be used to counteract the consequences of confinement and hospitalization, such as increased vulnerability, decreased functional capacity, and dependency. VITAAL may also find application in these contexts.

Lessons Learned

This study proved to be possible to incorporate multiple training components, specifically, balance, strength, cognition and pelvic floor muscle training, in a single exergame solution, relying on an interaction with multidirectional steps and inertial sensors placed on the feet. Although being simple, the interaction constrained game narrative and the evaluation of full-body movements. As a web-based solution, the exergame allowed cross-platform compatibility, and could communicate with Bluetooth devices without any noticeable delay. A vaginal dynamometer could be integrated to provide feedback to older women wanting to confirm pelvic floor muscle contractions. The connection with a clinician portal allows clinicians to remotely follow patient training at home, as well as prescribe and change interventions. These functionalities may support better access to services, e.g., in the context of a pandemic. The game mechanics allows adaptation to different training requirements, and ensures automatic control of training times as prescribed by the therapist. The game design and mechanics can be adapted to additional interventions.

5. Conclusions

Exergames are a promising approach to counteract age-related impairments such as mobility limitations, cognitive impairment, and urinary incontinence. To optimally address these conditions, exergames should include interventions for strength, balance, cognition and pelvic floor muscle training, in one single session. To address this requirement, we developed the VITAAL exergame, a solution for the geriatric rehabilitation of mobility limitations, cognitive impairment, and urinary incontinence. The solution incorporates a game mechanics that ensures the fulfilment of training needs as specified by the therapist. By personalizing the training times of each component, and adjusting its load, individual training needs should be optimally addressed. The exergame is cross-platform compatible, includes automatic progression adaptation, and novel means of interaction with wearable sensors.

Future work should assess interaction, usability and game experience of the newly developed exergame. These aspects shall be assessed with prospective users in a future study, ensuring the continuity of the iterative design process. The feasibility of the intervention shall be explored in a subsequent study.

Author Contributions: Conceptualization, V.G., E.O., A.C., N.C. and E.D.d.B.; methodology, V.G., E.O., A.C., N.C., J.E., C.D., N.S. and J.D.J.; software, V.G., E.O., A.C., N.C. and J.E.; investigation, V.G., E.O., C.D. and E.D.d.B.; writing—original draft preparation, V.G., E.O., A.C. and N.C; writing—review and editing, J.E., C.D., N.S. and E.D.d.B.; visualization, E.O.; supervision, V.G.; project administration, V.G.; funding acquisition, V.G. All authors have read and agreed to the published version of the manuscript.

Funding: This work has been performed in the context of the project VITAAL AAL-2017-066, funded under the AAL Joint Program and co-funded by the European Commission and the National Funding Authorities of Portugal, Switzerland, and Belgium.

Institutional Review Board Statement: Not applicable.

Informed Consent Statement: Not applicable.

Data Availability Statement: Data sharing not applicable.

Acknowledgments: We thank all older adults who informally provided feedback about exergame development. We thank Juarez Souza, who created the main game character and produced all animations within the game. We thank Mariana Pereira for supporting the creation of video contents within the game. We thank Ana Pereira for supporting game design on the first stages of the project. We thank all the partners within the VITAAL project for their valuable inputs and feedback.

Conflicts of Interest: The authors declare no conflict of interest.

References

1. Morley, J.E. The New Geriatric Giants. *Clin. Geriatr. Med.* **2017**, *33*, xi–xii. [CrossRef]
2. Rubenstein, L.Z. Falls in older people: Epidemiology, risk factors and strategies for prevention. *Age Ageing* **2006**, *35* (Suppl 2), ii37–ii41. [CrossRef]
3. Yu, W.C.; Chou, M.Y.; Peng, L.N.; Lin, Y.T.; Liang, C.K.; Chen, L.K. Synergistic effects of cognitive impairment on physical disability in all-cause mortality among men aged 80 years and over: Results from longitudinal older veterans study. *PLoS ONE* **2017**, *12*, e0181741. [CrossRef] [PubMed]
4. Li, H.; Chen, K.; Hsu, H. Modelling factors of urinary incontinence in institutional older adults with dementia. *J. Clin. Nurs.* **2019**, *28*, 4504–4512. [CrossRef]
5. Grande, G.; Triolo, F.; Nuara, A.; Welmer, A.K.; Fratiglioni, L.; Vetrano, D.L. Measuring gait speed to better identify prodromal dementia. *Exp. Gerontol.* **2019**, *124*, 110625. [CrossRef] [PubMed]
6. Kim, K.J.; Shin, J.; Choi, J.; Park, J.M.; Park, H.K.; Lee, J.; Han, S.H. Association of Geriatric Syndromes with Urinary Incontinence according to Sex and Urinary-Incontinence–Related Quality of Life in Older Inpatients: A Cross-Sectional Study of an Acute Care Hospital. *Korean J. Fam. Med.* **2019**, *40*, 235–240. [CrossRef]
7. Le Berre, M.; Morin, M.; Corriveau, H.; Hamel, M.; Nadeau, S.; Filiatrault, J.; Dumoulin, C. Characteristics of Lower Limb Muscle Strength, Balance, Mobility, and Function in Older Women with Urge and Mixed Urinary Incontinence: An Observational Pilot Study. *Physiother. Can.* **2019**, *71*, 250–260. [CrossRef]
8. Wagg, A.; Lee, R. Urinary Incontinence in People Living with Cognitive Impairment. *Curr. Geriatr. Rep.* **2021**, 1–8 [CrossRef]
9. Sadjapong, U.; Yodkeeree, S.; Sungkarat, S.; Siviroj, P. Multicomponent Exercise Program Reduces Frailty and Inflammatory Biomarkers and Improves Physical Performance in Community-Dwelling Older Adults: A Randomized Controlled Trial. *Int. J. Environ. Res. Public Health* **2020**, *17*, 3760. [CrossRef]
10. Kim, H.; Suzuki, T.; Yoshida, Y.; Yoshida, H. Effectiveness of multidimensional exercises for the treatment of stress urinary incontinence in elderly community-dwelling Japanese women: A randomized, controlled, crossover trial. *J. Am. Geriatr. Soc.* **2007**, *55*, 1932–1939. [CrossRef]
11. Park, H.; Kim, K.J.; Komatsu, T.; Park, S.K.; Mutoh, Y. Effect of combined exercise training on bone, body balance, and gait ability: A randomized controlled study in community-dwelling elderly women. *J. Bone Miner. Metab.* **2008**, *26*, 254–259. [CrossRef] [PubMed]
12. Baker, M.K.; Atlantis, E.; Fiatarone Singh, M.A. Multi-modal exercise programs for older adults. *Age Ageing* **2007**, *36*, 375–381. [CrossRef] [PubMed]
13. Wang, R.Y.; Wang, Y.L.; Cheng, F.Y.; Chao, Y.H.; Chen, C.L.; Yang, Y.R. Effects of a multicomponent exercise on dual-task performance and executive function among older adults. *Int. J. Gerontol.* **2018**, *12*, 133–138. [CrossRef]
14. Song, D.; Yu, D.S.; Li, P.W.; Lei, Y. The effectiveness of physical exercise on cognitive and psychological outcomes in individuals with mild cognitive impairment: A systematic review and meta-analysis. *Int. J. Nurs. Stud.* **2018**, *79*, 155–164. [CrossRef]
15. Sáez de Asteasu, M.L.; Martínez-Velilla, N.; Zambom-Ferraresi, F.; Casas-Herrero, A.; Izquierdo, M. Role of physical exercise on cognitive function in healthy older adults: A systematic review of randomized clinical trials. *Ageing Res. Rev.* **2017**, *37*, 117–134. [CrossRef]

16. Penedo, F.J.; Dahn, J.R. Exercise and well-being: A review of mental and physical health benefits associated with physical activity. *Curr. Opin. Psychiatry* **2005**, *18*, 189–193. [CrossRef]
17. Matsuda, P.N.; Shumway-Cook, A.; Ciol, M.A. The effects of a home-based exercise program on physical function in frail older adults. *J. Geriatr. Phys. Ther.* **2010**, *33*, 78–84.
18. Law, L.L.F.; Barnett, F.; Yau, M.K.; Gray, M.A. Effects of combined cognitive and exercise interventions on cognition in older adults with and without cognitive impairment: A systematic review. *Ageing Res. Rev.* **2014**, *15*, 61–75. [CrossRef] [PubMed]
19. Fritz, N.E.; Cheek, F.M.; Nichols-Larsen, D.S. Motor-Cognitive Dual-Task Training in Persons With Neurologic Disorders: A Systematic Review. *J. Neurol. Phys. Ther. JNPT* **2015**, *39*, 142–153. [CrossRef]
20. Ogawa, E.F.; You, T.; Leveille, S.G. Potential Benefits of Exergaming for Cognition and Dual-Task Function in Older Adults: A Systematic Review. *J. Aging Phys. Act.* **2016**, *24*, 332–336. [CrossRef]
21. Amjad, I.; Toor, H.; Niazi, I.K.; Pervaiz, S.; Jochumsen, M.; Shafique, M.; Haavik, H.; Ahmed, T. Xbox 360 Kinect Cognitive Games Improve Slowness, Complexity of EEG, and Cognitive Functions in Subjects with Mild Cognitive Impairment: A Randomized Control Trial. *Games Health J.* **2019**, *8*, 144–152. [CrossRef]
22. Bettez, M.; Tu, L.M.; Carlson, K.; Corcos, J.; Gajewski, J.; Jolivet, M.; Bailly, G. 2012 update: Guidelines for adult urinary incontinence collaborative consensus document for the canadian urological association. *Can. Urol. Assoc. J.* **2012**, *6*, 354–363. [CrossRef]
23. Dumoulin, C.; Cacciari, L.P.; Hay-Smith, E.J.C. Pelvic floor muscle training versus no treatment, or inactive control treatments, for urinary incontinence in women. *Cochrane Database Syst. Rev.* **2018**, *10*, CD005654. [CrossRef]
24. World Health Organization. *WHO Guidelines on Physical Activity and Sedentary Behaviour*; Guideline; World Health Organization: Geneva, Switzerland, 2020; ISBN 9789240015128.
25. Valenzuela, T.; Okubo, Y.; Woodbury, A.; Lord, S.R.; Delbaere, K. Adherence to Technology-Based Exercise Programs in Older Adults: A Systematic Review. *J. Geriatr. Phys. Ther.* **2018**, *41*, 49–61. [CrossRef]
26. Meekes, W.; Stanmore, E.K. Motivational Determinants of Exergame Participation for Older People in Assisted Living Facilities: Mixed-Methods Study. *J. Med. Internet Res.* **2017**, *19*. [CrossRef]
27. Stanmore, E.; Stubbs, B.; Vancampfort, D.; de Bruin, E.D.; Firth, J. The effect of active video games on cognitive functioning in clinical and non-clinical populations: A meta-analysis of randomized controlled trials. *Neurosci. Biobehav. Rev.* **2017**, *78*, 34–43. [CrossRef]
28. Gerling, K.; Mandryk, R. Custom-designed motion-based games for older adults: A review of literature in human-computer interaction. *Gerontechnology* **2014**, *12*, 68–80. [CrossRef]
29. Silva, L.M.d.; Flôres, F.S.; Matheus, S.C. Can exergames be used as an alternative to conventional exercises? *Motriz Rev. Educ. FíSica* **2021**, *27*, e1021020197. [CrossRef]
30. Piech, J.; Czernicki, K. Virtual Reality Rehabilitation and Exergames—Physical and Psychological Impact on Fall Prevention among the Elderly—A Literature Review. *Appl. Sci.* **2021**, *11*, 4098. [CrossRef]
31. Liao, Y.Y.; Chen, I.H.; Lin, Y.J.; Chen, Y.; Hsu, W.C. Effects of Virtual Reality-Based Physical and Cognitive Training on Executive Function and Dual-Task Gait Performance in Older Adults With Mild Cognitive Impairment: A Randomized Control Trial. *Front. Aging Neurosci.* **2019**, *11*, 162. [CrossRef]
32. Zhao, Y.; Feng, H.; Wu, X.; Du, Y.; Yang, X.; Hu, M.; Ning, H.; Liao, L.; Chen, H.; Zhao, Y. Effectiveness of Exergaming in Improving Cognitive and Physical Function in People With Mild Cognitive Impairment or Dementia: Systematic Review. *JMIR Serious Games* **2020**, *8*, e16841. [CrossRef]
33. Soares, V.N.; Yoshida, H.M.; Magna, T.S.; Sampaio, R.A.C.; Fernandes, P.T. Comparison of exergames versus conventional exercises on the cognitive skills of older adults: A systematic review with meta-analysis. *Arch. Gerontol. Geriatr.* **2021**, *97*, 104485. [CrossRef] [PubMed]
34. Alhagbani, A.; Williams, A. Home-Based Exergames for Older Adults Balance and Falls Risk: A Systematic Review. *Phys. Occup. Ther. Geriatr.* **2021**, 1–17. [CrossRef]
35. Pacheco, T.B.F.; de Medeiros, C.S.P.; de Oliveira, V.H.B.; Vieira, E.R.; de Cavalcanti, F.A.C. Effectiveness of exergames for improving mobility and balance in older adults: A systematic review and meta-analysis. *Syst. Rev.* **2020**, *9*, 163. [CrossRef]
36. Viana, R.B.; Oliveira, V.N.; Dankel, S.J.; Loenneke, J.P.; Abe, T.; Silva, W.F.; Morais, N.S.; Vancini, R.L.; Andrade, M.S.; Lira, C.A.B. The effects of exergames on muscle strength: A systematic review and meta-analysis. *Scand. J. Med. Sci. Sport.* **2021**, *31*, 1592–1611. [CrossRef] [PubMed]
37. Botelho, S.; Martinho, N.M.; Silva, V.R.; Marques, J.; Carvalho, L.C.; Riccetto, C. Virtual reality: A proposal for pelvic floor muscle training. *Int. Urogynecol. J.* **2015**, *26*, 1709–1712. [CrossRef] [PubMed]
38. Kappen, D.L.; Mirza-Babaei, P.; Nacke, L.E. Older Adults' Physical Activity and Exergames: A Systematic Review. *Int. J. Hum. Comput. Interact.* **2019**, *35*, 140–167. [CrossRef]
39. Choi, S.D.; Guo, L.; Kang, D.; Xiong, S. Exergame technology and interactive interventions for elderly fall prevention: A systematic literature review. *Appl. Ergon.* **2017**, *65*, 570–581. [CrossRef] [PubMed]
40. Skjæret, N.; Nawaz, A.; Morat, T.; Schoene, D.; Helbostad, J.L.; Vereijken, B. Exercise and rehabilitation delivered through exergames in older adults: An integrative review of technologies, safety and efficacy. *Int. J. Med. Inform.* **2016**, *85*, 1–16. [CrossRef]
41. Gerling, K.; Schild, J.; Masuch, M. Exergaming for Elderly: Analyzing Player Experience and Performance. In Proceedings of the Mensch & Computer 2011, Oldenbourg Verlag, Chemnitz, Germany, 11–14 September 2011; pp. 401–411 [CrossRef]

42. Bleakley, C.M.; Charles, D.; Porter-Armstrong, A.; McNeill, M.D.J.; McDonough, S.M.; McCormack, B. Gaming for health: a systematic review of the physical and cognitive effects of interactive computer games in older adults. *J. Appl. Gerontol. Off. J. South. Gerontol. Soc.* **2015**, *34*, NP166–NP189. [CrossRef]
43. Martinho, D.; Carneiro, J.; Corchado, J.M.; Marreiros, G. A systematic review of gamification techniques applied to elderly care. *Artif. Intell. Rev.* **2020**, *53*, 4863–4901. [CrossRef]
44. Chen, M.; Tang, Q.; Xu, S.; Leng, P.; Pan, Z. Design and Evaluation of an Augmented Reality-Based Exergame System to Reduce Fall Risk in the Elderly. *Int. J. Environ. Res. Public Health* **2020**, *17*, 7208. [CrossRef] [PubMed]
45. Guimarães, V.; Pereira, A.; Oliveira, E.; Carvalho, A.; Peixoto, R. Design and evaluation of an exergame for motor-cognitive training and fall prevention in older adults. In Proceedings of the 4th EAI International Conference on Smart Objects and Technologies for Social Good—Goodtechs'18, Bologna, Italy, 28–30 November 2018; ACM Press: Bologna, Italy, 2018; pp. 202–207 [CrossRef]
46. Marston, H.R.; Woodbury, A.; Gschwind, Y.J.; Kroll, M.; Fink, D.; Eichberg, S.; Kreiner, K.; Ejupi, A.; Annegarn, J.; de Rosario, H.; et al. The design of a purpose-built exergame for fall prediction and prevention for older people. *Eur. Rev. Aging Phys. Act.* **2015**, *12*, 13. [CrossRef]
47. Zhang, H.; Shen, Z.; Liu, S.; Yuan, D.; Miao, C. Ping Pong: An Exergame for Cognitive Inhibition Training. *Int. J. Hum. Comput. Interact.* **2021**, *37*, 1104–1115. [CrossRef]
48. Fraser, S.A.; Elliott, V.; de Bruin, E.D.; Bherer, L.; Dumoulin, C. The Effects of Combining Videogame Dancing and Pelvic Floor Training to Improve Dual-Task Gait and Cognition in Women with Mixed-Urinary Incontinence. *Games Health J.* **2014**, *3*, 172–178. [CrossRef] [PubMed]
49. Adcock, M.; Fankhauser, M.; Post, J.; Lutz, K.; Zizlsperger, L.; Luft, A.R.; Guimarães, V.; Schättin, A.; de Bruin, E.D. Effects of an In-home Multicomponent Exergame Training on Physical Functions, Cognition, and Brain Volume of Older Adults: A Randomized Controlled Trial. *Front. Med.* **2020**, *6*, 321. [CrossRef]
50. Gschwind, Y.J.; Eichberg, S.; Ejupi, A.; de Rosario, H.; Kroll, M.; Marston, H.R.; Drobics, M.; Annegarn, J.; Wieching, R.; Lord, S.R.; et al. ICT-based system to predict and prevent falls (iStoppFalls): Results from an international multicenter randomized controlled trial. *Eur. Rev. Aging Phys. Act.* **2015**, *12*, 10. [CrossRef]
51. VITAAL. VITAAL Website. Available online: https://vitaal.fit/ (accessed on 10 May 2021).
52. Ryselis, K.; Petkus, T.; Blažauskas, T.; Maskeliūnas, R.; Damaševičius, R. Multiple Kinect based system to monitor and analyze key performance indicators of physical training. *Hum. Centric Comput. Inf. Sci.* **2020**, *10*, 51. [CrossRef]
53. Elliott, V.; de Bruin, E.D.; Dumoulin, C. Virtual reality rehabilitation as a treatment approach for older women with mixed urinary incontinence: A feasibility study: Virtual Reality to Treat Mixed Urinary Incontinence. *Neurourol. Urodyn.* **2015**, *34*, 236–243. [CrossRef]
54. Seifert, A.; Schlomann, A. The Use of Virtual and Augmented Reality by Older Adults: Potentials and Challenges. *Front. Virtual Real.* **2021**, *2*, 639718. [CrossRef]
55. Herold, F.; Hamacher, D.; Schega, L.; Müller, N.G. Thinking While Moving or Moving While Thinking—Concepts of Motor-Cognitive Training for Cognitive Performance Enhancement. *Front. Aging Neurosci.* **2018**, *10*, 228. [CrossRef]
56. Okubo, Y.; Schoene, D.; Lord, S.R. Step training improves reaction time, gait and balance and reduces falls in older people: A systematic review and meta-analysis. *Br. J. Sport. Med.* **2017**, *51*, 586–593. [CrossRef]
57. Giannouli, E.; Morat, T.; Zijlstra, W. A Novel Square-Stepping Exercise Program for Older Adults (StepIt): Rationale and Implications for Falls Prevention. *Front. Med.* **2019**, *6*, 318. [CrossRef]
58. Buskard, A.N.L.; Jacobs, K.A.; Eltoukhy, M.M.; Strand, K.L.; Villanueva, L.; Desai, P.P.; Signorile, J.F. Optimal Approach to Load Progressions during Strength Training in Older Adults. *Med. Sci. Sport. Exerc.* **2019**, *51*, 2224–2233. [CrossRef]
59. de Bruin, E.D.; Schmidt, A. Walking behaviour of healthy elderly: Attention should be paid. *Behav. Brain Funct. BBF* **2010**, *6*, 59. [CrossRef] [PubMed]
60. Dumoulin, C.; Glazener, C.; Jenkinson, D. Determining the optimal pelvic floor muscle training regimen for women with stress urinary incontinence. *Neurourol. Urodyn.* **2011**, *30*, 746–753. [CrossRef]
61. Schoene, D.; Valenzuela, T.; Lord, S.R.; de Bruin, E.D. The effect of interactive cognitive-motor training in reducing fall risk in older people: A systematic review. *BMC Geriatr.* **2014**, *14*, 107. [CrossRef]
62. Segev-Jacubovski, O.; Herman, T.; Yogev-Seligmann, G.; Mirelman, A.; Giladi, N.; Hausdorff, J.M. The interplay between gait, falls and cognition: Can cognitive therapy reduce fall risk? *Expert Rev. Neurother.* **2011**, *11*, 1057–1075. [CrossRef]
63. Bamidis, P.D.; Vivas, A.B.; Styliadis, C.; Frantzidis, C.; Klados, M.; Schlee, W.; Siountas, A.; Papageorgiou, S.G. A review of physical and cognitive interventions in aging. *Neurosci. Biobehav. Rev.* **2014**, *44*, 206–220. [CrossRef]
64. Healy, A.F.; Kole, J.A.; Bourne, L.E. Training principles to advance expertise. *Front. Psychol.* **2014**, *5*, 131. [CrossRef]
65. Dormans, J. Engineering Emergence: Applied Theory for Game Design. Ph.D. Thesis, University of Amsterdam, Amsterdam, The Netherlands, 2012.
66. Weisman, S. Computer games for the frail elderly. *Gerontologist* **1983**, *23*, 361–363. [CrossRef]
67. Flores, E.; Tobon, G.; Cavallaro, E.; Cavallaro, F.I.; Perry, J.C.; Keller, T. Improving patient motivation in game development for motor deficit rehabilitation. In Proceedings of the 2008 International Conference in Advances on Computer Entertainment Technology—ACE'08, Yokohama, Japan, 3–5 December 2008; ACM Press: Yokohama, Japan, 2008; p. 381. [CrossRef]

68. Marston, H.R. Design Recommendations for Digital Game Design within an Ageing Society. *Educ. Gerontol.* **2013**, *39*, 103–118. [CrossRef]
69. Thiebes, S.; Lins, S.; Basten, D. Gamifying Information Systems—A synthesis of Gamification mechanics and Dynamics. In Proceedings of the ECIS 2014 Proceedings—22nd European Conference on Information Systems, Tel Aviv, Israel, 9–11 June 2014.
70. Silva, J.; Oliveira, E.; Moreira, D.; Nunes, F.; Caic, M.; Madureira, J.; Pereira, E. Design and Evaluation of a Fall Prevention Multiplayer Game for Senior Care Centres. In *Entertainment Computing—ICEC 2018*; Clua, E., Roque, L., Lugmayr, A., Tuomi, P., Eds.; Lecture Notes in Computer Science; Springer International Publishing: Cham, Switzerland, 2018; Volume 11112, pp. 103–114. [CrossRef]
71. Robertson, M.C.; Campbell, A.J. *Otago Exercise Programme to Prevent Falls in Older Adults*; ACC Thinksafe: Wellington, New Zealand, 2003.
72. Guimarães, V.; Sousa, I.; Correia, M.V. Detection and classification of multidirectional steps for motor-cognitive training in older adults using shoe-mounted inertial sensors. In Proceedings of the 2019 41st Annual International Conference of the IEEE Engineering in Medicine and Biology Society (EMBC), Berlin, Germany, 23–27 July 2019; pp. 6926–6929. ISSN 1558-4615. [CrossRef]
73. El-Sayegh, B.; Dumoulin, C.; Ali, M.; Assaf, H.; Sawan, M. A Dynamometer-based Wireless Pelvic Floor Muscle Force Monitoring. In Proceedings of the Annual International Conference of the IEEE Engineering in Medicine and Biology Society, Montreal, QC, Canada, 20–24 July 2020; Volume 2020, pp. 6127–6130. [CrossRef]
74. Web Bluetooth Community Group. Web Bluetooth API. Available online: https://webbluetoothcg.github.io/web-bluetooth/ (accessed on 10 May 2021).
75. Dividat AG. Dividat Senso. Available online: https://dividat.com/en/senso (accessed on 10 May 2021).
76. Jachan, D.E.; Müller-Werdan, U.; Lahmann, N.A. Impaired Mobility and Urinary Incontinence in Nursing Home Residents: A Multicenter Study. *J. Wound, Ostomy Cont. Nurs.* **2019**, *46*, 524–529. [CrossRef] [PubMed]
77. Carvalho, R.N.S.d.; Ishitani, L. Motivational Factors for Mobile Serious Games for Elderly Users. In Proceedings of the SBGames 2012, Brasilia, Brasil, 2–4 November 2012.
78. Zhao, Z.; Arya, A.; Whitehead, A.; Chan, G.; Etemad, S.A. Keeping Users Engaged through Feature Updates: A Long-Term Study of Using Wearable-Based Exergames. In Proceedings of the 2017 CHI Conference on Human Factors in Computing Systems, Denver Colorado USA, 6–11 May 2017; ACM: Denver, CO, USA, 2017; pp. 1053–1064. [CrossRef]
79. Adcock, M.; Sonder, F.; Schättin, A.; Gennaro, F.; de Bruin, E.D. A usability study of a multicomponent video game-based training for older adults. *Eur. Rev. Aging Phys. Act.* **2020**, *17*, 3. [CrossRef] [PubMed]
80. Hayes, D. Telerehabilitation for Older Adults. *Top. Geriatr. Rehabil.* **2020**, *36*, 205–211. [CrossRef]
81. Corregidor-Sánchez, A.I.; Polonio-López, B.; Martin-Conty, J.L.; Rodríguez-Hernández, M.; Mordillo-Mateos, L.; Schez-Sobrino, S.; Criado-Álvarez, J.J. Exergames to Prevent the Secondary Functional Deterioration of Older Adults during Hospitalization and Isolation Periods during the COVID-19 Pandemic. *Sustainability* **2021**, *13*, 7932. [CrossRef]

Article

Biofeedback Applied to Interactive Serious Games to Monitor Frailty in an Elderly Population

Serhii Shapoval [1,2], Begoña García Zapirain [2], Amaia Mendez Zorrilla [2,*] and Iranzu Mugueta-Aguinaga [3]

1. "Kharkiv Polytechnic Institute", National Technical University, 61000 Kharkiv, Ukraine; s.shapoval@deusto.es
2. eVida Research Group, Faculty of Engineering, University of Deusto, 48007 Bilbo, Spain; mbgarciazapi@deusto.es
3. Biocruces Health Research Institute, Cruces University Hospital, 48903 Barakaldo, Spain; iranzu.muguetaaguinaga@osakidetza.eus
* Correspondence: amaia.mendez@deusto.es

Citation: Shapoval, S.; García Zapirain, B.; Mendez Zorrilla, A.; Mugueta-Aguinaga, I. Biofeedback Applied to Interactive Serious Games to Monitor Frailty in an Elderly Population. *Appl. Sci.* **2021**, *11*, 3502. https://doi.org/10.3390/app11083502

Academic Editor: Marco Gesi

Received: 15 March 2021
Accepted: 12 April 2021
Published: 14 April 2021

Publisher's Note: MDPI stays neutral with regard to jurisdictional claims in published maps and institutional affiliations.

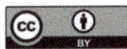

Copyright: © 2021 by the authors. Licensee MDPI, Basel, Switzerland. This article is an open access article distributed under the terms and conditions of the Creative Commons Attribution (CC BY) license (https://creativecommons.org/licenses/by/4.0/).

Abstract: This article proposes an example of a multiplatform interactive serious game, which is an additional tool and assistant used in the rehabilitation of patients with musculoskeletal system problems. In medicine, any actions and procedures aimed at helping the rehabilitation of patients should entail the most comfortable, but at the same time, effective approach. Regardless of how these actions are orientated, whether for rehabilitation following surgery, fractures, any problems with the musculoskeletal system, or just support for the elderly, rehabilitation methods undoubtedly have good goals, although often the process itself can cause all kinds of discomfort and aversion among patients. This paper presents an interactive platform which enables a slightly different approach to be applied in terms of routine rehabilitation activities and this will help make the process more exciting. The main feature of the system is that it works in several ways: for normal everyday use at home, or for more in-depth observation of various biological parameters, such as heart rate, temperature, and so on. The basic component of the system is the real-time tracking system of the body position, which constitutes both a way to control the game (controller) and a means to analyze the player's activity. As for the closer control of rehabilitation, the platform also provides the opportunity for medical personnel to monitor the player in real time, with all the data obtained from the game being used for subsequent analysis and comparison. Following several laboratory tests and feedback analysis, the progress indicators are quite encouraging in terms of greater patient interest in this kind of interaction, and effectiveness of the developed platform is also on average about 30–50% compared to conventional exercises, which makes it more attractive in terms of patient support.

Keywords: serious games; rehabilitation; elderly; body tracking; exercise games

1. Introduction

T Rehabilitation procedures in various aspects of medicine are one of the most important and time-consuming treatment processes for patients with various diseases [1–3]. According to the World Health Organization, there are 2.4 billion people who are living with a health condition that depend on rehabilitative measures. Unfortunately, there is quite a pressing demand for rehabilitation procedures. This is especially true in countries with a low or near-average standard of living, where about 40–50% of patients cannot gain access to rehabilitative medicine. In this regard, the situation with COVID-19 has only exacerbated this situation. Depending on the focus of the procedure, the measures used in the patient's recovery can vary considerably, from simple physical exercises [4] to the use of various kinds of additional technical aids [5]. This is especially true for the rehabilitation process of people with musculoskeletal system problems, such as injuries, mild, partial, or complete muscle atrophy, deterioration or loss of motor control, or the usual support for the physical condition of the elderly [6–11].

The application of different sets of exercises that are used in these procedures can vary depending on the type of the problem and the extent of it. They can also be divided into different categories, depending on the place, time, or environment in which they are applied, the means used during the procedures, and so on. It is also important to understand that different categories of such rehabilitative measures may have different degrees of effectiveness for different characteristics of patients' problems and are often only applicable in their own specific area [12–14]. This can be especially seen in the presence of additional conditions and means.

Over time, each of the methods used as rehabilitation measures has undergone constant checks and improvements, and become more effective. Nevertheless, due to different technical features or the way in which rehabilitation procedures are carried out, there are cases in which patients may experience various kinds of discomfort during their recovery. This discomfort can be caused by various factors from both physical and emotional aspects [15–18].

For quite a long time now, the medical field has been researching the possibility of applying various additional remedies to the rehabilitation process, among which there is such a trend known as Serious Games [19–21]. This is due to the fact that over the past 20 years, computer technology has made impressive leaps in terms of development, which has expanded the technical capabilities of modern computer equipment, as well as its availability. Modern game making technology enables not only almost any real process to be reproduced within a virtual simulation, but also impresses with its graphic and visual level of elaboration and detail.

Therefore, the idea emerges of finding rehabilitative tasks that could include the additional integration of various game mechanics and devices. Because patients may often encounter all sorts of emotional problems during long rehabilitation courses, this game innovation can help to get rid of this aspect [22–25]. All problems should be understood to mean that long and even more monotonous exercises or activities over time mean that patients become used to the process, which reduces the motivation to do them each subsequent time. Although this situation does not arise often or in all patients, providing routine activities with a bit of interactivity can have a definite positive effect [26,27].

The introduction of interactive game features makes the patient's recovery process more meaningful [28]. Even though those actions prescribed by the attending physician are obligatory and indisputable, in some cases they are perceived as "I was told so, so it is necessary". That is certainly true, but it does not always work with certain age groups, such as children and the elderly. In the case of both the former and the latter, engagement is necessary, and the action process itself is important [29]. If a person finds any kind of activity, including rehabilitation activities, attractive and interesting, then he or she will be more motivated to perform them [30].

This makes even the simplest and most boring physical exercises, such as regular exercise, much more appealing to the patient, but the point is that these kinds of game require special conditions under which they can be used in this way. One of the main problems is how to manage such games—in other words, gameplay [31–33]. Firstly, it should be as accurate as possible so as to repeat the actions that the patient needs to perform during rehabilitation procedures. Put another way, in-game levels or activities should essentially take the form of a complete or at least partial substitute for the prescribed exercises. Secondly, it is important that the game should somehow recognize the player's movements and respond to them correctly. If the first case is quite simple to implement, then the second will cover the more complex and important spectrum of these kinds of computer games.

The purpose of this article is to research the effectiveness of using an interactive game platform as an additional tool for rehabilitation and support for the elderly, or patients with musculoskeletal system problems. An additional goal is to compare how effective the system developed is compared to conventional physical exercises, both in terms of rehabilitation and recovery, as well as in terms of motivation and overall moral satisfaction.

This article is divided into five sections. The first is a literature review. This part is Section 2: a review of articles featuring similar solutions that can be compared to the platform presented in this article. Section 3, titled Materials and Methods, includes a description of the tools and algorithms that were used to develop the system. Section 4 presents the results obtained from the system, as well as examples of analysis and comparison of results. Sections 5 and 6, titled Discussion and Conclusions, provide a direct discussion of the results obtained from the study and their subsequent prospects, as well as a comparison with similar solutions.

2. Literature Review

With a suitable player tracking system, several technical approaches can be used. For example, in such systems as Kinect [34] or VR-technology [35], body recognition is undertaken by means of several cameras and additional controllers, which together form a kind of coordinate system, in which the player is located [36]. Another option is systems based on neural network algorithms, examples of such systems being OpenPose [37] or PoseNet [38]. In short, it cannot be said which method is better or worse, as both categories have their advantages and disadvantages, such as being dependent on image quality accuracy for recognition of the body in systems based on neural networks, or the need for a large amount of additional equipment and special space requirements in VR-systems.

Whatever the case may be, there are many factors to consider when developing a Serious Games product [39–41], although it is most important to understand how effective this or that solution will be. In terms of effectiveness, we mean not only the therapeutic and rehabilitative effect, but also the player's interest. It is this aspect that will be explored in this article.

The goal was to test the effectiveness of interactive computer games in the rehabilitation of patients with musculoskeletal system problems. The game platform being developed will be compared under real conditions to a set of conventional physical exercises. One of the conditions for development will be the need to ensure the minimum requirements of the system to the players. This means that for a basic game, the number of additional tools should be limited to a personal computer and a webcam. This condition will expand the likely audience, thereby allowing the platform to be used not only for medical purposes, but also as an everyday leisure activity.

The platform being developed was also tested in two stages. At the first stage, the players being tested performed the usual physical exercises for a certain time over a fixed number of times. Then the same players played the game developed directly. After the testing phase, both the body recognition system performance and the emotional aspect of each player was then analyzed. The results obtained from this study will help to determine the effectiveness of the system developed in relation to the rehabilitation process, as well as the relevance of the application using this method in general.

Table 1 shows similar studies and their results below. Some of them are compared to the results obtained from our studies in the Discussion section.

Table 1 provides 10 references to articles that describe similar research to the one proposed. It briefly describes the main purpose of the description, and the methods and means used, as well as the result.

After studying the articles in the table, it was decided to use the simplest sensor system (webcam in this proposal). This decision was made in order to make the platform as accessible as possible to older people, both economically and technically. As one of the aims of the study is to create a system that is as accessible as possible, unlike solutions with additional VR peripherals, consoles or other additional equipment, the use of a webcam reduces the list of requirements. In addition, the system becomes accessible not only, for example, in the doctor's office, but also at the patient's home.

Table 1. Comparison between similar approaches.

Reference	Aim of the Article	Hardware Used	Algorithm	Measurements	Results
[42]	Present low-cost full body rehabilitation framework for the generation of 3D immersive serious games	Camera system: ToF camera IR camera HDM device (Virtual Reality helmet)	GRU-RNN Virtual Reality algorithms	Track position of the body in space.	Increase in rehabilitation rates by an average 15%
[43]	Introduce a smart rehabilitation system for the elderly, without requiring physical contact with traditional control systems.	Webcam	TANGO:H 2d representation system	The method used in the study is based on the evaluation of a vision-based gesture interface by measuring effectiveness, efficiency, and satisfaction.	Gestural exercises yielded higher percentages of task completion (>83%) and task effectiveness (>63%). Eye fatigue($x = 3.15$; SD = 0.37). Accurate point is above average ($x = 2.57$; SD = 0.60)
[44]	Improvement in the balance and postural control of adults.	Webcam + markers Vision-based interaction sensor Wii mote	Modified algorithm based on Kinect body tracking technology	Body position Balance indicators	Usage of interaction objects related to patient interests; patients performed the rehabilitation activity 13.5% faster than when the objects did not represent such interests
[45]	Assess the effects on functional outcomes and treatment adherence of wearable technology and serious games currently used in physical rehabilitation of patients following traumatic bone and soft tissue injuries.	-	Comparison methods of serious games with standard therapy	The search yielded 2704 eligible articles, which were screened by 2 independent reviewers.	Serious games seem a safe alternative or addition to conventional physiotherapy following traumatic bone and soft tissue injuries.
[46]	Describe of newly-developed platform of Remote Monitoring Validation Engineering System for motion rehabilitation.	Microsoft Kinect V2 Microsoft Band 2	Leap Motion Cloud back-end	Different aspects of upper and lower limbs movement, balance, heart rate and electrodermal activity, balance shift.	Most games within this system are nearly useless for supervised analysis.

Table 1. *Cont.*

Reference	Aim of the Article	Hardware Used	Algorithm	Measurements	Results
[47]	Research into the effectiveness of SGs in motor rehabilitation for upper limb and movement/balance	-	Rehabilitation games and systems data systematizing and comparison	Meta-analysis including 61 studies reporting randomized controlled trials in which at least one intervention for motor rehabilitation is included.	Overall moderate effect of SGs on motor indexes, d = 0.59, [95% CI, 0.48, 0.71], $p < 0.001$
[48]	Evaluate the effects of novel immersive virtual reality technology used for serious games (Oculus Rift 2 plus leap motion controller—OR2-LMC) for upper limb outcomes.	Virtual Reality kit	Mixed methods intervention (MMI)	A mixed methods intervention study, with a qualitative design following technology intervention.	Good result in strength improvements, coordination and dexterity, and speed of participants. No side effects.
[49]	Implement and tests of a system for assessment and monitoring movements, which includes the sensors from Kinect and Leap Motion Controller devices	Microsoft Kinect Leap Motion Controller Kinect	Leap Motion	Using additional motion capture tools along with the virtual game environment.	A study of the feasibility and effectiveness of supplementary remedies on the results of rehabilitation of upper limb problems. Verification of further effectiveness.
[50]	The aim is to evaluate the Fietsgame (Dutch for cycling game), which translates existing rehabilitation exercises into fun exercise games	Control system based on Raspberry Pi Kinect v2 IoT platform	Kinect body tracking system	The study is conducted in a rehabilitation center with 9 participants, including 2 physiotherapists and 7 patients. 6 exercise games under the guidance of a physiotherapist. The mean age of the patients was 74.57 years; all the patients were in the recovery process following hip surgery.	The results showed that 75% to 100% of the patients experienced high levels of enjoyment in all the games except the squats game
[51]	Present a rehabilitation system based on a customizable exergame protocol to prevent falls in the elderly population	Web Camera	Self-developed body tracking platform KINOPTIM	System based on depth sensors and exergames. Measuring of physical abilities and emotional reaction	Performance of the postural response is improved by an average of 80%

3. Materials and Methods

3.1. Materials

The game platform is an additional tool to improve the effectiveness of rehabilitation activities, or to spend leisure time. The main purpose of this study is to test the effectiveness of additional interactive tools and means in the field of rehabilitation and support for the elderly, or people who have received various kinds of injuries to the musculoskeletal system. This study includes both the direct development of the interactive platform itself and the process involved in testing it.

The main task will be to study the effectiveness of rehabilitation procedures using the platform being developed in relation to the usual standard physical exercises. In the long term, a positive result is expected to be seen from the tests, namely a greater efficiency in terms of the interactive way of performing medical rehabilitation exercises, and most importantly, a greater motivational indicator for these actions. The main aspects and parameters of the system developed, as well as testing procedures, will be described below.

3.1.1. Hardware Used

The development and testing process took place on multiple platforms, to maximize the possible devices being supported. The equipment included the following samples, which are shown in Table 2.

Table 2. Equipment for developing and testing.

Element	Characteristics
Desktop PC	
CPU	Ryzen 7 3700x, s-AM4 3.6 GHz/32 Mb
GPU	NVidia GeForce RTX 2070 Super, 8 Gb
RAM	DDR4 32 Gb 2888 GHz
HDD	Seagate Barracuda 1 Tb
Web Camera	InnJoo FHD1080p (1920 × 1080) 60 fps
Laptop Lenovo LEGION Y-540-IPS15i	
CPU	Intel(R) Core(TM) i7-9750H CPU@ 2.60 GHz
GPU	NVidia GeForce GTX 1660 Ti, 6 Gb
RAM	DDR4 16 Gb 2888 GHz
SSD	INTEL SSD PEKKW010T8L 1Tb
Web Camera	Integrated Web Camera 720p (1080 × 720) 30 fps

This system is designed for use on personal computers or laptops running Windows 10 operating systems. A version for Android 5 and higher is being developed parallel to this, although this variation is reduced in some features.

3.1.2. Inclusion and Exclusion Criteria

For this experiment the inclusion criteria are as follows:

- The user must have a personal computer or laptop and a webcam
- The user must be between the ages of 12 and 85
- The user must be in a spacious room during the game to avoid hitting their surroundings
- The playing room should be well lit with natural or voluminous artificial light
- It is desirable that there be at least one other person next to the user while they are playing
- People with vestibular problems and those who are sensitive to light should only use the system in the presence of others
- People who currently have minor musculoskeletal problems or have had them before.

The authors excluded blind people during the tests because they must read the instructions from the tutorials. Additionally, the user must not have had any serious problems or injuries to the musculoskeletal system, such as, for example, complete or partial paralysis. The room in which the system will be used should be well lit with natural or artificial light.

3.1.3. Experimental Features

(a) *Information about testers*

Ten volunteers were selected for the experiment, in the age range from 21 to 42 years. The main data pertaining to the players are shown in Table 3 and Figure 1.

Table 3. Players main parameters.

№	Gender	Age	Height	Weight	Spine or Limbs Problems	Country
1	Male	26	182	72	Left clavicle fracture	Ukraine
2	Female	25	179	89	-	Morocco
3	Male	26	178	77	Left arm fracture	Pakistan
4	Female	42	167	55	Right wrist injury	Spain
5	Male	27	170	65	-	Spain
6	Male	25	178	72	Left shoulder injury	Spain
7	Male	31	173	78	-	Pakistan
8	Male	25	169	69	-	Colombia
9	Female	21	159	50	Right hip fracture	Czech Republic
10	Male	22	176	63	-	Italy

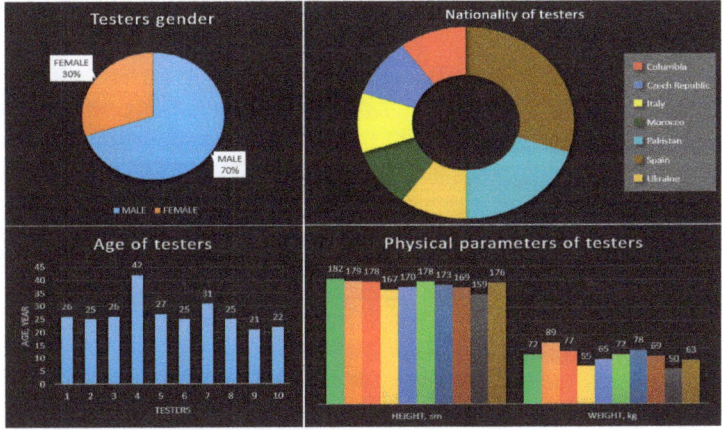

Figure 1. Main information about test participants.

As can be seen in Figure 1 and Table 3, the data provided show information on both physical parameters (height, weight and age, and the presence of any injuries) and social parameters. In the case of the latter, specifically which country the player is from, will help to better understand the results obtained by each of the players during the game.

At the same time, information about the presence or absence of injuries will also help to understand whether injuries in the past have an impact on current results. The data in the column "Spine or limb problems" are information about injuries that occurred before the tests, in order to determine the possible effects of these injuries on the players' performance. At the time of the tests, all patients were healthy and feeling well.

The choice of this set of players was due in large part to the current situation at the time of the study with the pandemic COVID-2019. Ideally, all tests should be conducted with participants within the age range of 60 to 85 years. Nevertheless, the data that were obtained with the set of players provided will help to qualitatively evaluate the results and more accurately adjust the system for the target age category.

(b) *Testing plan and regulations*

As mentioned earlier, the procedure for testing the system was divided into two stages: obtaining players' performance during normal exercises and obtaining performance during direct play. During both phases, a total of six tests were conducted in each. The testing interval ranged from 5 to 15 min, depending on the test stage. The time interval between tests was 12 h.

In the first stage, the players took turns performing five exercises while standing in front of the camera. The only information available was the task for the exercise, the number of repetitions required, and the distance to the camera in order to obtain the data as accurately as possible. During this phase, the system recorded the values necessary for each specific exercise, as well as the time of the exercise. The values were saved as a data set for each of the categories of interest.

The second stage differs from the first in that the players now directly used the game platform as a guide for action and exercise. All information about the latter was provided through the user interface. In this case, there was also a record of the parameters that were key for each level-exercise.

It is also important to note that this project was approved and accepted by the Deusto University Ethics Committee.

3.2. Methods

This section will describe in detail the main aspects of the game, such as technical information about the game client itself, the data handled, the exercises, the optional tracker systems, etc.

3.2.1. Overall View

In general, the platform developed is a computer game client, which includes a wide range of features. Figure 1 shows a general diagram of the game platform, which includes the following elements.

Three basic conditions had to be fulfilled in order to create this platform: Condition 1—to create a stable system for tracking player movements, Condition 2—to create a gaming platform that allows the player to perform activities, and Condition 3—to ensure that the data collected during the game are processed and stored. Figure 2 is a general schematic representation of the system. Each of the conditions will be discussed below.

(a)   Gaming platform

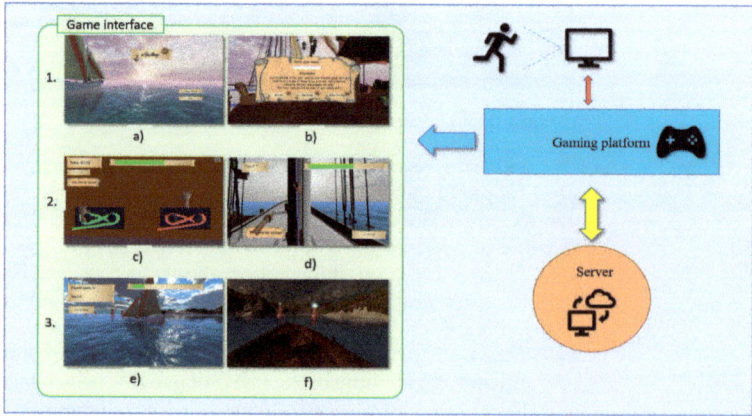

Figure 2. General introduction to the gaming platform. Of the 3 sections in the game platform block: 1—example of the initial information levels such as (**a**) main menu, (**b**) difficulty selection menu and profile creation; 2—example of the first exercise block for upper body, (**c**) Level 1, (**d**) Level 2; 3—example of exercises for lower body and general mobility, (**e**) Level 4, (**f**) Level 5.

The gaming platform is a game client, a computer game. Structurally, it is divided into levels, which are in turn divided into 3 categories:
- Levels of settings
- Levels for the upper body
- Levels for the lower body.

Each of the categories includes several levels of exercises that are responsible for a specific exercise and, respectively, for a specific muscle and joint group. This system has two main functions. The first is visual and involves providing the player with visual information about what is happening now and what the player should do. In addition to the visual instructions for each exercise, the game interface provides the player with a visual representation of their actions, whether it be interactions with objects, the environment, etc. The second function is to collect information regarding the player's movements and activity. For each level, the system registers certain indicators, whether it be arm movements or general body position. In general, the platform consists of three functional blocks; more information about which will be given in Sections 3.2.2–3.2.5. In this Section 3.2.1 is a description of the game client.

The total game interface consists of 7 levels, which are divided into different categories, depending on the focus and purpose of the exercise, which it simulates. It is important to note that all game levels have been created to simulate different kinds of physical exercise as accurately as possible.

(b) Exercises used

The exercises chosen to develop of the system are some of the basic strengthening physical activities. Each was integrated into the game in a specific order, and the choice of each was coordinated with the therapist. There are 5 exercises in total, including the following:

(1) **"The sign of infinity"**. This exercise is a simple activity for the upper extremities. The task involves putting your hands with the palms in front of you, bending your hands at the elbows, and describing the "sign of infinity" in the air. This exercise should be repeated 10 times for each hand, keeping in mind that the right hand moves clockwise and the left counterclockwise. The purpose of this exercise is to assess the player's motor skills and coordination.

(2) **"Rope Pull"**. This level is a movement that is exactly the same as a top-down rope pull, repeated 10 times overall. The goal is to assess the overall mobility of the upper extremities, as well as the accuracy and simultaneity of the movements.

(3) **"Inflating the lifejacket"**. This exercise is similar to the previous one, but also involves the shoulder girdle. The activity is also aimed at assessing the synchronicity of actions and the general condition of the upper body.

(4) **"Sailing on a yacht"**. The essence of this exercise is to steer the boat and pass through 10 control points, by moving the hips left and right. It is necessary to perform 10 repetitions in each direction. The purpose is to assess the general mobility of the joints of the pelvic area, and condition of the lumbar spine, as well as to train balance.

(5) **"Dinghy Control"**. Conceptually, this exercise is similar to the previous one. The only difference is that this time, the movement is not with the hips but with the shoulder girdle. In this case, the main purpose of the exercise is to support and warm up the spine and examine its condition.

Before choosing a set of exercises for the platform, this issue was discussed with the therapist. In the process, it was discovered that for the category of elderly people, the most optimal set of activities would be one that could engage all major muscle groups in a single play session. As such, the order and specificity of each exercise allows you to work on all the major groups, from the upper limbs to the back and hips.

Thus, the order of the exercises described in Section 3.2.1 (b) corresponds to the order that was recommended by the therapist and is integrated into the game. In this way, the player engages the different parts of the musculoskeletal system on a "from lesser to greater" basis: upper limbs, shoulder joints, pelvic girdle, lower back. In addition, coordination (The sign of infinity) and balance (Dinghy Control) are trained.

These exercises are intended solely for the general warm-up and support of players whose age range is between 60 and 85 years.

(c) *Game Interface*

The game itself is a visual user shell made in 3D style. The main message and design of the game involves a maritime theme, namely traveling on a personal yacht on the ocean. This is due to the relatively low mobility of the target audience; at the same time, the theme of travel is one of the most appealing. At the first stages of the system development, we also considered the 2D version, but it was decided to abandon this concept in favor of a greater visual immersion.

The game is also divided into 5 main levels, which comprise essentially an interactive visualization of the physical exercises used and several additional levels, such as the main menu, the level of profile creation and the results table. At each exercise level, the player's body tracking system is connected, allowing the collection of movement data from different parts of the player's body. For the latter, this system is invisible and works in the background, allowing sole focus on the game. The algorithm for obtaining these data is described further in Sections 3.2.5 and 3.2.6.

3.2.2. Architecture Explanation

The architecture of the system is quite simple. It consists of 3 interconnected functional blocks, which perform different kinds of functions. The architecture diagram itself is shown in Figure 3.

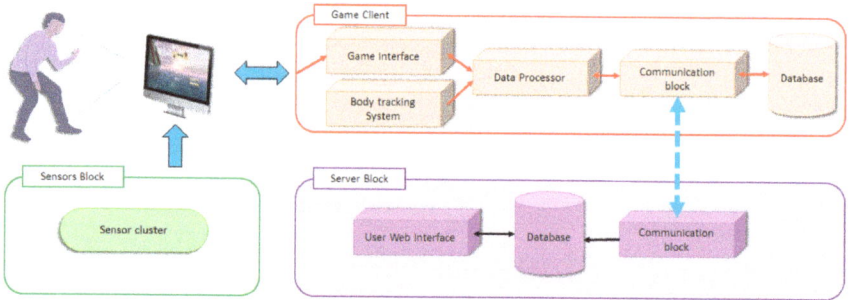

Figure 3. Main system architecture.

The order is next. The sensor connection block is responsible for direct communication of additional sensors or devices with the game platform client. This is done either by using the usual USB protocols, Bluetooth connection, or by using additional tools (expansion boards, Arduino boards, Raspberry Pi boards, and so on). The main sensor required, without which the system loses its efficiency and usefulness in general, is a USB webcam. More about this device will be described later.

The server unit is a remote repository where each player's progress during the game is saved. There is also the possibility of remote access to a special page, which shows the statistics pertaining to the player, their main indicators, and progress in rehabilitation over a certain period. Demonstrating this information is intended solely for the attending physician, but where necessary, access can also be given to the players themselves. Any information received from the player is not confidential but falls under the rule of medica confidentiality.

The Game Client block is the game client itself, which the player or doctor installs on their personal or hospital computer, and through which the player's medical data are received and processed. It also includes local data storage, which is essentially a backup copy of the data sent to the server. It is important to note that data processing in the game client, as well as sending them to the server, is carried out in real time.

3.2.3. Body Tracking System Description

The main feature of the platform being developed is a real-time motion tracking system. During the first stages of development, several different systems were tested that can produce human recognition in images, with both machine-learning and neural network-based algorithms having been tested. In the end, the choice fell on the OpenPose system. Even though this algorithm was most suitable for the task at hand, it still required a lot of tweaking, and is based on a trained Convolutional Neural Network (CNN). The system works with both single images and video. In the second case, the load on the system is somewhat greater, as a continuous storyboard with a rate of 30 frames per second (fps) is used. During adaptation of the OpenPose system to our platform, several functional changes were made to the algorithm, without changing the neural network itself:

- The hand recognition module has been reduced (fingers, palm).
- The face recognition module (eyes, mouth, nose, ears, eyebrows) was reduced.
- The storyboarding process was optimized, which allowed a stable 30 fps to be obtained (in the original state the rate was 18–24 fps).

It is worth providing more detail on the features of the finalized OpenPose. As mentioned above, during testing it was found that at this stage, all motion tracking functions are redundant. Therefore, the system was simplified which improved performance. Initially, the system was designed for 25 key points for the body, 21 for the arms, and 70 for the face, although in the modified system, there are only 21 points for the body. A view of the tracker is shown in Figure 4.

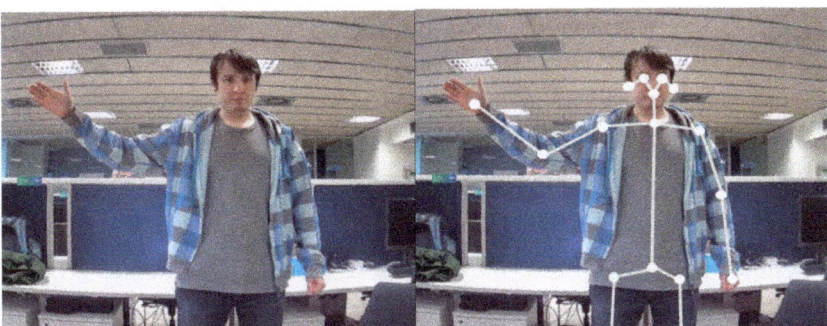

Figure 4. Example of body tracking system.

In a nutshell, the Body Position Algorithm works by selecting each frame individually from the video stream. The neural network then creates a kind of confidence map on the frame, which creates key points on it. From these points, the direction of the found body parts and their connections are calculated. After that, the points are "assembled" depending on the direction, and finally a "body map" is assigned to the frame. The result is a "skeleton" which is created directly in the production environment, and with which further manipulations can be carried out.

As the algorithm uses a storyboard of the received image, the efficiency and accuracy of the system directly depends on the quality of the incoming video (cropped images). The system is, therefore, highly dependent on the ambient light factor. The accuracy and speed of the algorithm is also affected by the resolution of the source image. The higher it is, the more accurately the neural network detects the key points of the body, which increases the overall accuracy, but at the same time, the speed of rendering these points decreases.

Body tracking algorithm was also integrated into the Unity game engine environment with the functions being based on the generation of 3D objects, which are tied to 2D image coordinates. This image is obtained from the output of the neural network. Then the X and Y coordinates are mapped, which allows binding objects within the system.

For the system to work correctly in a game engine, the main task for the algorithm is to ensure the highest possible accuracy at the highest possible framerate. The modifications we made allowed us to achieve 30 frames per second, with a sufficiently high accuracy.

It is important to note that the accuracy is also affected by the frequency of the incoming video stream. At 25, 30 and 60 fps (camera parameters), the rate of change in the position of key body points in subsequent frames decreases as the number of frames increases. Therefore, during the neural network operation for each frame, there may be "oscillations" of these points on the rendered skeleton. In the game itself, this translates into a fluctuation of the coordinates of each of the points being created. This optimization has reduced these oscillations to 0.4–0.9% of the error between frames.

A more detailed description of the features of the OpenPose algorithm is presented in reference [37].

3.2.4. Game Structure

This section will describe the general structure of the levels, as well as a description of each of them individually. It should be said right away that all available game levels were based on the therapist's recommendations.

As mentioned above, the main task of the platform is to help in the player's rehabilitation. Therefore, the main point and main challenge was precisely the need to disguise the usual routine physical exercises in such a way that they would be as difficult to recognize as possible.

At this stage in the game there are 5 levels, which are lined up in a clear sequence, and serve a certain function. The structure of each of the levels is quite simple, including the following elements:

- A level guide with a description of the task, and a demonstration of the movement to be performed by the player
- The actual playing process (performing the exercise)
- The result window, where the player sees how well they did, and the transition window to the next activity (level).

Each level is also divided into two parts: the game interface visible to the player, as well as a function block, which is responsible for obtaining game session data. What these data are and how they are obtained will be described later. Now, it is worth going to each of the levels separately.

A sailboat ride was adopted as a game theme. Considering the target audience, and the relaxing and interesting process in general, this solution proved to be the most appropriate both in terms of activity and level of interest, and in terms of adaptability of the proposed exercises.

One of the main features of the game platform is that, thanks to the work done to integrate the tracking system into the Unity environment, the player does not need any kind of controllers. All control in the game is assured by their movement. The control points, which are responsible for the hands, are essentially analogous to the mouse cursor of a personal computer and allow not only performance of the task to control, but also to the game menu. The usual mouse control is also considered standard.

3.2.5. Data Collection Method

As mentioned earlier, the platform has two methods of collecting information about the player. The first involvers the collection of game information (run time, points, reps), while the second involves the collection of information about the activity of the movements of individual body parts, as well as the player. This system takes the form of a built-in algorithm, which works regardless of the difficulty selected by the player and does not imply a shutdown function.

Although this information about movement activity is not confidential, notification about its collection for purely medical needs is provided before the start of the game. The movement data may be subject to medical secrecy rules and will not be available to anyone other than the treating physician and the player themselves.

Now here is more about the functions of the system, with the general principle for obtaining data being shown in Figure 5.

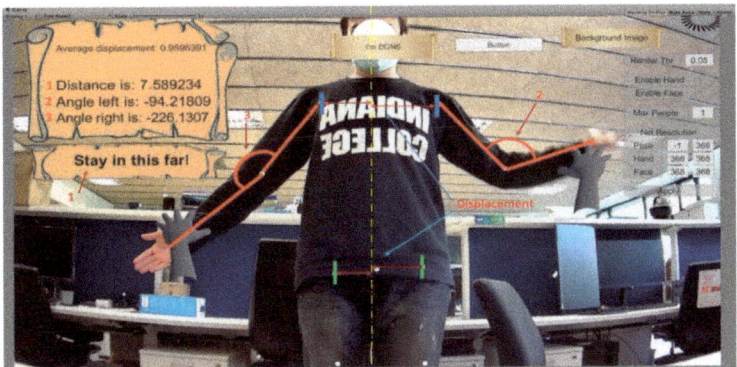

Figure 5. Visual example of activity system parameters.

In total, the algorithm receives data on the following parameters:

- Angle between shoulder and left hand forearm
- Angle between shoulder and right hand forearm
- Left hand position
- Right arm position
- Hip position
- Shoulder position
- Head position
- Head rotation angle.

It all works as follows. Inside the Unity environment, each of the key points, which are created by a neural network (OpenPose algorithm), are tied to the coordinates of the 3D space of the game scene. When fixing the player's movement, these coordinates change, but only in two directions, X and Y, while the Z coordinate always remains unchanged. Using this, each of the game scenes is constructed in such a way that when linking 3D objects to points of the neural network, these objects will also change only 2 coordinates. This method has both advantages and disadvantages.

The main disadvantage of the system is that it cannot correctly track complex movements in 3 planes. For example, the difference between the arm outstretched forward and outstretched to the side is tracked by the difference in distance between the arm outstretched forward and outstretched sideways, tracked by the straight-line distance between the key points of that arm. Thus, technically, there is a distortion of the limb length in the system, which can also affect the angle at certain positions.

An important aspect when gathering the above information on the indicators is that it is affected by the general lighting of the room which the player is in, as well as the camera position. It may be that lighting reduces the accuracy of body recognition by the neural network and at some moments, it may affect the objects inside the game scene in the form of objects "twitching" (each frame from the camera may give different coordinate positions of key points). In the second case, if the webcam is installed incorrectly, when the lens is excessively raised, lowered, or directed more forcefully to one side, the position may be detected with an error. To avoid this, a calibration level was created, whereby the player must set the lens and lighting correctly.

Despite the disadvantages of the system, it is not intended to obtain accurate values, but rather to track the player's activity. The main purpose of these indicators is to record activity and provide data for further evaluation and comparison of progress.

Next, we shall look at the way the system works. When you load a level and activate the body tracking algorithm, the activity logging system starts recording the key point coordinate readings for all tracked indicators. The recording frequency is 1 coordinate value every 1 centisecond, and the method for obtaining this coordinate for each of the parameters is different. Table 4 shows the algorithms for obtaining these values.

Table 4. Parameters recording methods.

Parameter	Title 2
Left arm position	Object X. and Y.properties coordinate recording
Right arm position	Object X. and Y.properties coordinate recording
Head rotation angle	Function of coordinates transform + Vector angle calculation
Head position	Object X.properties coordinate recording
Shoulder position	Object X.properties coordinate recording
Hip position	Object X.properties coordinate recording

The resulting values are written in the form of a data array, which, after the level is completed, is written in a separate file format—json. This method of saving makes it convenient to work with data both in a manual format and for algorithm processing on the server side of the platform. Next, Figure 6 shows an example of the graphical representation of the resulting data.

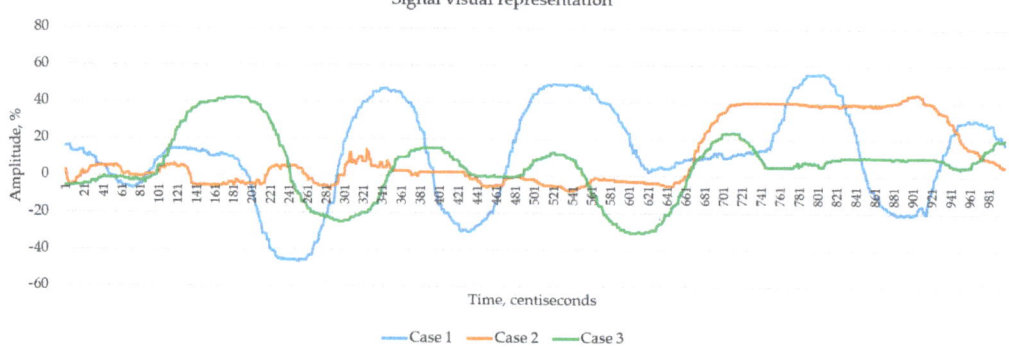

Figure 6. Visual representation of the data received.

Figure 6 shows the dataset of the hip position of one person in 3 different cases: Case 1—normal pace of movement; Case 2—the pace of movement is reduced; and Case 3—the player was inactive most of the time. The task was set for 10 repetitions of hip movement (5 to the left and 5 to the right). The amount of time spent on the exercise in both cases was 10 s. The values on the Y-axis are the deviation coordinate values and are shown in the form of positive and negative values, which also characterizes the deviation side: positive values refer to the right deviation, whereas negative values refer to the left deviation. Based on the information provided in Figure 6, it is possible to draw several conclusions in terms of physical activity:

- The timing of the player's movements, both the total number and each repetition individually
- The maximum value of the deviation amplitude, which indicates the intensity of the exercise
- The activity as a whole, based on the number of peak values of the deviation amplitude

- The evaluative characteristic of motor skills, based on the direction in which there is a greater number of peak values of the deviation amplitude.

Thus, the parameters obtained from a player's activity make it possible to evaluate both their current activity during a given game session and to obtain an evaluation over time by comparing their motor characteristics. This information, in theory, should help physicians and the patients themselves to monitor the outcome and progress of the rehabilitation process for different degrees and types of musculoskeletal problems.

3.2.6. Data Saving and Interpretation

As a result of each of the tasks, the system stored all the data obtained in a special .json file, the information from which was used to process the results. All indicators obtained are shown in the form of a data array for each of the categories. An example of such a file is shown in Table 5.

Table 5. Example of retrieved data cluster.

Body Parameter	Point 1	Point 2	Point 3	Point 4	Point 5	Point 6	Point 7	Point 8	Point 9	Point 10
rightAngelData	−3.660	−3.660	−8.564	−8.564	−8.564	−7.300	−5.835	−5.835	−4.547	−4.547
leftAngelData	−82.022	−82.042	−82.006	−81.974	−81.974	−82.679	−82.825	−82.789	−83.523	−83.467
HeadAngelData	179.786	179.780	179.791	179.784	179.805	179.794	179.795	179.789	179.792	179.785
HipsData	8.276	6.507	7.878	7.878	5.987	4.728	6.099	4.788	6.159	6.159
HeadData	179.788	179.786	179.780	179.791	179.784	179.805	179.794	179.795	179.789	179.792
rangeData	6.908	6.965	6.997	7.054	7.043	7.039	7.091	7.139	7.150	7.209
shoulderData	−0.037	0.862	−0.509	−0.509	0.318	0.095	−1.276	−1.336	−2.707	−2.707
leftMoveData	−58.095	−58.103	−58.103	−58.103	−58.128	−58.115	−58.115	−58.138	−58.138	−58.138
rightMoveData	−56.344	−56.381	−56.383	−56.383	−56.145	−55.957	−55.951	−56.100	−56.107	−56.107
averageArmLData	60.127	−57.823	−58.518	−50.405	6.438	−19.626	−49.406	48.971	−53.573	−41.703
averageArmRData	77.494	−49.893	−56.770	15.153	−12.699	−33.412	27.298	−55.278	2.442	−2.859
averageHipsData	95.968	4.780	7.458	8.700	8.086	8.137	8.336	6.683	8.547	8.080
averageShouldersData	47.749	−3.716	−0.577	−0.610	−0.642	−0.603	−1.873	−0.038	−2.035	−1.135

There are 13 parameters in total:

- Right- and left-hand angle data—information that allows you to assess the overall movement activity of the player when performing upper limb exercises
- Head angle and head displacement data—allow tracking the degree of rotation of the player's head. Useful for understanding the approximate direction of the player's gaze, as well as problems with general motor skills (for problems with the cervical spine
- Range data—show the general dynamics of the player's position in space. Useful for evaluating general activity, as well as for evaluating the player's movement during game activities
- Hips and shoulders displacement data—show the dynamic displacement of the player's shoulders and hips, as well as the degree of this displacement
- Left and right arm displacement data—the activity of the player's hand movement. Characteristics of upper and lower maximum deflection, smoothness, and accuracy of the movements
- Average arm, hip, and shoulder movements—characteristics that allow the average position of the body to be estimated, as well as individual areas of the body. Useful when researching into temporary or permanent partial atrophy, palsy, or dysfunction of the muscles of a particular area of the body.

It is important to note that all parameters saved in the file refer to the value of the coordinate of a particular point, which is created by the motion tracking system. By default, the screen coordinate system in the Unity environment is [0%, . . . , 100%] vertically and [0%, . . . , 100%] horizontally, from the current screen resolution, which is set to 1080p (1920 × 1080 pixels) in the system by default. Given that all parameters are calculated relative to the median line on the X or Y axis, which is 50% and 50%, respectively, it appears that the screen space is divided into 4 segments, in which, depending on the exercise, the coordinates may record both positive and negative values. This indicates only the direction of movement (in the case of the hips or shoulders, "+" means right and "−" means left.

3.2.7. Data Visualization

To assess exercise performance, it is necessary to select a benchmark example by means of which one can judge not only the correctness of a single activity, but also the quality of progress and how close it is to the desired result. In this regard, a "benchmark characteristic" was created for each of the exercises, which will serve as a reference point in the evaluation of results. For this purpose, each exercise was performed 5 times at the correct tempo and with the correct amplitude of movement, naturally as much as possible. Then, a general result was obtained from the 5 results, which became the "reference" for the system being developed. The following were chosen as the key parameters of these signals:

- Time to complete each task
- Amplitude of the received signal (by means of direct Fourier transform);
- Frequency of repetitions
- Repetition period
- Jitter and shimmer.

As an example, how to check and parse the signal parameters with their subsequent evaluation is shown in Figure 7 with the parameters providing referring to the reference result obtained for Exercise 3.

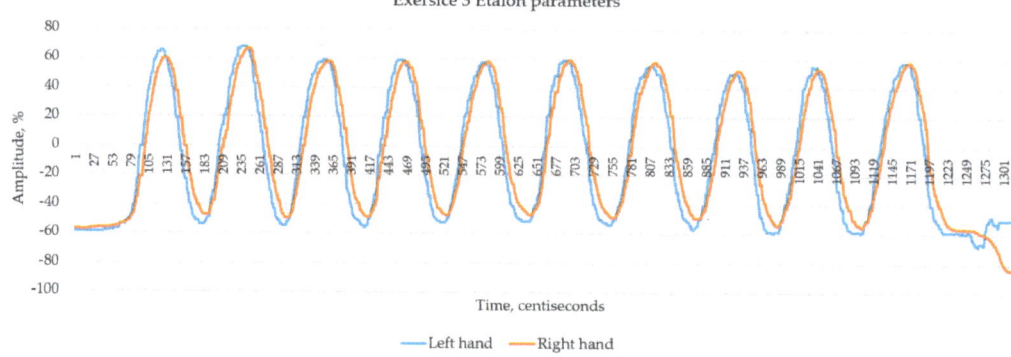

Figure 7. Etalon parameters for Exercise 3.

Additionally, to gain a clearer picture and better assessment of the results, it was decided to obtain a signal that corresponds to a very bad version of the exercise—namely, poor timing, incorrect amplitude, and speed of repetitions, as well as the presence of external factors that could disrupt the procedure involved in obtaining results. An example of this exercise is shown in Figure 8.

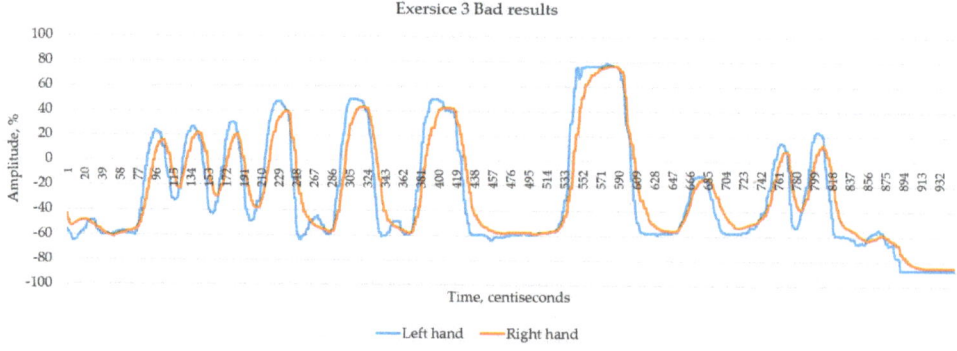

Figure 8. The result of incorrect performance of Exercise 3.

Even a visual analysis of the two graphs shows that Figure 8 provides a clear difference in amplitude and repetition time. To describe this example more accurately, Figures 9 and 10 are shown below, which show the results obtained from Exercise 3 in the normal view, and immediately after passing the game level.

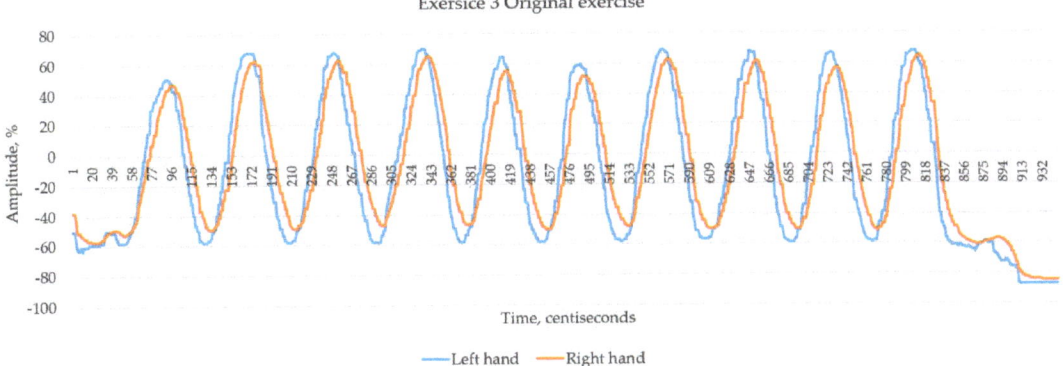

Figure 9. Result of normal performance in Exercise 3.

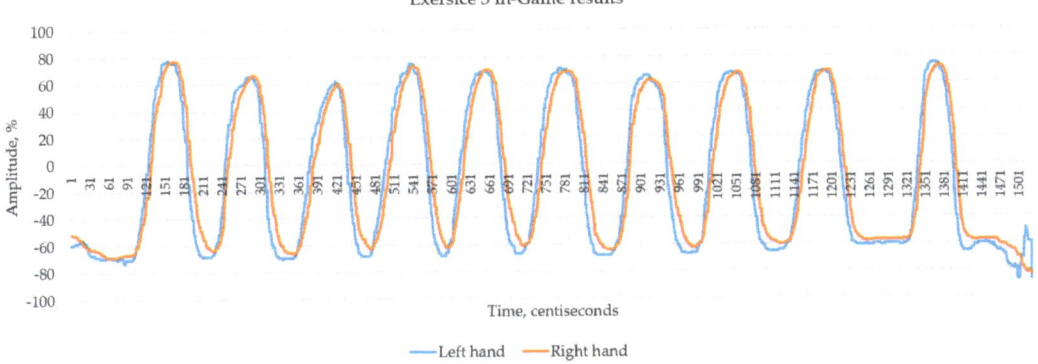

Figure 10. Result of game performance in Exercise 3.

In Figure 9 you can see that the graph referring to this signal already more accurately resembles the reference signal. We can clearly see the even level of amplitude and time of each repetition.

Figure 10 directly shows the result obtained during the passage of the level on the game platform.

3.2.8. Data Comparison

As described in Section 3.2.5, the signals received must be processed and certain characteristic data must be obtained from them. Therefore, the following parameters must be extracted from each signal:

(a) *Time parameter:*

This is the exercise time in total. This characteristic helps to ascertain how fast or slow the player performed a particular exercise.

(b) *Amplitude parameter:*

This includes the value of the minimum and maximum amplitude of the signal. The main purpose of the measurement is to represent the player's activity during the exercise, namely to understand the spatial characteristic of the activity. Given that the amplitude value obtained during the analysis of the player's movements is shown in the percentage value of the deviation of the key points from the central plane lines on the screen, by obtaining this value, it is possible to judge, for example, how high the player raised their arms, how much they deflected when moving their hips, or how actively they moved in front of the camera.

(c) *Frequency of repetitions:*

It is also important to understand the frequency with which the player performed a particular exercise. This parameter can be obtained by several methods, but since the data obtained in the time and graphical representation are a sinusoidal signal, the most convenient method is the application of the direct Fourier transform, the formula for which is shown below.

$$f(t) = \frac{1}{2\pi} \int_{-\infty}^{\infty} F(j\omega) e^{j\omega t} d\omega \tag{1}$$

Obtaining this parameter will help to keep track of how often the player is performing the exercise. This parameter is also important for understanding the quality of the exercise (whether it is too slow or too fast), and therefore its effectiveness.

(d) *Shimmer and Jitter:*

Shimmer and jitter values are an estimative characteristic of the quality of exercise performance. Thanks to these parameters, we can judge the quality of the periodicity of movements, both in terms of the difference in time of each repetition and the difference in the amplitude of the movements.

Jitter absolute: Variation of fundamental frequency. The average absolute difference between consecutive periods:

$$jitter\ (a) = \frac{1}{N-1} \sum_{i}^{N-1} |T_i - T_{i+1}| \tag{2}$$

Jitter relative: Average absolute difference between consecutive periods, divided by the average period:

$$jitter\ (r) = \frac{\frac{1}{N-1} \sum_{i}^{N-1} |T_i - T_{i+1}|}{\frac{1}{N} \sum_{i=1}^{N} T_i} \tag{3}$$

where T_i is the extracted period lengths and N is the number of extracted periods.

Shimmer dB: Expressed as the variability of the peak-to-peak amplitude in decibels, average absolute base-10 logarithm of the difference between the amplitudes of consecutive periods.

$$shimmer\ (a) = \frac{1}{N-1} \sum_{i=1}^{N-1} \left| 20 \log \left(\frac{A_{i+1}}{A_i} \right) \right| \tag{4}$$

Shimmer relative: Defined as the average absolute difference between the amplitudes of consecutive periods, divided by the average amplitude, and expressed as a percentage.

$$shimmer\ (r) = \frac{\frac{1}{N-1} \sum_{i}^{N-1} |A_i - A_{i+1}|}{\frac{1}{N} \sum_{i=1}^{N} A_i} \tag{5}$$

where A_i are the extracted peak-to-peak amplitude data and N is the number of extracted fundamental frequency periods.

Having obtained all of the above parameters, it is possible to compare the results obtained, as well as judge the quality of the exercise. Table 6 directly shows the results obtained from four cases of Exercise 3.

Table 6. Example of comparing the results of one iteration in Exercise 3.

Result	Time, s	Min. Amplitude, %	Max. Amplitude, %	Frequency, Hz	Shimmer Absolute, dB	Shimmer Relative	Shimmer, %	Jitter Absolute	Jitter Relative	Jitter, %
				LEFT HAND						
Etalon	13.01	−68.15	67.52	0.859	11.78	0.029	2.886	0.076	0.064	5.344
Bad	9.46	−87.34	77.69	1.025	25.14	0.318	31.827	0.414	0.512	63.168
Exercise	9.41	−87.37	69.75	1.297	10.59	0.042	4.241	0.067	0.080	9.701
InGame	15.26	−87.34	77.55	0.806	16.29	0.033	3.280	0.164	0.118	8.438
				RIGHT HAND						
Etalon	13.01	−84.37	66.29	0.8591	8.69	0.029	2.940	0.091	0.076	6.380
Bad	9.46	−85.22	76.35	1.025	25.04	0.373	37.262	0.389	0.477	58.548
Exercise	9.41	−85.04	64.78	1.297	16.67	0.056	5.568	0.084	0.102	12.228
InGame	15.26	−83.75	76.99	0.806	13.00	0.035	3.483	0.196	0.140	9.997

The data in Table 6 refer to measurements of a single exercise performed once. Figure 11 shows a graphical analysis of the data obtained.

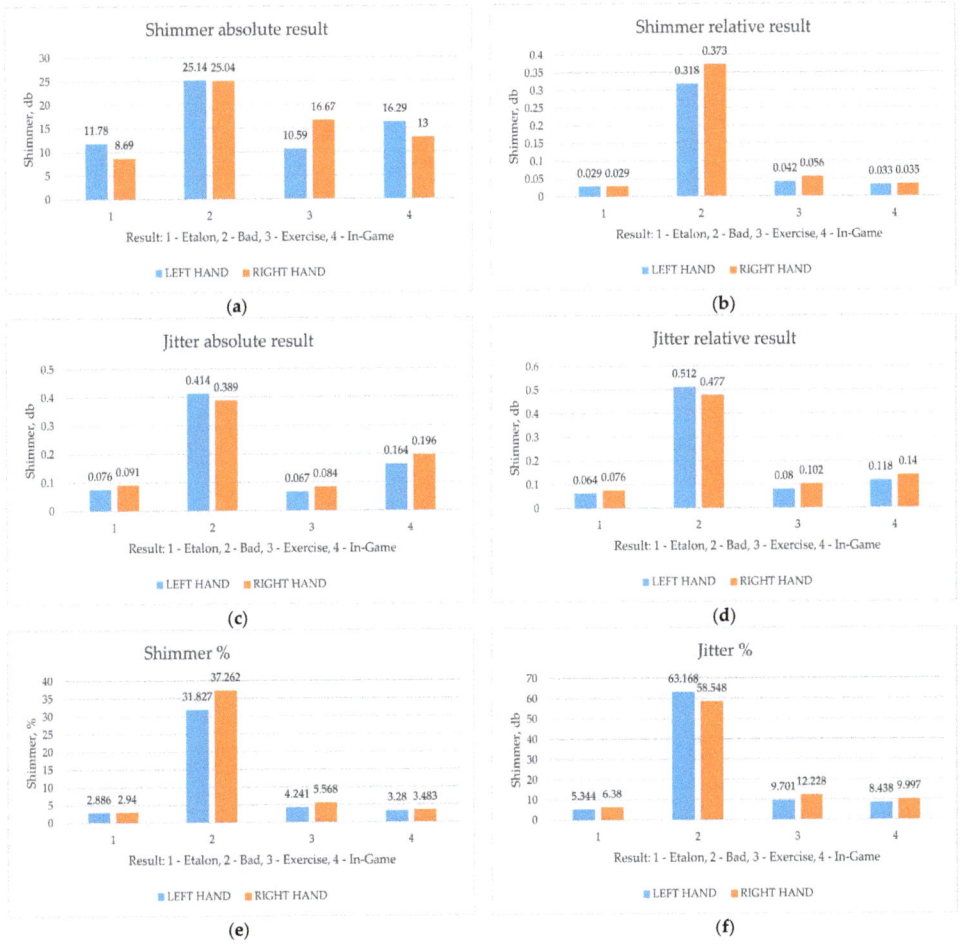

Figure 11. Visualization of the parameters of the result obtained. Where (**a**)—shimmer absolute result for Exercise 3, (**b**)—shimmer relative result for Exercise 3, (**c**)—jitter absolute result for Exercise 3, (**d**)—jitter relative result for Exercise 3, (**e**)—percent of shimmer value in signal, (**f**)—percent of jitter value in signal.

As for the jitter and shimmer parameters, it is worth noting that the lower their values, the better the result obtained in the end. This will mean that the player performed the game exercise as clearly and correctly as possible.

Additionally, the time and amplitude parameters should be compared in a different way. The reference point is the value of the repetition amplitude of the reference signal, in this case, the distance between the maximum and minimum amplitude of each repetition and the entire signal (values in Table 6).

4. Results

4.1. Comparison of Results

In addition to comparing the results obtained from a single exercise, it is also important to understand the dynamics of those results. This is necessary in order to understand the efficiency of the system in repeated use, as well as to ascertain the parameter of overall efficiency. Table 7 shows the results obtained from Exercise 4 over six days with a 12-h interval between exercises for one person. The exercises are performed in normal exercise mode and directly in the game. The comparison is made according to the same parameters that were shown in Table 6. The results presented are the specific case of a particular player. The results of other players are treated in the same way and according to the same methodology as presented below.

Table 7. The results obtained from Exercise 4 in its two interpretations: game and usual.

Result	Time, s	Min. Amplitude, %	Max. Amplitude, %	Frequency, Hz	Shimmer Absolute, dB	Shimmer Relative	Shimmer, %	Jitter Absolute	Jitter Relative	Jitter, %
				Ordinary Exercise						
Etalon	25.39	−19.4	19.7	28.55	0.44	7.91	0.044	4.398	0.590	0.241
Bad	12.41	−11.92	28.67	31.01	0.82	13.54	0.198	19.77	0.229	0.201
Try 1	11.24	−19.04	11.15	24.75	0.91	10.76	0.120	12	0.158	0.140
Try 2	10.94	−9.46	22.86	29.12	0.93	7.91	0.057	5.731	0.142	0.130
Try 3	10.61	−15.16	18.98	27.66	0.96	10.38	0.112	11.241	0.108	0.096
Try 4	10.54	−12.28	17.88	26.72	1.06	4.94	0.055	5.498	0.100	0.095
Try 5	10.44	−10.96	20.92	28.09	0.98	11.04	0.090	8.955	0.082	0.083
Try 6	9.18	−13.81	17.58	26.824	1.12	7.82	0.092	9.233	0.128	0.139
				In-Game Exercise						
Etalon	19.27	−37.20	41.82	70.35	0.31	15.41	0.084	8.422	0.508	0.155
Bad	29.79	−38.53	38.27	63.08	0.28	17.85	0.178	17.770	2.758	0.484
Try 1	28.00	−45.05	58.12	80.16	0.21	19.83	0.136	13.585	0.330	0.077
Try 2	25.69	−45.06	46.28	76.19	0.23	13.40	0.092	9.168	0.223	0.050
Try 3	25.72	−39.05	49.01	83.95	0.19	18.02	0.182	18.24	0.545	0.127
Try 4	23.17	−42.46	44.82	70.47	0.3	21.70	0.196	19.573	0.368	0.105
Try 5	22.88	−43.91	46.9	74.81	0.26	21.39	0.162	16.153	0.952	0.254
Try 6	22.09	−22.68	26.4935	43.81	0.23	15.76	0.153	15.327	0.778	0.187

Table 7 shows the results obtained from Exercise 4 in two different interpretations: as a game level performance and as a normal physical exercise. Figure 12 shows a visual representation of the results.

The effectiveness of the system can be judged following the first tests. One of the indicators of the system is time, which shows how fast the player completes a level. From this, it is possible to compile statistics on the player's progress, and this can be done by comparing it to the normal way of performing the exercise. In the example of the results obtained from Exercise 4 in Table 7 and Figure 12, the time value decreases in both cases of normal exercise and the in-game level. In essence, however, the time values for both cases mean a different situation. Figure 13 and Table 8 shows the progression of the results as a percentage.

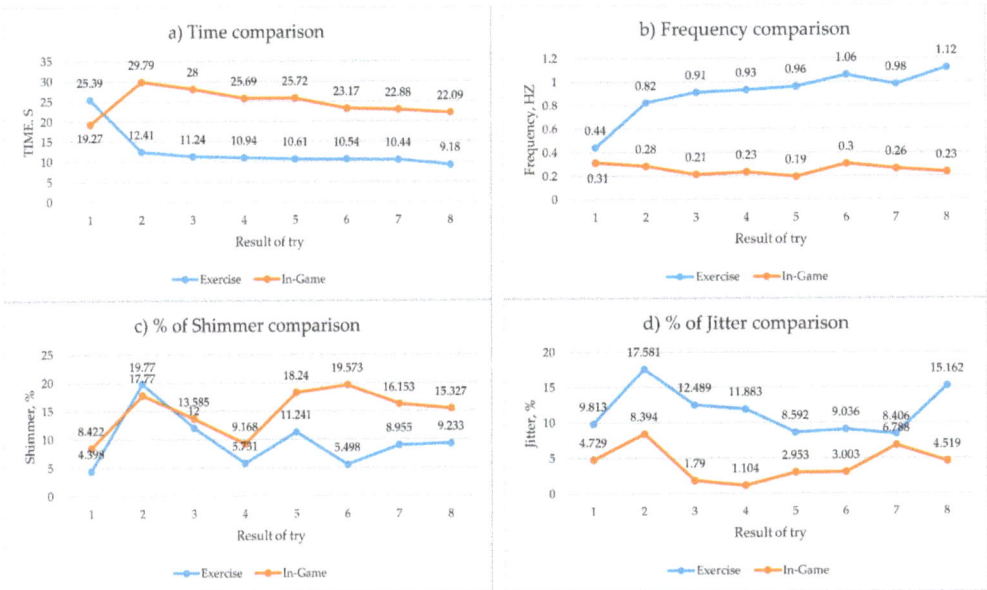

Figure 12. Visual representation of Exercise 4 result comparison in time, frequency, % of Shimmer and Jitter. Where (**a**)—time value for each try of Exercise 4, (**b**)—frequency value of each Exercise 4 try, (**c**)—percent of shimmer value influence on signal for each Exercise 4 try, (**d**)—percent of jitter value influence on signal for each Exercise 4 try.

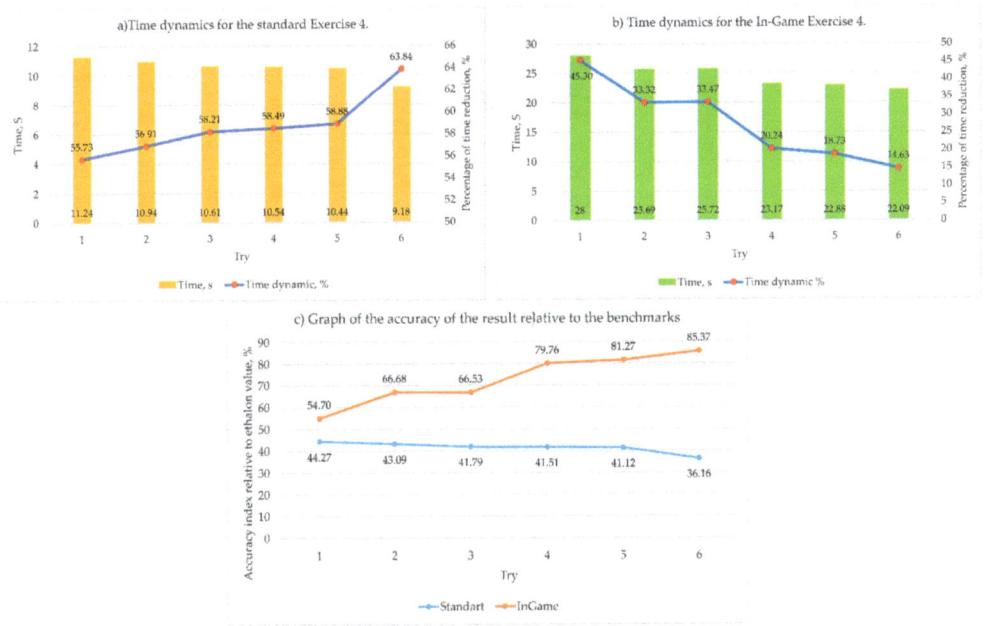

Figure 13. Comparison of both variations of Exercise 4. Where (**a**)—characteristic of the change in the time result indicator for the usual form of Exercise 4, (**b**)—characteristic of the change in the time result indicator for In-Game interpretation of the Exercise 4, (**c**)—characteristic of the closeness of the obtained time to the etalon time in percent (higher is better).

Table 8. Players time parameters.

Result	Time Standard, s	Time Standard Error, %	Time In-Game, s	Time In-Game Error, %	Percentage of Standard Accuracy, %	Percentage of In-Game Accuracy, %
Etalon	25.39	0	19.27	0	100	100
Try 1	11.24	55.73	29.79	45.30	44.27	54.70
Try 2	10.94	56.91	28	33.32	43.09	66.68
Try 3	10.61	58.21	25.69	33.47	41.79	66.53
Try 4	10.54	58.49	25.72	20.24	41.51	79.76
Try 5	10.44	58.88	23.17	18.73	41.12	81.27
Try 6	9.18	63.84	22.88	14.63	36.16	85.37

The data in Table 8 are obtained from the percentage ratio between the values of the reference and received signals. The table shows the difference in the main indicators of the signals in terms of time and accuracy. This is clearly expressed in the fact that the time of the standard execution of Exercise 4 decreases with each new attempt (column "Time Standard, s"). At the same time, the "Time Standard error, %" column shows the percentage of deviation of the obtained time for each try from the "Etalon" value. Time indicators are taken as an example as one of the main evaluation parameters.

Figure 13a,b shows the difference in time needed to complete Exercise 4 for each trial. In the first case, the Try 1 result differs from the reference by 14.15 s, which is 44.27%. This gap then increases with each new trial to 9.18 s, i.e., 63.84%. This indicates that this examinee is trying to finish the exercise quickly (there is no question as to the correctness of the exercise at this point).

The second case is exactly the opposite. This time difference is 10.52 s (45.3%), and the time difference decreases to 3.61 s, which is only 14.63%, unlike in the case of the standard exercise. Based on this result, we can conclude that by choosing an interpretation of the exercise based on the platform developed, the player will have a greater motivation and desire to perform the exercise more correctly.

Even though in both cases the exercise time is reduced, the case of the in-game result shows that the platform developed justifies itself as an additional tool for rehabilitation proposes. This is due to the fact that by introducing a certain kind of activity, such as, in this case, steering the ship through the control points, the person focuses not just on completing the exercise, but also on performing it as correctly as possible. This is also greatly helped by the presence of a visual response to the player's actions.

The same pattern is observed in the case of the frequency of exercise. In Figure 12, the frequency response of both cases shows that while in the case of the normal exercise, the player tries to perform the exercise faster each time, the in-game case allows to regulate the tempo of the movements at the same level.

The jitter and shimmer values are also indicative of a certain kind of result. Due to the peculiarities of the game level for Exercise 4, there is a need to control the period of each repetition by the game itself, which allows you to bring the time of each repetition to the median value. Calculation these parameters is an important part of the system because they mainly control and regulate the dynamics of the player's movements, which allows monitoring and regulating the rehabilitation process more accurately.

4.2. Explanations of Results

As can be seen in Figure 12, in general, both interpretations of Exercise 4 evidence a similar progression of results. Nevertheless, it should be noted that with respect to some specifics, Exercise 4 is somewhat different in nature in these two interpretations. While in the case of the simple hip movement, the main goal is the precision of the movement—namely, the most similar values of the amplitude of the movement, the period of each repetition and the total time of the movement—in the game version, the key goals are somewhat different.

Based on the peculiarities of Level 4 (which is the interpretation of the Exercise 4), the number of repetitions is 10, with 5 hip movements on each side, while for normal performance it is 20, with 10 movements on each side. However, this reduction in repetition is compensated by the fact that the player is not limited to this number. Since the goal of the game level is to steer the boat through 10 gates, and not just 20 moves, the player can do more to achieve this. An example of how this works is shown in Figure 13.

Unlike the usual physical interpretation of Exercise 4, the in-game version forces the player to focus more on the quality of the exercise. Considering that the boat is steered directly with the hips, the number of repetitions will be determined by the player's level of dexterity and control. In the "ideal" performance of this exercise, the movement pattern (Figure 13b) is similar to the physical performance movement pattern (Figure 14a). As you can see in Figure 14c, the first attempt to pass the level required far more movement for the player, although after passing the same level on the 6th attempt (Figure 14d), player significantly improved their score. Instead of 18 moves, they needed 10, which is a 44.4% increase. At the same time, the level completion time also improved, whereby the score improved from 28 s to 22.09, which is 21.1% better than the 1st try.

In the case of a normal exercise, the time score indicates that the exercise was performed faster with each new time, to perform it faster. These rules of analysis also apply to Exercise 5 since they are similar in their nature and the way they are performed. At the same time, the game interpretation of the first three exercises does not differ in mechanics from the physical one, and so in this case, a direct comparison of the indexes given in Tables 6 and 7 is provided.

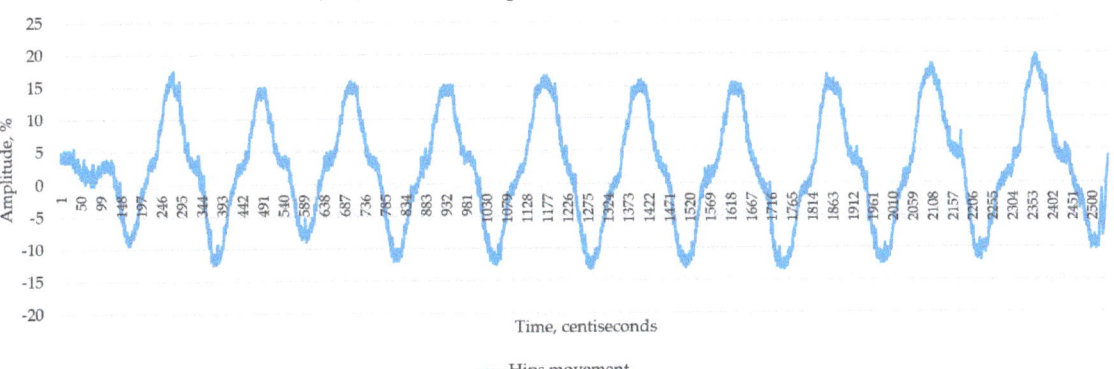

Figure 14. Cont.

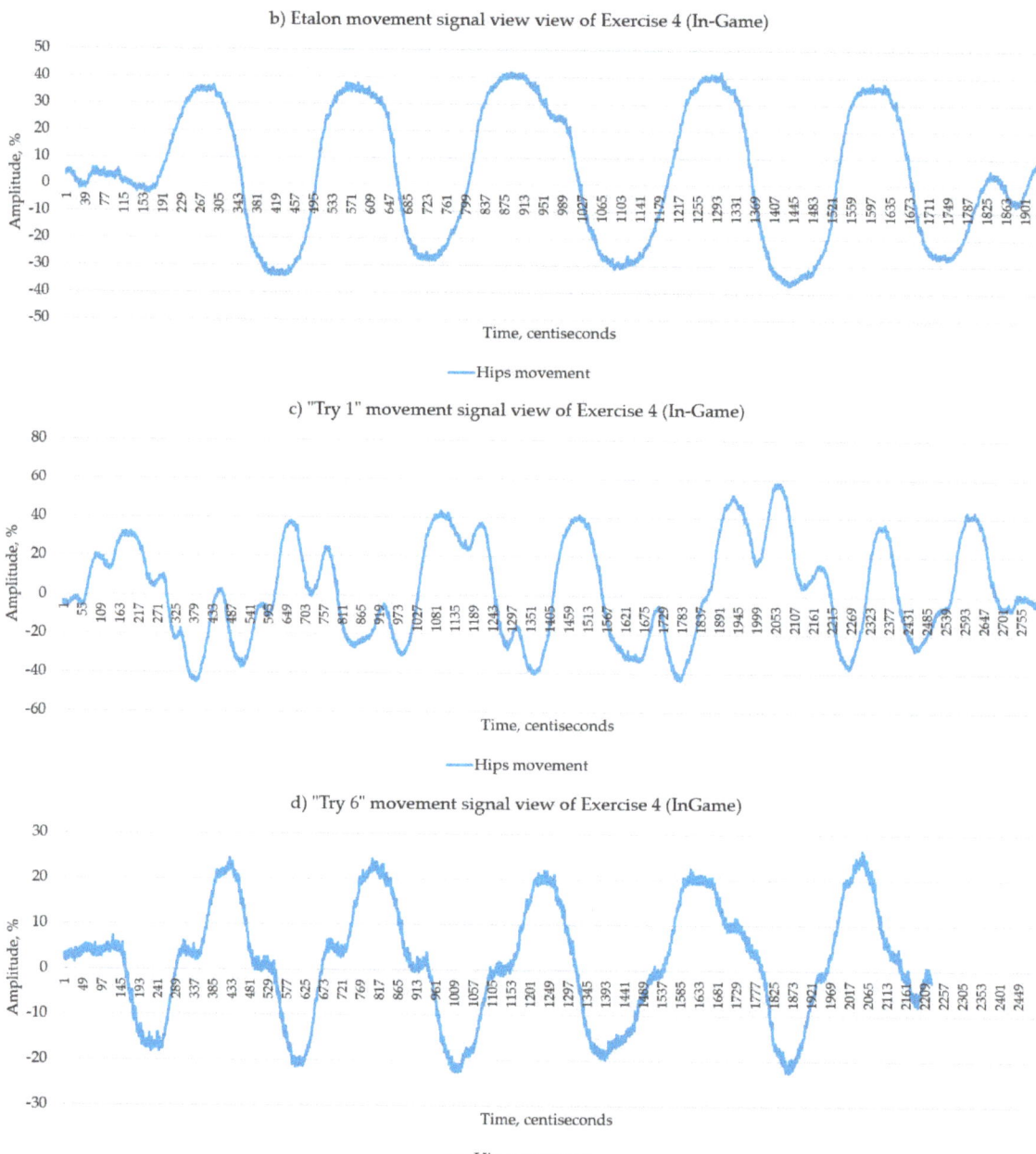

Figure 14. Example of the difference in the pattern of movements for different interpretations of Exercise 4. Where (**a**)—etalon signal view for standard exercise interpretation, (**b**)—etalon signal view for In-Game exercise interpretation, (**c**)—example of In-Game signal view of Ty 1, (**d**)—example of In-Game signal view of Try 6.

5. Discussion

Even though, based on the results, the system shows its effectiveness, additional checks and evaluations are required. Having analyzed those articles that are listed in

Table 1, as well as other similar studies, it was concluded that, in general, the effectiveness of introducing additional systems, such as computer games, into the rehabilitation process is quite effective at present. Thanks to the variability of technical and software solutions, it is possible to choose the activity for almost any types of rehabilitation procedure. This includes, for example, assistance with problems with the upper extremities [44,47,49], lower extremities [47,50], or for the whole body [42,43,51]. The variability in the methods used in these studies also allows the rehabilitation process to be tailored as effectively as possible. These include the use of special tracking tools, such as the Kinect system or Virtual reality interfaces [42,44,46,49,50], and neural networks to avoid the need for additional sensors [43,51].

Since the system presented in this article also has its own characteristics, it is possible to compare it to the above solutions. This should be undertaken in terms of several aspects that affect different sides of the platforms.

Technical side: Includes additional peripherals or technical devices. If we refer to that case, then it is worth comparing the additional tools and sensors that were used in different approaches, and what the reason for this decision was. The purpose of the platform described in this article is to create the most convenient and simple system, which does not require any additional handling by the doctor or players. This technical solution already offers certain kinds of advantages, in contrast to the variants where a virtual reality system was used [42,48]: the Kinect platform or Wii [46,49], additional camera systems and additional technical means [42,50]. Disregarding additional sensors offers you an advantage in terms of accessibility, as well as in terms of the longer-term relevance of the platform. For example, Microsoft Kinect and Nintendo Wii have been out of production and without support since 2017 and 2013, respectively.

The platform presented here does not require any additional peripherals other than the webcam, which is a very common and cheap device. This makes the system not only as affordable as possible from the financial standpoint, but also easy to install and use.

Visual side: Undoubtedly, the visual part of the platform has a very important function, namely, to attract the player and motivate them to return to the game. In the case of the platform developed, it was decided to make the player part of a certain little story in which they are directly involved. Unlike other solutions [44,48–50] where the player simply performs tasks and activities related only to one general style, or has no thematic activities at all [43,50] our platform offers a small adventure, which makes the system more interesting.

In addition, this kind of exercise presentation, which has a beginning and an end goal, is designed to help the player, mentally. The theme of travel is chosen precisely because of the possible limited mobility of the players, given the age category in addition to the peculiarities of the location, and thus helps to try out activities that are not normally available to a person, even if not to the fullest extent. This, in turn, has a positive effect on their mental state.

Algorithm used: The built-in motion recognition algorithm is based on a neural network, and this solution has both pluses and minuses. Unlike the Kinect technologies [46,49], where the 3D image is built using a system of depth cameras, or the Virtual Reality system [42,48], in which the work is based on a constant reading of the position of sensors inside the helmet and controllers in addition to building a volumetric image with the camera system, solutions based on neural networks depend quite heavily on external parameters. These include the quality of lighting, positioning of the player in front of the camera, and quality of the processed image. In this regard, and in order to obtain the most correct data, it is necessary to introduce and observe additional rules of work with systems based on neural networks [43,51].

Bearing in mind that the main task was to make the platform as accessible and simple as possible, it was decided in this study to take the neural network algorithm as a basis. Consequently, use of the platform allows you to apply the principle of "install–run–use".

Medical focus and value to physicians: The system proposed is designed to help support and rehabilitate predominantly the elderly, although it can also be applied to patients with minor musculoskeletal system problems. The focus of the choice of exercises and their direction is based on the principle of "a little of everything", in contrast to the systems aimed at working with a particular part of the body, such as the upper extremities [44,46,48] or the lower extremities [42,50,51].

In terms of the value of the system to medical staff, the platform acts as a tool for systematizing information, which allows the doctor to monitor progress of the patient's recovery and their overall activity indices more accurately and qualitatively. The main feature is that, unlike some similar systems [43,48,50], direct participation by the attending physician in the game process is not required. All the data obtained can be viewed and examined at any time, thanks to the cloud interface where this information is duplicated, as seen, for example, in the solution [43].

Results and effectiveness: Given the specific nature of the study presented, it is rather difficult to compare it to the results obtained from similar solutions. Although the effectiveness of the gaming platform increases the patient's outcome from 30% to 50% depending on the level and activity, the value in this case does not show the specific rehabilitative potential of the system. There are several reasons for this.

Firstly, while in studies like ours, the main parameters for assessing the effectiveness of the system were precisely the rehabilitation indicators, and it was the result of rehabilitation actions that was compared and evaluated, in our case, the signals into which the system converts the player's performance are researched. Therefore, in this case, it is the indicators of the received signals, such as jitter, shimmer, amplitude–frequency response, and so on, that are important for the study presented here. It is on this comparison that the working principle of the platform presented is based.

Secondly, because of the situation regarding the COVID-19 pandemic, it was not possible to conduct tests with the target audience. Bearing in mind that young people (from 21 to 42 years old) took part in the study, the results obtained from them are not entirely accurate, albeit at the same time, proving extremely useful for further research purposes.

Thirdly, which follows on from the first point, based on the results obtained, it turned out to be a wrong solution to study such indicators as the Activities of Daily Living (ADLs), Cognitive Function Scale (CFS), Nottingham Health Profile (NHP) [45] score. The reason for this is that it would be incorrect to compare the performance of healthy young people to results from elderly people.

Fourthly, one of the main tasks at this stage of research was to find out the value of the system's effectiveness, as well as its capabilities as an additional module for rehabilitation procedures, which, unfortunately, we were unable to fully test at the time of writing this article due to the COVID-19 pandemic.

Emotional component. While testing the platform, most of the players noted that performing physical activities in the form of a computer game was a more interesting experience for them, as opposed to conventional physical activities. In this study, we did not test participants on their emotional state after the game, as the data obtained would not have been entirely correct. The explanation for this is that older people react differently to computer games than the age group that took part in the test. Therefore, the estimated results would have been different.

Nevertheless, the feedback provided a certain kind of information that will help to further develop the system.

6. Conclusions and Future Plans

This article presents an interactive system developed to help rehabilitate and support the elderly, as well as patients with musculoskeletal system problem. The main idea was to create an additional tool that would be as simple as possible and would not require any additional material resources, designed to improve the rehabilitation process, and to make it more interesting. At this stage, the developed platform is an independent gaming platform, which includes a set of tools and algorithms aimed at improving the rehabilitation process itself, as well as aspects of it. During the development and testing of the system, there were certain questions that needed to be addressed, as follows.

Question 1: Technical Basis. Given that the original goal was to create a system that can be used by different users, it was decided to create an interactive gaming platform, in other words, a serious game that the user can install easily and use at any time.

The main point was that the player's indicators should be recorded in real time with the use of a minimum number of additional means. That is why a body tracking system was used with only a webcam, while providing the maximum level of functionality.

Question 2: Medical rationale. That set of 5 basic exercises that were integrated into the platform form part of a set of rehabilitative activities specified by a physiotherapist. Considering the specific target population, namely, elderly people from 60 to 85 years old, as well as people with minor musculoskeletal system problems, the set of exercises used can support the user in physical terms in a complex way, similar to the usual exercise. The only difference is that the interpretation of these exercises and the presence effect make physical activity more meaningful and visually attractive to the user.

Question 3: How valuable is the system, and how can it be used? In addition to its use in the home as a regular entertainment system, it is also of medical value. Thanks to the built-in player tracking and analysis system, all player results are stored and can be viewed immediately after the game or after a period of time. Furthermore, these results can be used as a record of the rehabilitation process, owing to data systematization. This feature is very useful for doctors because it allows them to monitor the patient's progress not only in the hospital, but also remotely.

Limitations: Unfortunately, owing to the situation regarding the pandemic, it is not possible at present to compare the results of the effect of the system developed directly on the target audience. This is also because those subjects who participated in this study do not have any problems with the musculoskeletal system, and their ages are lower than the target age. Nevertheless, the results clarify many aspects and allow us to draw conclusions about the effectiveness of the platform.

Future plans: There are also plans to improve the system. In view of the current situation regarding the COVID-19 pandemic, the testing process was unfortunately deprived of the opportunity to obtain results directly from the target audience. Nevertheless, we plan to test elderly people in the near future.

We also plan to expand the set of integrated exercises, and their different gradation in terms of complexity and orientation. At present, research is underway on the use of additional material aids, such as smart bands, balance sensors, and so on. Work is also already underway to connect additional tools and sensors, although first and foremost, the plan is to implement and connect levels that will be aimed at analyzing and training the player's balance.

Author Contributions: Conceptualization, I.M.-A.; methodology, B.G.Z. and A.M.Z.; software, S.S.; validation, S.S.; investigation, S.S., B.G.Z. and A.M.Z.; resources, B.G.Z. and A.M.Z.; writing—original draft preparation, S.S.; writing—review and editing, B.G.Z. and A.M.Z.; visualization, S.S.; supervision, A.M.Z.; project administration, B.G.Z., funding acquisition, B.G.Z. All authors have read and agreed to the published version of the manuscript.

Funding: That this study forms part of a European research program and is partially funded by the AAL Programme—Project FrAAgile. It is a part of a large set of game and visual platforms for different needs, such as memory and logic training, physical training, support of visual functions, etc.

Institutional Review Board Statement: The study was conducted according to the guidelines of the Declaration of Helsinki and approved by the Ethics Committee of University of Deusto.

Informed Consent Statement: Informed consent was obtained from all subjects involved in the study.

Data Availability Statement: Used data is a private medical data and could not be published anywhere accept this article.

Conflicts of Interest: There are no conflict of interest with this study.

References

1. Tscheikner-Gratl, F.; Egger, P.; Rauch, W.; Kleidorfer, M. Comparison of multi-criteria decision support methods for integrated rehabilitation prioritization. *Water* **2017**, *9*, 68. [CrossRef]
2. Bisio, I.; Delfino, A.; Lavagetto, F.; Sciarrone, A. Enabling IoT for in-home rehabilitation: Accelerometer signals classification methods for activity and movement recognition. *IEEE Internet Things J.* **2016**, *4*, 135–146.
3. Faria, A.L.; Andrade, A.; Soares, L.; i Badia, S.B. Benefits of virtual reality based cognitive rehabilitation through simulated activities of daily living: A randomized controlled trial with stroke patients. *J. Neuroeng. Rehabil.* **2016**, *13*, 1–12. [CrossRef]
4. Bush, M.L.; Dougherty, W. Assessment of vestibular rehabilitation therapy training and practice patterns. *J. Community Health* **2015**, *40*, 802–807. [CrossRef]
5. Tsoupikova, D.; Stoykov, N.S.; Corrigan, M.; Thielbar, K.; Vick, R.; Li, Y.; Kamper, D. Virtual immersion for post-stroke hand rehabilitation therapy. *Ann. Biomed. Eng.* **2015**, *43*, 467–477. [CrossRef]
6. Röijezon, U.; Clark, N.C.; Treleaven, J. Proprioception in musculoskeletal rehabilitation. Part 1: Basic science and principles of assessment and clinical interventions. *Man. Ther.* **2015**, *20*, 368–377. [CrossRef]
7. Tannous, H.; Istrate, D.; Benlarbi-Delai, A.; Sarrazin, J.; Gamet, D.; Ho Ba Tho, M.C.; Dao, T.T. A new multi-sensor fusion scheme to improve the accuracy of knee flexion kinematics for functional rehabilitation movements. *Sensors* **2016**, *16*, 1914. [CrossRef]
8. Grooms, D.; Appelbaum, G.; Onate, J. Neuroplasticity following anterior cruciate ligament injury: A framework for visual-motor training approaches in rehabilitation. *J. Orthop. Sports Phys. Ther.* **2015**, *45*, 381–393.
9. Sánchez-Rodríguez, D.; Miralles, R.; Muniesa, J.M.; Mojal, S.; Abadía-Escartín, A.; Vázquez-Ibar, O. Three measures of physical rehabilitation effectiveness in elderly patients: A prospective, longitudinal, comparative analysis. *BMC Geriatr.* **2015**, *15*, 1–11. [CrossRef] [PubMed]
10. Lohse, K.; Shirzad, N.; Verster, A.; Hodges, N.; Van der Loos, H.M. Video games and rehabilitation: Using design principles to enhance engagement in physical therapy. *J. Neurol. Phys. Ther.* **2013**, *37*, 166–175. [CrossRef] [PubMed]
11. Mugueta-Aguinaga, I.; Garcia-Zapirain, B. Is technology present in frailty? Technology a back-up tool for dealing with frailty in the elderly: A systematic review. *Aging Dis.* **2017**, *8*, 176. [CrossRef] [PubMed]
12. Chaparro-Cárdenas, S.L.; Lozano-Guzmán, A.A.; Ramirez-Bautista, J.A.; Hernández-Zavala, A. A review in gait rehabilitation devices and applied control techniques. *Disabil. Rehabil. Assist. Technol.* **2018**, *13*, 819–834. [CrossRef] [PubMed]
13. Babaiasl, M.; Mahdioun, S.H.; Jaryani, P.; Yazdani, M. A review of technological and clinical aspects of robot-aided rehabilitation of upper-extremity after stroke. *Disabil. Rehabil. Assist. Technol.* **2016**, *11*, 263–280. [CrossRef]
14. Ward, T.; Heffernan, R. The role of values in forensic and correctional rehabilitation. *Aggress. Violent Behav.* **2017**, *37*, 42–51. [CrossRef]
15. Wade, D. Rehabilitation—A new approach. Overview and part one: The problems. *Sage J.* **2015**, *29*, 1041–1050. [CrossRef]
16. Frutos-Pascual, M.; Zapirain, B.G.; Zorrilla, A.M. Adaptive tele-therapies based on serious games for health for people with time-management and organisational problems: Preliminary results. *Int. J. Environ. Res. Public Health* **2014**, *11*, 749–772. [CrossRef]
17. Khan, F.; Amatya, B. Refugee health and rehabilitation: Challenges and response. *J. Rehabil. Med.* **2017**, *49*, 378–384. [CrossRef]
18. Christiansen, B.; Feiring, M. Challenges in the nurse's role in rehabilitation contexts. *J. Clin. Nurs.* **2017**, *26*, 3239–3247. [CrossRef] [PubMed]
19. Rikkers, W.; Lawrence, D.; Hafekost, J.; Zubrick, S.R. Internet use and electronic gaming by children and adolescents with emotional and behavioural problems in Australia–results from the second Child and Adolescent Survey of Mental Health and Wellbeing. *BMC Public Health* **2016**, *16*, 1–16. [CrossRef] [PubMed]
20. Bonnechère, B. *Serious Games in Physical Rehabilitation*; Springer International Publishing: Berlin/Heidelberg, Germany, 2018; pp. 72–78.
21. Ortiz-Vigon Uriarte, I.D.L.; Garcia-Zapirain, B.; Garcia-Chimeno, Y. Game design to measure reflexes and attention based on biofeedback multi-sensor interaction. *Sensors* **2015**, *15*, 6520–6548. [CrossRef]
22. Ushaw, G.; Davison, R.; Eyre, J.; Morgan, G. Adopting best practices from the games industry in development of serious games for health. In Proceedings of the 5th International Conference on Digital Health, Florence, Italy, 18–20 May 2015; pp. 1–8.
23. de Urturi Breton, Z.S.; Hernández, F.J.; Zorrilla, A.M.; Zapirain, B.G. Mobile communication for intellectually challenged people: A proposed set of requirements for interface design on touch screen devices. *Commun. Mob. Comput.* **2012**, *1*, 1–4. [CrossRef]
24. Ricotti, V.; Mandy, W.P.; Scoto, M.; Pane, M.; Deconinck, N.; Messina, S.; Muntoni, F. Neurodevelopmental, emotional, and behavioural problems in Duchenne muscular dystrophy in relation to underlying dystrophin gene mutations. *Dev. Med. Child Neurol.* **2016**, *58*, 77–84. [CrossRef] [PubMed]
25. Edgren, J.; Salpakoski, A.; Sihvonen, S.E.; Portegijs, E.; Kallinen, M.; Arkela, M.; Sipilä, S. Effects of a home-based physical rehabilitation program on physical disability after hip fracture: A randomized controlled trial. *J. Am. Med. Dir. Assoc.* **2015**, *16*, 350-e1. [CrossRef] [PubMed]
26. Goršič, M.; Cikajlo, I.; Novak, D. Competitive and cooperative arm rehabilitation games played by a patient and unimpaired person: Effects on motivation and exercise intensity. *J. Neuroeng. Rehabil.* **2017**, *14*, 1–18. [CrossRef]
27. Bonnechère, B.; Jansen, B.; Omelina, L.; Van Sint Jan, S. The use of commercial video games in rehabilitation: A systematic review. *Int. J. Rehabil. Res.* **2016**, *39*, 277–290. [CrossRef]
28. Hocine, N.; Gouaïch, A.; Cerri, S.A.; Mottet, D.; Froger, J.; Laffont, I. Adaptation in serious games for upper-limb rehabilitation: An approach to improve training outcomes. *User Model. User Adapt. Interact.* **2015**, *25*, 65–98. [CrossRef]

29. Nguyen TT, H.; Ishmatova, D.; Tapanainen, T.; Liukkonen, T.N.; Katajapuu, N.; Makila, T.; Luimula, M. Impact of serious games on health and well-being of elderly: A systematic review. In Proceedings of the 50th Hawaii International Conference on System Sciences, Hilton Waikoloa Village, HI, USA, 4–7 January 2017.
30. Howard, M.C. A meta-analysis and systematic literature review of virtual reality rehabilitation programs. *Comput. Hum. Behav.* **2017**, *70*, 317–327. [CrossRef]
31. Kawagoshi, A.; Kiyokawa, N.; Sugawara, K.; Takahashi, H.; Sakata, S.; Satake, M.; Shioya, T. Effects of low-intensity exercise and home-based pulmonary rehabilitation with pedometer feedback on physical activity in elderly patients with chronic obstructive pulmonary disease. *Respir. Med.* **2015**, *109*, 364–371. [CrossRef] [PubMed]
32. Madani, K.; Pierce, T.W.; Mirchi, A. Serious games on environmental management. *Sustain. Cities Soc.* **2017**, *29*, 1–11. [CrossRef]
33. Rego, P.; Moreira, P.M.; Reis, L.P. Serious games for rehabilitation: A survey and a classification towards a taxonomy. In Proceedings of the 5th Iberian Conference on Information Systems and Technologies, Santiago de Compostela, Spain, 16–19 June 2010; IEEE: Piscataway, NJ, USA, 2010; pp. 1–6.
34. Loh, C.S.; Sheng, Y.; Ifenthaler, D. Serious games analytics: Theoretical framework. In *Serious Games Analytics*; Springer: Cham, Switzerland, 2015; pp. 3–29.
35. Lun, R.; Zhao, W. A survey of applications and human motion recognition with Microsoft kinect. *Int. J. Pattern Recognit. Artif. Intell.* **2015**, *29*, 1555008. [CrossRef]
36. Anthes, C.; García-Hernández, R.J.; Wiedemann, M.; Kranzlmüller, D. State of the art of virtual reality technology. In Proceedings of the 2016 IEEE Aerospace Conference, Big Sky, MT, USA, 5–12 March 2016; IEEE: Piscataway, NJ, USA; pp. 1–19.
37. Cao, Z.; Hidalgo, G.; Simon, T.; Wei, S.E.; Sheikh, Y. OpenPose: Realtime multi-person 2D pose estimation using Part Affinity Fields. *IEEE Trans. Pattern Anal. Mach. Intell.* **2019**, *43*, 172–186. [CrossRef] [PubMed]
38. Kendall, A.; Grimes, M.; Cipolla, R. Posenet: A convolutional network for real-time 6-dof camera relocalization. In Proceedings of the IEEE International Conference on Computer Vision, Santiago, Chile, 7–13 December 2015; pp. 2938–2946.
39. Carvalho, M.B.; Bellotti, F.; Berta, R.; De Gloria, A.; Sedano, C.I.; Hauge, J.B.; Rauterberg, M. An activity theory-based model for serious games analysis and conceptual design. *Comput. Educ.* **2015**, *87*, 166–181. [CrossRef]
40. Lopez-Basterretxea, A.; Mendez-Zorrilla, A.; Garcia-Zapirain, B. A telemonitoring tool based on serious games addressing money management skills for people with intellectual disability. *Int. J. Environ. Res. Public Health* **2014**, *11*, 2361–2380. [CrossRef]
41. Sáenz-de-Urturi, Z.; García Zapirain, B.; Méndez Zorrilla, A. Elderly user experience to improve a Kinect-based game playability. *Behav. Inf. Technol.* **2015**, *34*, 1040–1051. [CrossRef]
42. Avola, D.; Cinque, L.; Foresti, G.L.; Marini, M.R. An interactive and low-cost full body rehabilitation framework based on 3D immersive serious games. *J. Biomed. Inform.* **2019**, *89*, 81–100. [CrossRef] [PubMed]
43. González-González, C.S.; Toledo-Delgado, P.A.; Muñoz-Cruz, V.; Torres-Carrion, P.V. Serious games for rehabilitation: Gestural interaction in personalized gamified exercises through a recommender system. *J. Biomed. Inform.* **2019**, *97*, 103266. [CrossRef]
44. Amengual Alcover, E.; Jaume-i-Capó, A.; Moyà-Alcover, B. PROGame: A process framework for serious game development for motor rehabilitation therapy. *PLoS ONE* **2018**, *13*, e0197383. [CrossRef]
45. Meijer, H.A.; Graafland, M.; Goslings, J.C.; Schijven, M.P. Systematic review on the effects of serious games and wearable technology used in rehabilitation of patients with traumatic bone and soft tissue injuries. *Arch. Phys. Med. Rehabil.* **2018**, *99*, 1890–1899. [CrossRef]
46. Morando, M.; Ponte, S.; Ferrara, E.; Dellepiane, S. Definition of motion and biophysical indicators for home-based rehabilitation through serious games. *Information* **2018**, *9*, 105. [CrossRef]
47. Tăut, D.; Pintea, S.; Roovers, J.P.W.; Mañanas, M.A.; Băban, A. Play seriously: Effectiveness of serious games and their features in motor rehabilitation. A meta-analysis. *NeuroRehabilitation* **2017**, *41*, 105–118. [CrossRef]
48. Sánchez-Herrera-Baeza, P.; Cano-de-la-Cuerda, R.; Oña-Simbaña, E.D.; Palacios-Ceña, D.; Pérez-Corrales, J.; Cuenca-Zaldivar, J.N.; Cuesta-Gomez, A. The Impact of a Novel Immersive Virtual Reality Technology Associated with Serious Games in Parkinson's Disease Patients on Upper Limb Rehabilitation: A Mixed Methods Intervention Study. *Sensors* **2020**, *20*, 2168. [CrossRef] [PubMed]
49. Postolache, G.; Carry, F.; Lourenço, F.; Ferreira, D.; Oliveira, R.; Girão, P.S.; Postolache, O. Serious Games Based on Kinect and Leap Motion Controller for Upper Limbs Physical Rehabilitation. In *Modern Sensing Technologies*; Springer: Cham, Switzerland, 2019; pp. 147–177.
50. Ling, Y.; Ter Meer, L.P.; Yumak, Z.; Veltkamp, R.C. Usability test of exercise games designed for rehabilitation of elderly patients after hip replacement surgery: Pilot study. *JMIR Serious Games* **2017**, *5*, e19. [CrossRef] [PubMed]
51. Palestra, G.; Rebiai, M.; Courtial, E.; Koutsouris, D. Evaluation of a rehabilitation system for the elderly in a day care center. *Information* **2019**, *10*, 3. [CrossRef]

Article

Target Maintenance in Gaming via Saliency Augmentation: An Early-Stage Scotoma Simulation Study Using Virtual Reality (VR)

Alexandra Sipatchin [1,*], Miguel García García [1] and Siegfried Wahl [1,2]

[1] Institute for Ophthalmic Research, 72076 Tübingen, Germany; miguel.garcia-garcia@uni-tuebingen.de (M.G.G.); siegfried.wahl@zeiss.com (S.W.)
[2] Carl Zeiss Vision International GmbH, 73430 Aalen, Germany
* Correspondence: alexandra.sipatchin@uni-tuebingen.de

Abstract: This study addresses the importance of salience placement before or after scotoma development for an efficient target allocation in the visual field. Pre-allocation of attention is a mechanism known to induce a better gaze positioning towards the target. Three different conditions were tested: a simulated central scotoma, a salience augmentation surrounding the scotoma and a baseline condition without any simulation. All conditions were investigated within a virtual reality VR gaming environment. Participants were tested in two different orders, either the salient cue was applied together with the scotoma before being presented with the scotoma alone or the scotoma in the wild was presented before and, then, with the augmentation around it. Both groups showed a change in gaze behaviour when saliency was applied. However, in the second group, salient augmentation also induced changes in gaze behaviour for the scotoma condition without augmentation, gazing above and outside the scotoma following previous literature. These preliminary results indicate salience placement before developing an advanced stage of scotoma can induce effective and rapid training for efficient target maintenance during VR gaming. The study shows the potential of salience and VR gaming as therapy for early AMD patients.

Keywords: AMD; salience; virtual reality; VR; preventive care

1. Introduction

The macula is the human eye's richest area in terms of photoreceptors. This part of the retina is endeavoured to produce a sharp image of the objects we gaze upon. Hence, deterioration of this area may lead to the formation of scotomas or areas with partial or complete diminished visual acuity.

Amid the different conditions that can deteriorate the status of the macula, two are the conditions that appear more often: the myopic macular degeneration, which occurs in the presence of high myopia [1], and the age-related macular degeneration (AMD), which usually appears in the last decades of life [2]. Myopic macular degeneration and AMD combined affect approximately 11% of the world's population [1,3].

Patients with macular degeneration are known to adapt to the central visual loss by modifying the so-called foveated behaviour, i.e., objects of interest will no longer be fixated within the macula. A peripheral behaviour substitutes this foveation, meaning that patients will learn to fixate away from the target of interest so that the target can be positioned on a healthy retinal location, and consequently acknowledged. This technique is called eccentric viewing, and the healthy part of the retina used to look at objects is referred to as the preferred retinal locus (PRL). This peripheral gaze behaviour is known to be the only way that patients have to continue their daily life [4].

However, the peripheral retina has a poor visual resolution [5], and it is not intended to acknowledge details in focused objects. It takes time to adapt and modify the natural foveation behaviour, but in the end, one or more eccentric PRLs develop naturally [6–10]. Correct adaptation and use of the retinal areas with intact visual quality are a key part of safely continuing day-life activities such as safely crossing the street [11,12].

New technologies such as virtual reality (VR) and augmented reality (AR) have recently proposed new assisting tools for patients suffering from macular degeneration [13–15]. These tools aim to improve the quality of life of patients by improving the eccentric viewing and assisting patients specifically during critical tasks.

Embracing these new technologies and applying them to patients can assist them in improving eccentric fixation. Likewise, these technologies can be used with healthy subjects to study improvements in gaze behaviour under simulated visual loss conditions.

Standardised gaze-contingent scotoma simulations can change gaze behaviour in healthy participants in the same way as patients do [16–20] and scotoma simulations can replicate visual loss in a standardised manner with a well-defined area and filling [21–23]. Thanks to this standardization, there is the advantage to overcome the variability of different shapes and positions the scotoma patients bring into studies [16,17] and investigate augmentations in a generalized manner that can get later validated when applied to patients [24].

In this study, a standardised gaze-contingent scotoma simulation was used to occlude the central vision bilaterally to test, for the first time, the effects of gaze placement before and after salience application. The study's purpose was to test the hypothesis according to which preventive attention placement can lead to a better target positioning in relation to scotomas [4,25].

An augmented peripheral cue was designed to be perceived as salient, and induce the eyes to position a moving target outside the central occluded area. The circular cue was applied to the dominant eye only, in the periphery and gaze-contingent. A unique-eye-of-origin stimulus presented in the periphery is known to attract the gaze towards its position; it induces a popping-out effect, known as saliency [26]. Furthermore, the augmentation was gaze-contingent, with a constant position in the peripheral visual field. It is known that peripheral cues have an automatic component of attention allocation that once they have triggered it, its focus is preserved in that location [27,28]. For the present study, this means that once the eyes were attracted towards the peripheral cue, the target would start to be positioned in an annulus area where automatic attention is known to be focused [27].

Traditional tasks used for PRL development studies and therapy can be repetitive, exhaustive, and tedious, ending in a decrease in the subject's motivation [29]. For the current study, a VR game that involved tracking and detecting changes in a moving object was introduced to re-definite these traditional tasks. Gamification, in this context, was intended as a leap from those training sessions to more engaging experiment blocks.

2. Materials and Methods

2.1. Participants

Thirteen participants took part in the study (7 females and 6 males, mean age 29, standard deviation (SD) ± 3 years, only one subject wearing eye-correction, eye contact lenses).

2.2. Set-Up

For the virtual experiment, the Unity 2019.3.0a5 version was used as a design tool, with C# as a programming language, running on a PC with Windows 10 Home, having a 64-bit operating system, an Intel Core i7 -7700HQ, 2.8 GHz, 16 GB RAM, and an NVIDIA GeForce GTX 1070 GDDR5 graphics card.

The HTC Vive Pro Eye [30] headset was used to present the virtual environment. This headset has an integrated eye tracker with a sampling frequency of 120 Hz and a known latency between 58 ms and 80 ms [31,32]. This HMD also has two AMOLED screens, with a resolution of 1.440 × 1.600 pixels to each eye (pixel density of 615 pixels per inch (PPI)), and a refresh rate of 90 Hz. Tobii Pro SDK v1.7.1.1081 [33] and Vive SRanipal

SDK v1.0.3.0 [34] were used to save eye-tracking data and to present the gaze-contingent simulations, respectively. A Microsoft Xbox wireless controller was used for subject input.

2.3. Calibration Procedure

An initial semi-automated inter-pupillary distance (IPD) adjustment and a calibration of five points (SRAnipal) was carried out for all participants at the beginning of each condition. The participant sets the IPD through a knob that can be rotated to adjust the lenses distance. Based on the pupil position, the SRAnipal system provides feedback to the subject when the distance has been set correctly. Only after a correct IPD adjustment, the eye-tracking calibration can start. After a correct calibration output offered by the software, the subject could start with each condition type.

2.4. Experimental Procedure

Participants were asked to pursuit a moving target with unrestricted head movement while playing a 2-D Pong game in VR. The playing area covered ±28° horizontally by ±26° vertically. The moving target consisted of a 3° ball moving at an average velocity of 21.74 ° s^{-1} (SD: ±0.63 ° s^{-1}) from one side to the other of the screen following a randomised triangular trajectory. The subjects controlled two paddles to keep the moving ball inside the playing area. If the ball left the playing area, the trial was re-started by the participant.

During the Pong game, the ball changed colour at random intervals. Participants were asked to press a button whenever they acknowledged that the ball stimulus changed colour, which, if recognised, it would increase their score. During the session, the participants could move their heads freely. In addition, a head-fixed rectangle of ±14.25° horizontally and vertically was presented to motivate the subjects to move their heads.

2.4.1. Conditions

All participants were tested in three (3) conditions: normally sighted, central scotoma, and salience augmentation of scotoma simulation. In the normal condition, no simulation was used while playing the game. During the central scotoma condition, eye-tracking was used to simulate a 12° circular scotoma occluding the central visual field. In the augmented central scotoma condition, a 2° circular augmentation, with a diameter of 27° was implemented around the simulated scotoma and applied to the dominant eye.

Figure 1 shows of how the simulations in the scotoma and augmented condition looked like. Each condition was measured in three blocks of five (5) minutes. Before each block, a manual drift correction had to be performed by the subject.

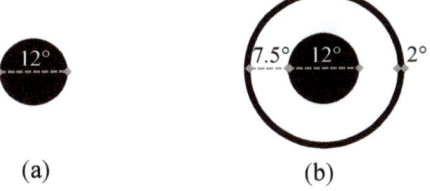

Figure 1. (**a**) Specifications of the central scotoma (CS) and (**b**) augmented scotoma (AS) condition. In the CS condition the scotoma (**a**) had a diameter of 12°. In the AS condition (**b**) there was an concentric augmentation of 2° around the scotoma and an annulus area extending 7.5°.

2.4.2. Manual Drift Correction

A manual drift correction was applied at the beginning of each block for all conditions. The manual drift correction (Figure 2) consisted of a manual scotoma adjustment performed by the participant. Each subject was presented with a scotoma simulation for each eye and a central red dot, attached to the eye camera. The red dot was used as a reference to centre the scotoma. Participants could correct the scotoma position using the Xbox controller. After the scotoma was correctly centred and checked by the experimenter, the experimenter pressed a key to start the next block. These offset values were then applied throughout the block session. The drift correction was designed to compensate for eye-tracking data quality decay in VR due to the movement of the participant, which is known to induce drifts into the precision of the eye tracker [35]. These drifts can influence scotoma positioning.

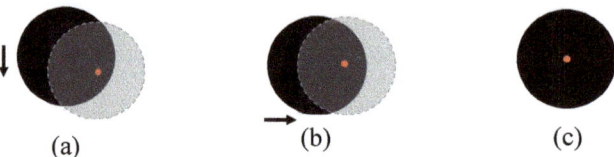

(a)   (b)   (c)

Figure 2. Drift correction was performed manually by the subject to have a centralized scotoma around the red dot at the beginning of each block. In the figure above, a hypothetical example of how a decentralized scotoma (in black) might look like (**a**) and hypothetical stages of position correction (**b**,**c**), black arrows, performed to have a concentric positioning of the scotoma around the red dot (**c**). The grey circle is used as a reference for this figure to indicate where the simulated scotoma should be positioned.

2.5. Groups

The participants were separated into two groups, defined by the order in which the different conditions were presented. Although the augmentation and scotoma conditions were randomized, all subjects started playing the game without any applied simulation first (normally sighted condition) (Figure 3).

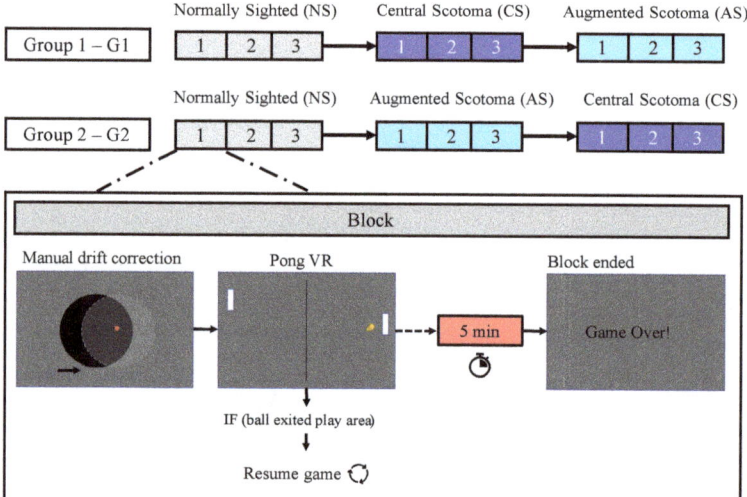

Figure 3. Scheme of the experimental procedure. Participants were divided into two groups (G1 and G2). Both groups initiated playing the Pong game under normal vision conditions (normally sighted, NS). The difference between groups was defined by the order by which the scotoma (CS) and augmented scotoma (AS) simulations were presented. In group 1, the scotoma simulation followed the augmentation, in group 2 the opposite. During each condition, three blocks (1, 2, and 3) were tested. Each block was the same for all conditions. It started with a manual drift correction followed by a 5-min timer playtime. During the game, the ball could have exited the play area. In that case, the timer was frozen and the game re-started. When the timer ended, a new block started.

3. Data Processing

3.1. Data Pre-Processing

3.1.1. Noise Cancellation: Fluctuation in the Sampling Data

Eye-tracking data were first checked for fluctuations in the sampling rate which can lead to noise in the eye-tracking data introducing spurious variation into the eye movements [36,37]. Sampling rate fluctuations were found if the time that passed between two samplings were bigger than the known inter-sample range (8.3 ms, with an error margin of ±0.4 ms). Following common practice [37], when fluctuations were detected, two data points before, and two data points after the identified fluctuation were deleted from the dataset. After this filter, a percentage of total data exclusion was calculated.

3.1.2. Latency Error Correction

All gaze-contingent paradigms are always subject to a lag between where the participant's current eye position is and where the rendering of the scotoma is shown on display. This latency is related to the system's processes to display the image based on the eye position. First, it needs to record the eye position and transmit it to the computer; the computer would receive it and shift the scotoma position, render the new image, and finally, it displays the new image on the headset screen [38]. This delay in the scotoma presentation means for the current experiment that the scotoma might not cover the exact 6° radius of the central vision at all time.

To account for the latency error between the actual eye's position and the actual recording of the eye, the target position was used as an indicator of where the recording of the eye should have been. This error can be approximated in the distance between the gaze and target positions measured during the normal condition.

For every frame, the normalised target (re-referenced to the eye) and the dominant eye's normalised gaze were transformed into two-dimensional Cartesian coordinates. Then, the eye-target distance was calculated using the Pythagorean theorem. For every target data sample, twenty-one eye data points (ten previous to the matching timestamp and ten forward) were registered. The median in the distances between these 21 points and the target position was considered the system standard error.

A mean and the standard deviation [39] for this error were calculated for each subject and assumed as the time delay between the recorded eye position and the actual eye location.

3.1.3. Eye-Tracking Data Filtering

The Nyström and Holmqvist [40] velocity-based algorithm was used to filter the high jumps in eye velocity caused by missing eye data. These jumps occur above the normal velocity of the eye during a saccade ($300°\,s^{-1}$). The *sgolay* function in Matlab based on Savitzky and Golay [41] was used over the 3D raw gaze coordinates. Sample-to-sample velocity between two consecutive gaze coordinates in degrees was calculated for the raw and filtered data. These velocities were compared to observe the filtering effect of this algorithm.

3.1.4. Saccades Smoothing: Moving Median Window

As described by Shanidze et al. [42], to calculate the gaze-target distance, saccade information is usually kept. To smooth the saccade's data and look for trends that could otherwise be overlooked due to a high number of saccades that occur during the initial phases of scotoma habituation [43], a moving median window was used. Different sliding windows of 5, 10, 20, and 40 s were compared until saccades smoothing was achieved, and a more clear trend with less volatility in gaze-target distance was observed.

3.1.5. Colour Change Recognition Sub-Task and Scotoma Radius as Cutoff for the Maximum Positive and Negative Predictive Values

Bayes' theorem was applied to test the probability of colour recognition due to scotoma coverage. The distance between gaze and the edge of the target and whether it was above the scotoma's radii were used to indicate seen or not seen, and the colour change detection to determine correct or wrong.

Seen and correctly recognised was defined as true-positive, while non-seen and detected was false-positive. Similarly, if the colour change was not detected but the target was visible, it was considered a false-negative. If it was not visible and not detected, it counted as a true-negative. The probability of the positive and the negative predictive value were then calculated for the group and individually, and can indicate that the central vision might not be correctly occluded due to eye movements such as saccades and blinks [44,45]. Hence, the subject could have seen the target outside the intended radius of occlusion partially or entirely when he/she was not supposed to, influencing the correct and incorrect colour recognition task ratio. To test for possible errors in scotoma occlusion, five different scotoma radii extensions were considered, from 6° to 4°, in steps of 0.5°. Suppose an actual error due to partial occlusion of the central visual field was present. In that case, all subjects should present a low positive predictive value and a high negative predictive value for the 6° scotoma radii.

The lower the margin for the scotoma radii, the higher number of positive predictive values are expected. This increase will occur until the positive predictive value would reach a plateau. The opposite would be observed for the negative predictive value. Furthermore, this test allows us to identify the subjects who performed the task correctly from those who did not. Each subject was looked at individually to observe the trend. If the positive and negative predictive values did not show the same trend as the majority did, they were identified as having a bad performance, not in line with the experiment and therefore excluded.

3.2. Data Analysis

3.2.1. Gaze-Target Distancing: Condition Type Influence over Eye Position

After data pre-processing, the effect of the independent variable, condition type, was investigated over the dependant variable, the median distance between the gaze and the centre of the target. The normality of the sample was tested with the Kolmogorov–Smirnov one-sample test ($p < 0.001$). Given the absence of a normal distribution in our data, the non-parametric Kruskal–Wallis test was used. These results were further compared with an FWER test (Dunn–Šidák).

3.2.2. Gaze-Target Direction: Training Effect across Blocks

To examine whether there was a significant change in gaze behaviour, the gaze-target direction was plotted as a function of different blocks. Re-direction of eye positions in favour of the upper, lower, right, or leftwards hemifield indicated changes of gaze behaviour across time [18,25]. A polar histogram was used to look into the gaze direction and confront it to the target across blocks. Zittrell [46] polar histogram plot based on Berens [47] was used after calculating the wrap angle between gaze and target. Circular statistics were used, and the mean resultant vector (r) and the average direction were calculated for each block. The mean resultant vector values range between 0 and 1, where 0 indicates that data have a large spread while 1 means that the entire dataset is concatenated towards one point. This parameter was used to look into the spread of the gaze direction with respect to the target. The average angle indicates the potential directionality for the tested block.

4. Results

4.1. Data Pre-Processing

4.1.1. Noise Cancellation: Fluctuation in the Sampling Data

Only 0.83% of the data were omitted due to fluctuations in the sampling rate, meaning that these points had a sampling rate outside the normal range of sampling.

4.1.2. Latency Error Correction

The best gaze-target distance was found to be when gaze data points were 3 position updates behind the target data. Considering the sampling frequency of 120 Hz, in terms of latency, this indicates that the recorded eye position and the actual eye position had a delay error of 25 ms (Figure 4).

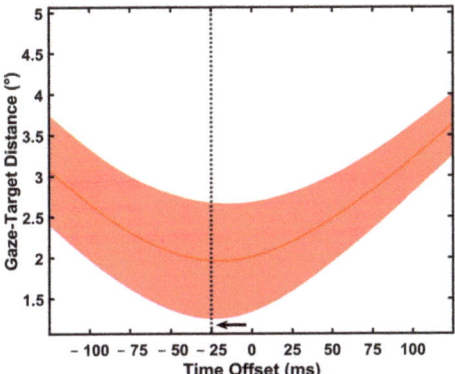

Figure 4. Latency offset for best gaze-target distance across all subjects. The red line indicates the mean tested for all the different time offsets, and the shading red represented the SD around the mean. The black arrow indicates that the best gaze-target distance is at its lowest when gaze data are sifted by 25 ms.

4.1.3. Eye-Tracking Data Filtering

A 24 sample Savitzky and Golay [41]'s algorithm was found to effectively refine the velocity between successive gaze data. This second-order polynomial interpolation smooths the gaze data gaps, where the velocity was above the normal saccades velocity, as reported by Nyström and Holmqvist [40]. The result of the filter can be seen in Figure 5 when comparing filtered data with raw data, sample-by-sample.

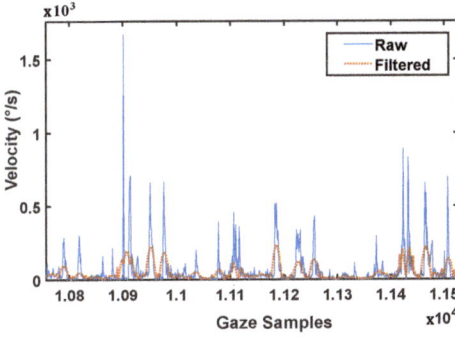

Figure 5. Gaze samples were filtered using the Savitzky–Golay filter, with second-order polynomials and 24 filter length. In the dataset, the effect (red) on simple, raw (blue), sample-to-sample velocity.

4.1.4. Saccades Smoothing: Moving Median Window

Four different moving median windows were tested to the gaze-target distance to de-noise it. In comparison to the original data, every sliding window proved to improve and smooth the gaze-target distance (Figure 6). Out of the four tested ones, the 40 s centred moving average window presented less volatility induced by saccadic behaviour and best smoothing in the data.

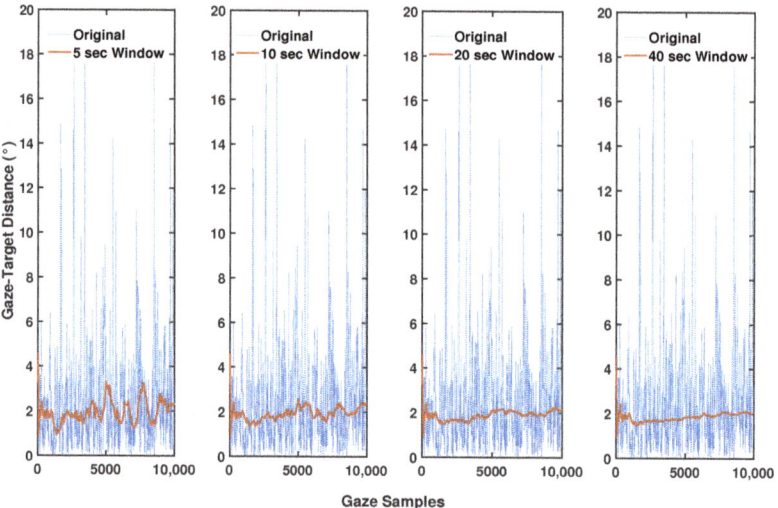

Figure 6. Original gaze samples (blue) and different moving window medians applied to the original data smoothing the saccades (red).

4.1.5. Colour Change Recognition Sub-Task and Scotoma Radius as Cutoff for the Maximum Positive and Negative Predictive Values

The test revealed that indeed there was a big variability when comparing positive and negative predictive values across different scotoma radii, starting already at 5.5° indicating that the actual radius of the coverage area was smaller than 6°. The probability of positive and negative predictive values had less considerable variability when reaching the 5° radius of scotoma coverage and started to reach a plateau (Figure 7). This indicated that the ball could have been perceived when the distance was ≤5°, and not 6° from the target.

On the other hand, it was observed that some subjects performed the task correctly across all conditions, while others did not. The probability of positive and negative predictive values did not show the same trend as the majority of subjects, with no plateau reached (Figure 8); those subjects were excluded from the analysis, as a poor performance in the test was suspected. A total of 5 subjects had to be excluded due to this criterion. For the analysis, a total of 8 subjects were included, four from each group.

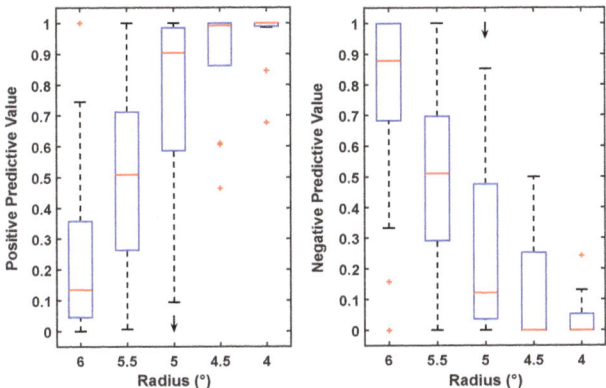

Figure 7. Bar plots of positive and negative predictive values of all subjects across different scotoma radii. The black arrow inside the box plots indicates the point from which a plateau is starting to emerge. The plateau is starting to emerge at 5°.

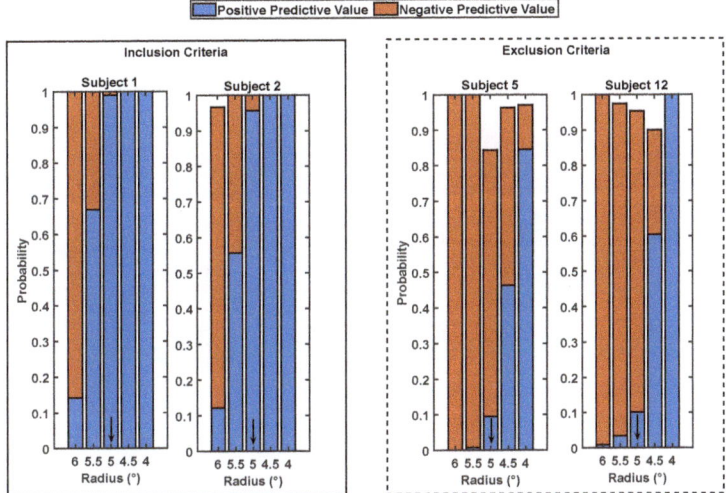

Figure 8. Inclusion and exclusion criteria for different subjects. Positive and negative predictive values were looked at to identify the trend where, irrespective of the scotoma radius, both values reached a plateau (the positive predictive value did not increase and the negative predictive value did not decrease anymore). The black arrow indicates where this plateau was reached for the majority of subjects. In this example, a demonstration is shown for subjects 1 and 2. For those where this trend was not observed, they were excluded. This was the case, for example, for subjects 5 and 12.

4.2. Data Analysis

4.2.1. Gaze-Target Distancing: Condition Type Influence over Eye Position

In the first group, salience was applied after subjects had to adapt for 15 min to an advanced scotoma simulation. The Kruskal–Wallis test found that there is a significant difference between the three conditions (χ^2 (2) = 7.19, p = 0.03) for the distance between gaze and target. The post-hoc Dunn's revealed that the cued scotoma induced significant changes in the gaze-target distance (p = 0.02) compared to the normal condition. No significant difference was found for the scotoma condition compared to the other two conditions (Figure 9, G1).

For the second group, where subjects were presented first with the scotoma simulation together with the cued salience, there was a significant effect between the three conditions as well (χ^2 (2) = 7.20, p = 0.03). The post-hoc Dunn's revealed that compared to the normal condition, the central scotoma changed significantly the gaze-target distance (p = 0.02, Figure 9, G2).

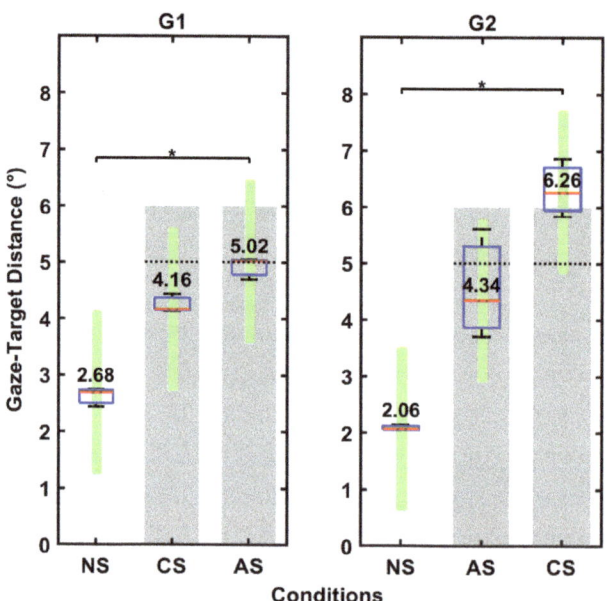

Figure 9. Box plots of the gaze-target distance for the two groups tested. A Kruskal–Wallis test indicated a significant difference between the three conditions for both groups. The post-hoc Dunn's indicated differences in gaze behaviour when comparing the normal condition to the augmented scotoma (AS) for group 1 (**G1**) and the scotoma condition (CS) for group 2 (**G2**). Both *p*-values were below 0.05 (indicated by the asterisk). The target cover area (in green) is both above the intended scotoma cover area (in gray) and the scotoma area with cover errors (scotoma trailing area, above the dotted lines). The values above the median line (red) of the box plots are the median value of the pre-processed gaze-target distance for all subjects across all three blocks.

4.2.2. Gaze-Target Direction: Training Effect across Blocks

Circular statistics revealed that gaze had a directional tendency above the target in the second group, where subjects started first with the augmented scotoma. For both groups, when the augmentation was present (during the three blocks), the gaze starts showing a preferred direction, with a less homogeneous distribution in the gaze directions, across blocks. For the second group, the gaze shifts upwards, and during the third block, the resultant mean vector doubles its size for the second block, meaning a greater bias in the directionality. An upper direction starts to emerge, with an average angle of 92° ± 2° of gaze with respect to target. This trend is maintained when the augmentation is removed (central scotoma condition), becoming more pronounced across blocks of this new condition, maintaining the gaze-target direction at 89° ± 1° and at 91° ± 1° for the second and third block, respectively (Figure 10). The bias strength also increased across blocks. No such trend was observed for group one.

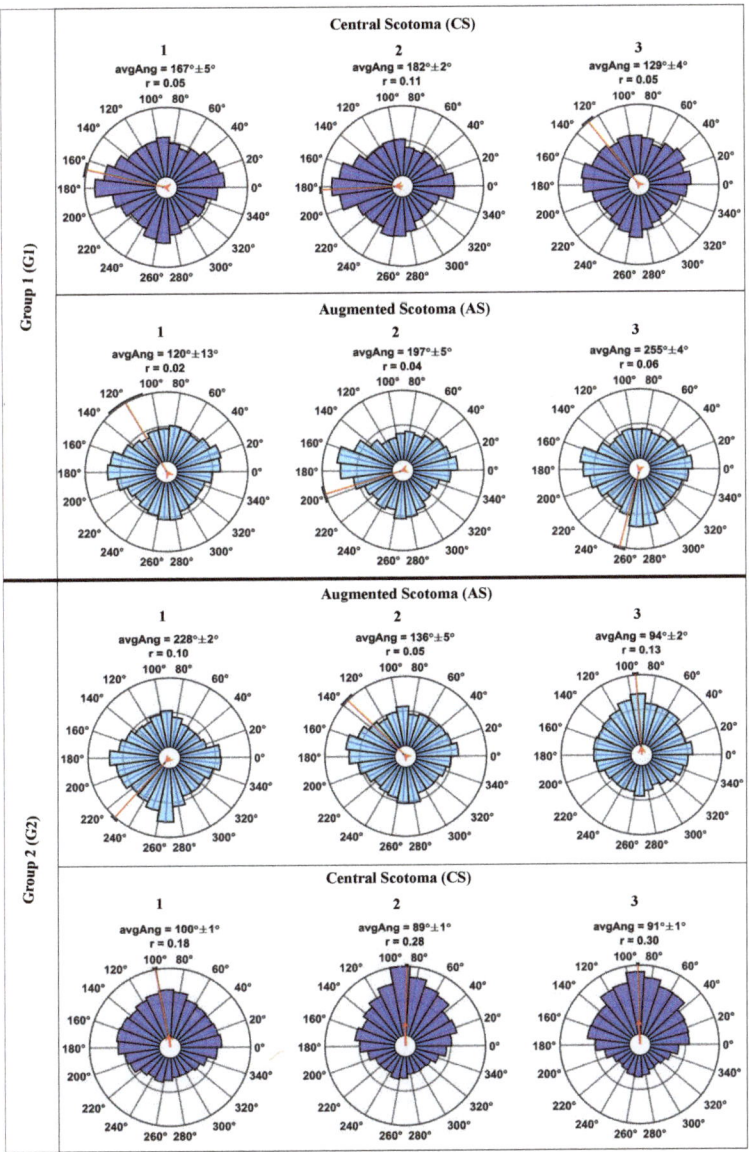

Figure 10. Polar histograms of gaze direction in respect to target for group 1 (**G1**) and group 2 (**G2**) across the blocks (1, 2, and 3). Above each polar histogram, the mean resultant length (r) and the average angle (avgAng) with the corresponding SD of gaze-target direction are represented. The long red line represents the average angle, the black bold semicircle at the end of the red line indicates the SD. The red arrow overlapped on top of the long red line is the mean resultant vector.

5. Discussion

Macular degeneration is a chronic disease that affects central vision; as the macular region deteriorates, it loses the ability to produce clear images of the focused objects. The visual system needs to re-adapt its behaviour to overcome this condition by shifting the gaze away from the object of interest and reallocating it in the periphery (outside the area of visual loss). Quickly developing a new adaptive mechanism is essential for patients suffering from macular degeneration to detect objects of interest, such as incoming cars or bicycles. Most patients with central visual loss take up to three (3) months to adapt, and only one out of three manages to direct their eyes correctly towards the object of interest [9,48].

Other authors have already used VR for rehabilitation and training of this eccentric fixation behaviour using patients [13–15]. However, one of the major challenges for these studies is that patients have different types of scotomas with different shapes and positions, and for this reason, patients require individualized augmentations. The mixed results obtained so far regarding individual augmentation on patients complicate its translation to clinical practice.

The current study investigates gaze behaviour during salience augmentation for standardised central scotoma simulation during tracking of a moving object. Previous studies only looked at changes in normally sighted participants with simulated scotomas without further testing how augmentations might change their behaviours. In our case, a modified version of a VR Pong game was presented to participants where they had to pursue a ball, stopping it from exiting the play area by moving the paddles, and they also had to acknowledge changes in the ball's colour.

The group whose participants initially experienced an advanced scotoma simulation, and only afterwards salience around the scotoma was presented, a significant change in gaze behaviour was observed. In comparison to the normal condition, during the salience augmented scotoma condition, the target was placed above the scotoma edge both when considering 5° as well as 6° radius (Figure 9, G1). Furthermore, the polar histograms show that, even if the mean resultant vector did not increase across blocks, gaze position started to be directed more and more towards the lower hemifield in the augmented condition. On the other hand, no such trend could be observed across blocks for the scotoma simulation condition (Figure 10, G1). The tendency observed for the salient augmented condition is in accordance with previous findings [4] where 57% of macula degeneration patients had better attention preference for the lower hemifield and where most patients with central visual loss direct their gaze [21,48–51].

For the second group, a change in gaze behaviour for both simulated conditions was also achieved. A significant change was observed during the scotoma simulation, with the target being placed further away from the scotoma edge when taking into account 5° and also 6° extension in the coverage range (Figure 9, G2), when compared with the baseline condition (normal). The polar histogram revealed a similar trend for the augmented condition to the one observed by the first group. The gaze's direction started having a specific directionality that was kept throughout the other two blocks. This direction was kept when scotoma simulated participants had to play the game without augmentation, and the value increased even more across the blocks. Additionally, by the end of the third block of the central scotoma condition, the bias strength tripled the value that subjects had when they finished the last block of the augmented condition (Figure 10, G2). The trend that emerged was to position the gaze above the target. However, even if in an uncommon position, the gaze position above the target was still in line with previous studies [25].

Based on the results, we hypothesise that presenting salient cues at the early stages of central visual loss can help build a preferred gaze location. In contrast, prior experiences of wild gazing in the presence of a scotoma may delay this choice. These results also point towards developing a preferred retinal locus (PRL) position for moving targets.

Subjects presented with advanced stages of a central scotoma who have not undergone any training and had not been presented with visual cueing usually develop an unclear and variable preferred gaze positioning. This variability is reduced when augmentation is implemented and the previously adopted positioning changes. However, this behavioural change might take longer due to this previously positioning that the subject already has.

Some potential limitations should be acknowledged, considering the pilot nature of the study. For instance, future studies will need to replicate our findings with greater samples.

Moreover, the present study indicates that different adjustments on the augmentation might be needed depending on the stage of the macular degeneration.

In this study, the HTC Vive Pro Eye, which is known to have an end-to-end latency between 58.1 ms [31] and 80 ms [32] was used. Thanks to the colour recognition subtask and the scotoma radii thresholding, the data were corrected for eye-tracking delays (25 ms). However, this end-to-end latency [31,32,44] is not stable as it can be seen in the results, and therefore may have influenced the scotoma positioning similarly to previous gaze-contingent paradigms [44,45].

After data pre-processing, a 1° error in scotoma coverage for the majority of subjects tested was found. This finding allowed a better understanding of the occluded area and allowed us to correct for it when analysing the results. However, it also decreased the area that was intended to be covered.

An additional limitation of the current system are errors in the IPD estimation. This type of error can lead to a breakdown of binocular fusion, with errors in correctly focusing on a target [52]. However, as calibrations were performed before each condition and manual adjustments of the scotoma were performed on a trial basis, this error can be neglected.

Despite the limitations discussed above, a standardised scotoma simulation of 5° was still achieved for eight subjects. The simulation changed the gaze behaviour compared to normal conditions. In general, our results confirm what was previously published [16–20,24], i.e., standardised scotoma simulations and augmentations help study and train gaze behaviours. Virtual reality gaming proved to be a more entertaining task, resulting in greater participants' engagement and rapid adaptation. The similar results obtained in a VR 2D world to previous literature is the first step for building a model for a future, more complex and immersive reference system. Once a model of PRL development with the key characteristics and behaviours has been established more immersive and realistic virtual scenarios can be used, such as, for example, crossing the street scenarios that involve tracking a moving target in the periphery.

6. Conclusions

Not only salience augmentation to standardised scotoma simulations in normally sighted participants was investigated for the first time in this study, but this study also looked and corrected for the latency effect these paradigms suffer from.

Displaying a gaze-contingent scotoma induces an eccentric gaze behaviour, and a ring augmentation on top of it can modify this behaviour. Early application of this augmentation enhances the gaze positioning and the development of a PRL, similar to what has been reported in the literature. Meanwhile, experiencing a scotoma without any cue can lead to a higher position disparity and may require more extended training periods.

This study needs to be replicated before clinical translation can be applied. Nonetheless, it shows potential for a new type of training for macular degeneration patients.

Author Contributions: Conceptualization, A.S., S.W., M.G.G.; methodology, A.S. and S.W.; formal analysis, A.S. and M.G.G.; investigation, A.S.; data curation, A.S.; writing—original draft preparation, A.S., M.G.G. and S.W.; writing—review and editing, A.S., M.G.G. and S.W.; visualization, A.S. and M.G.G.; supervision, S.W.; project administration, S.W. All authors have read and agreed to the published version of the manuscript.

Funding: The work of the authors is supported by the Institutional Strategy of the University Tübingen (Deutsche Forschungsgemeinschaft, ZUK 63), the German Excellence initiative from the Federal Ministry of Education and Research (BMBF) in the framework of IDeA (project number 16SV8104). This work was done in an industry on campus cooperation between the University of Tübingen and Carl Zeiss Vision International GmbH. The authors recognise intra-mutual funding of the University of Tübingen through the mini graduate school "Integrative Augmented Reality (I-AR)". There was no other additional external funding received for this study.

Institutional Review Board Statement: The Ethics Committee at the Medical Faculty of the Eberhard Karls University and the University Hospital Tübingen approved to carry out the study within its facilities (Institutional Review Board number: 986/2020BO2). The study followed the tenets of the Declaration of Helsinki.

Informed Consent Statement: Written informed consent was obtained from all participants after the content and possible consequences of the study had been explained.

Data Availability Statement: Data are available at the following doi:10.6084/m9.figshare.14810301 (accessed on 23 June 2021).

Acknowledgments: We would like to thank Tamás Borbáth and NMY Mixed-Reality Communication GmbH, Frankfurt am Main for technical assistance. The authors gratefully acknowledge the helpful support of Carl Zeiss Vision International GmbH, Aalen, Katharina Rifai and to all our colleagues for offering their help. We acknowledge support by Open Access Publishing Fund of University of Tübingen.

Conflicts of Interest: Author A.S. and M.G.G. declare no potential conflicts of interest regarding this study. S.W. is a scientist at the University of Tübingen and is employed by Carl Zeiss Vision International GmbH. There is no conflict of interest regarding this study.

References

1. Wong, W.L.; Su, X.; Li, X.; Cheung, C.M.G.; Klein, R.; Cheng, C.Y.; Wong, T.Y. Global prevalence of age-related macular degeneration and disease burden projection for 2020 and 2040: A systematic review and meta-analysis. *Lancet Glob. Health* **2014**, *2*, e106–e116. [CrossRef]
2. Harvey, P.T. Common Eye Diseases of Elderly People: Identifying and Treating Causes of Vision Loss. *Gerontology* **2003**, *49*, 1–11. [CrossRef]
3. Zou, M.; Wang, S.; Chen, A.; Liu, Z.; Young, C.A.; Zhang, Y.; Jin, G.; Zheng, D. Prevalence of myopic macular degeneration worldwide: A systematic review and meta-analysis. *Br. J. Ophthalmol.* **2020**, *104*, 1748–1754. [CrossRef] [PubMed]
4. Altpeter, E.; Mackeben, M.; Trauzettel-Klosinski, S. The importance of sustained attention for patients with maculopathies. *Vis. Res.* **2000**, *40*, 1539–1547. [CrossRef]
5. Curcio, C.A.; Sloan, K.R.; Kalina, R.E.; Hendrickson, A.E. Human photoreceptor topography. *J. Comp. Neurol.* **1990**, *292*, 497–523. [CrossRef] [PubMed]
6. Cummings, R.W.; Whittaker, S.G.; Watson, G.R.; Budd, J.M. Scanning characters and reading with a central scotoma. *Optom. Vis. Sci.* **1985**, *62*, 833–843. [CrossRef]
7. Timberlake, G.T.; Mainster, M.A.; Peli, E.; Augliere, R.A.; Essock, E.A.; Arend, L.E. Reading with a macular scotoma. I. Retinal location of scotoma and fixation area. *Investig. Ophthalmol. Vis. Sci.* **1986**, *27*, 1137–1147.
8. Timberlake, G.T.; Peli, E.; Essock, E.A.; Augliere, R.A. Reading with a macular scotoma. II. Retinal locus for scanning text. *Investig. Ophthalmol. Vis. Sci.* **1987**, *28*, 1268–1274.
9. White, J.M.; Bedell, H.E. The oculomotor reference in humans with bilateral macular disease. *Investig. Ophthalmol. Vis. Sci.* **1990**, *31*, 1149–1161.
10. Schuchard, R.A. Validity and Interpretation of Amsler Grid Reports. *Arch. Ophthalmol.* **1993**, *111*, 776–780. [CrossRef]
11. Hassan, S.E.; Snyder, B.D. Street-crossing decision-making: A comparison between patients with age-related macular degeneration and normal vision. *Investig. Ophthalmol. Vis. Sci.* **2012**, *53*, 6137–6144. [CrossRef] [PubMed]
12. Almutleb, E.S.; Hassan, S.E. The Effect of Simulated Central Field Loss on Street-crossing Decision-Making in Young Adult Pedestrians. *Optom. Vis. Sci. Off. Publ. Am. Acad. Optom.* **2020**, *97*, 229–238. [CrossRef]
13. Morales, M.U.; Limoli, P.G.; Limoli, C. Augmented reality eyewear for home-based vision training after biofeedback rehabilitation of eccentric fixation. *Investig. Ophthalmol. Vis. Sci.* **2015**, *56*, 548.
14. Pratt, J.D.; Stevenson, S.B.; Bedell, H.E. Scotoma Visibility and Reading Rate with Bilateral Central Scotomas. *Optom. Vis. Sci. Off. Publ. Am. Acad. Optom.* **2017**, *94*, 279. [CrossRef] [PubMed]
15. Deemer, A.D.; Swenor, B.K.; Fujiwara, K.; Deremeik, J.T.; Ross, N.C.; Natale, D.M.; Bradley, C.K.; Werblin, F.S.; Massof, R.W. Preliminary evaluation of two digital image processing strategies for head-mounted magnification for low vision patients. *Transl. Vis. Sci. Technol.* **2019**, *8*, 23. [CrossRef]
16. Bertera, J.H. Oculomotor adaptation with virtual reality scotomas. *Simulation* **1992**, *59*, 37–43. [CrossRef]
17. Bertera, J.H. The Effect of Simulated Scotomas on Visual Search in Normal Subjects. *Investig. Ophthalmol. Vis. Sci.* **1988**, *29*, 470–475.
18. Kwon, M.; Nandy, A.S.; Tjan, B.S. Rapid and persistent adaptability of human oculomotor control in response to simulated central vision loss. *Curr. Biol.* **2013**, *23*, 1663–1669. [CrossRef] [PubMed]
19. Wu, H.; Ashmead, D.H.; Adams, H.; Bodenheimer, B. Using Virtual Reality to Assess the Street Crossing Behavior of Pedestrians With Simulated Macular Degeneration at a Roundabout. *Front. ICT* **2018**, *5*, 27. [CrossRef]

20. Pidcoe, P.E.; Wetze, P.A. Oculomotor tracking strategy in normal subjects with and without simulated scotoma. *Investig. Ophthalmol. Vis. Sci.* **2006**, *47*, 169–178. [CrossRef] [PubMed]
21. Guez, J.E.; Le Gargasson, J.F.; Rigaudiere, F.; O'Regan, J.K. Is there a systematic location for the pseudo-fovea in patients with central scotoma? *Vis. Res.* **1993**, *33*, 1271–1279. [CrossRef]
22. Lewis, J.; Shires, L.; Brown, D.J. Development of a Visual Impairment Simulator Using the Microsoft XNA Framework. In Proceedings of the 9th International Conference on Disability, Virtual Reality and Associated Technologies (ICDVRAT), Laval, France, 10–12 September 2012.
23. Väyrynen, J.; Colley, A.; Häkkilä, J. Head mounted display design tool for simulating visual disabilities. In Proceedings of the ACM International Conference Proceeding Series, Association for Computing Machinery (MUM 2016), Rovaniemi, Finland, 13–15 December 2016; pp. 69–73. [CrossRef]
24. Kwon, M.; Ramachandra, C.; Satgunam, P.; Mel, B.W.; Peli, E.; Tjan, B.S. Contour enhancement benefits older adults with simulated central field loss. *Optom. Vis. Sci.* **2012**, *89*, 1374–1384. [CrossRef] [PubMed]
25. Barraza-Bernal, M.J.; Ivanov, I.V.; Nill, S.; Rifai, K.; Trauzettel-Klosinski, S.; Wahl, S. Can positions in the visual field with high attentional capabilities be good candidates for a new preferred retinal locus? *Vis. Res.* **2017**, *140*, 1–12. [CrossRef] [PubMed]
26. Zhaoping, L. Attention capture by eye of origin singletons even without awareness—A hallmark of a bottom-up saliency map in the primary visual cortex. *J. Vis.* **2008**, *8*, 1. [CrossRef] [PubMed]
27. Warner, C.B.; Juola, J.F.; Koshino, H. Voluntary allocation versus automatic capture of visual attention. *Percept. Psychophys.* **1990**, *48*, 243–251. [CrossRef] [PubMed]
28. Parr, T.; Friston, K.J. Attention or Salience? *Curr. Opin. Psychol.* **2019**, *29*, 1–5. [CrossRef] [PubMed]
29. Lumsden, J.; Edwards, E.A.; Lawrence, N.S.; Coyle, D.; Munafò, M.R. Gamification of Cognitive Assessment and Cognitive Training: A Systematic Review of Applications and Efficacy. *JMIR Serious Games* **2016**, *4*, e11. [CrossRef] [PubMed]
30. Vive Pro Eye, VIVE Pro Eye | The Professional-Grade VR Headset. Available online: https://www.vive.com/eu/product/vive-pro-eye/overview/ (accessed on 11 November 2020).
31. Sipatchin, A.; Wahl, S.; Rifai, K. Eye-Tracking for Clinical Ophthalmology with Virtual Reality (VR): A Case Study of the HTC Vive Pro Eye's Usability. *Healthcare* **2021**, *9*, 180. [CrossRef]
32. Stein, N.; Niehorster, D.C.; Watson, T.; Steinicke, F.; Rifai, K.; Wahl, S.; Lappe, M. A Comparison of Eye Tracking Latencies Among Several Commercial Head-Mounted Displays. *i-Perception* **2021**, *12*, 1–16. [CrossRef]
33. Tobii Pro SDK, Tobii Pro SDK v1.7.1.1081. Available online: https://www.tobiipro.com/product-listing/tobii-pro-sdk/ (accessed on 22 June 2020).
34. VIVE Eye Tracking SDK (SRanipal), SRanipal SDK v1.0.3.0. Available online: https://developer.vive.com/resources/vive-sense/sdk/vive-eye-tracking-sdk-sranipal/ (accessed on 23 September 2020).
35. Clay, V.; König, P.; König, S. Eye tracking in virtual reality. *J. Eye Mov. Res.* **2019**, *12*. [CrossRef]
36. Coey, C.A.; Wallot, S.; Richardson, M.J.; van Orden, G. On the structure of measurement noise in eye-tracking. *J. Eye Mov. Res.* **2012**, *5*, 5. [CrossRef]
37. Liu, B.; Zhao, Q.C.; Ren, Y.Y.; Wang, Q.J.; Zheng, X.L. An elaborate algorithm for automatic processing of eye movement data and identifying fixations in eye-tracking experiments. *Adv. Mech. Eng.* **2018**, *10*, 2018. [CrossRef]
38. Loschky, L.C.; Wolverton, G.S. How late can you update gaze-contingent multiresolutional displays without detection. *ACM Trans. Multimed. Comput. Commun. Appl.* **2007**, *3*. [CrossRef]
39. Musall, S. Stdshade, MATLAB Central File Exchange. Available online: https://www.mathworks.com/matlabcentral/fileexchange/29534-stdshade (accessed on 23 June 2021).
40. Nyström, M.; Holmqvist, K. An adaptive algorithm for fixation, saccade, and glissade detection in eyetracking data. *Behav. Res. Methods* **2010**, *42*, 188–204. [CrossRef]
41. Savitzky, A.; Golay, Marcel, J. Smoothing and Differentiation of Data by Simplified Least Squares Procedures. *Anal. Chem.* **1964**, *36*, 1627–1639. [CrossRef]
42. Shanidze, N.; Ghahghaei, S.; Verghese, P. Accuracy of eye position for saccades and smooth pursuit. *J. Vis.* **2016**, *16*. [CrossRef] [PubMed]
43. Whittaker, S.G.; Cummings, R.W.; Swieson, L.R. Saccade control without a fovea. *Vis. Res.* **1991**, *31*, 2209–2218. [CrossRef]
44. Saunders, D.R.; Woods, R.L. Direct measurement of the system latency of gaze-contingent displays. *Behav. Res. Methods* **2014**, *46*, 439–447. [CrossRef] [PubMed]
45. Aguilar, C.; Castet, E. Gaze-contingent simulation of retinopathy: Some potential pitfalls and remedies. *Vis. Res.* **2011**, *51*, 997–1012. [CrossRef] [PubMed]
46. Zittrell, F. CircHist—Circular/Polar/Angle Histogram. Available online: https://de.mathworks.com/matlabcentral/fileexchange/66258-circhist-circular-polar-angle-histogram (accessed on 23 June 2021).
47. Berens, P. CircStat : A MATLAB Toolbox for Circular Statistics . *J. Stat. Softw.* **2009**, *31*, 1–21. [CrossRef]
48. Crossland, M.D.; Culham, L.E.; Kabanarou, S.A.; Rubin, G.S. Preferred retinal locus development in patients with macular disease. *Ophthalmology* **2005**, *112*, 1579–1585. [CrossRef] [PubMed]
49. Sunness, J.S.; Applegate, C.A.; Haselwood, D.; Rubin, G.S. Fixation patterns and reading rates in eyes with central scotomas from advanced atrophic age-related macular degeneration and Stargardt disease. *Ophthalmology* **1996**, *103*, 1458–1466. [CrossRef]

50. Trauzettel-Klosinski, S.; Tornow, R.P. Fixation behavior and reading ability in macular scotoma. Assessed by Tuebingen manual perimetry and scanning laser ophthalmoscopy. *Neuro-ophthalmology* **1996**, *16*, 241–253. [CrossRef] [PubMed]
51. Fletcher, D.C.; Schuchard, R.A. Preferred retinal loci relationship to macular scotomas in a low-vision population. *Ophthalmology* **1997**, *104*, 632–638. [CrossRef]
52. Hibbard, P.B.; van Dam, L.C.; Scarfe, P. The implications of interpupillary distance variability for virtual reality. In Proceedings of the 2020 International Conference on 3D Immersion (IC3D), Brussels, Belgium, 15 December 2020; pp. 1–7.

Article

Evaluation of the Reaction Time and Accuracy Rate in Normal Subjects, MCI, and Dementia Using Serious Games

Yen-Ting Chen [1], Chun-Ju Hou [1,*], Natan Derek [1], Shuo-Bin Huang [1], Min-Wei Huang [2,3] and You-Yu Wang [4]

[1] Department of Electrical Engineering, Southern Taiwan University of Science and Technology, Tainan 701, Taiwan; ytchen@stust.edu.tw (Y.-T.C.); da62b206@stust.edu.tw (N.D.); ma520113@stust.edu.tw (S.-B.H.)
[2] Department of Psychiatry, Chiayi Bran Taichung Veterans General Hospital, Chiayi City 600, Taiwan; hminwei@gmail.com
[3] MOST AI Biomedical Research Center at NCKU, Tainan 701, Taiwan
[4] Department of Social Welfare, National Chung Cheng University, Chiayi City 620, Taiwan; jiay01516@gmail.com
* Correspondence: cjhou@stust.edu.tw; Tel.: +886-6-3310481; Fax: +886-6-3010073

Abstract: The main purpose of this research is to evaluate the differences in the reaction time and accuracy rate of three categories of subjects using our serious games. Thirty-seven subjects were divided into three groups: normal (n_1 = 16), MCI (Mild Cognitive Impairment) (n_2 = 10), and dementia—moderate-to-severe (n_3 = 11) groups based on the MMSE (Mini Mental State Examination). Two serious games were designed: (1) whack-a-mole and (2) hit-the-ball. Two dependent variables, reaction time and accuracy rate, were statistically analyzed to compare elders' performances in the games among the three groups for three levels of speed: slow, medium, and fast. There were significance differences between the normal group, the MCI group, and the moderate-to-severe dementia group in both the reaction-time and accuracy-rate analyses. We determined that the reaction times of the MCI and dementia groups were shorter compared to those of the normal group, with poorer results also observed in accuracy rate. Therefore, we conclude that our serious games have the feasibility to evaluate reaction performance and could be used in the daily lives of elders followed by clinical treatment in the future.

Keywords: reaction time; accuracy rate; serious game; PC-based game; MCI; dementia; elderly healthcare; cognitive function

Citation: Chen, Y.-T.; Hou, C.-J.; Derek, N.; Huang, S.-B.; Huang, M.-W.; Wang, Y.-Y. Evaluation of the Reaction Time and Accuracy Rate in Normal Subjects, MCI, and Dementia Using Serious Games. *Appl. Sci.* **2021**, *11*, 628. https://doi.org/10.3390/app11020628

Received: 23 December 2020
Accepted: 7 January 2021
Published: 11 January 2021

Publisher's Note: MDPI stays neutral with regard to jurisdictional claims in published maps and institutional affiliations.

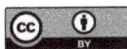

Copyright: © 2021 by the authors. Licensee MDPI, Basel, Switzerland. This article is an open access article distributed under the terms and conditions of the Creative Commons Attribution (CC BY) license (https://creativecommons.org/licenses/by/4.0/).

1. Introduction

The World Health Organization (WHO) estimates that around 50 million people have dementia, with nearly 10 million new cases every year [1]. Dementia refers to deterioration of cognitive function in the elderly. This syndrome affects memory, thinking, orientation, comprehension, calculations, learning capacity, language, and judgment. It also affects individual quality of life and is a financial burden for families due to expensive costs for healthcare [2]. According to the Alzheimer's association (2019), 36% of people aged 85 or older have Alzheimer's Disease (AD) [3]. Dementia and other cognitive impairment diseases have become an important global issue, as the number of elderly people is increasing. In 2025, it is predicted that Taiwan will become a super-aged society (National Development Council in Taiwan, 2016). As age increases, problems in cognitive abilities, such as divided attention, memory decline, etc., also increase [4].

Simple reaction times are valid for measuring cognitive function in both patients and normal subjects [5]. Furthermore, the authors in [6] also noted that accuracy rate can correlate significantly with episodic memory performance and other cognitive functions. Reaction time and accuracy rate are thus related to cognitive functions [5–7]. Most previous research used neuropsychological tests, such as the Flanker test, the Cambridge

Neuropsychological Test Automated Battery, and Repeatable Battery for the Assessment of Neuropsychological Status [6,7]. Therefore, in this study, our main objective is to determine the difference in the reaction time and accuracy rate between the aforementioned three categories of subjects (normal subjects, Mild Cognitive Impairment (MCI), and dementia) using our own designed serious games. We intended to determine whether the response performance (also mentioned in [7]) can differentiate between these three categories. A study by Phillips et al. [8] found that patients with MCI and Alzheimer's disease had significantly longer reaction times than normal aging control groups, with reaction times that did not eliminate individual differences. When the factors related to the different reaction times of individuals are excluded, patients with MCI actually behaved similarly to the normal aging control group, but the responses of patients with Alzheimer's disease, after excluding the effects of individual differences, were still not as good as those of the other two groups.

Numerous methods have been developed to examine Alzheimer's disease and MCI. Invasive methods are used to collect data from inside the human body and are not considered safe and comfortable for subjects [9]. Valladares-Rodriguez et al. [10] found that using noninvasive methods like serious games can detect the onset of MCI or Alzheimer's disease. In our study, we applied the same method noninvasively by designing PC-based serious games to evaluate the reaction times and accuracy rates related to the cognitive abilities among normal subjects, MCI subjects, and dementia subjects. Our approach was to compare the results of the performance of an elder individual when playing the game using neuropsychological tests of cognitive function based on the MMSE (Mini Mental State Examination).

There are many neuropsychological tests and clinical questionnaires used to assess dementia levels among the elderly. Clinical questionnaires, such as the Mini Mental State Examination (MMSE) [11] and the Montreal Cognitive Assessment (MoCA) [12], are a popular way to evaluate cognitive abilities via clinical measurements. Costaz et al. [13] used an Augmented Reality (AR) serious game called Smartkuber to perform cognitive screening among the elderly. To validate the relationship between game results and MoCa results, the authors used the Pearson correlation statistical method [13–15]. In our research, we use the MMSE to evaluate the level of dementia among the elderly due to the heterogeneity of the age-group. A study was conducted by the authors of [16] in Greece to validate the performance of the MMSE, and the result proved that an MMSE score of 23/24 is a credible test for diagnosis of dementia.

Several well-designed serious video games have been proposed and should be helpful for evaluating cognitive abilities [10,11,17–19]. Fontana, E et al. [19] developed a serious game called *TrainBrain*, designed to improve concentration and to minimize the effects of the cognitive decline in attention for the elderly and children with ADHD (Attention Deficit Hyperactivity Disorder). In recent years, the products currently on the mainstream market for video and mobile games were designed for young people to experience exciting sight and sound stimulation, which may not be adaptable for the elderly. The development of a serious game is very challenging, especially when addressing dementia patients. Many factors must be considered, such as the needs of the subjects, human–computer interactions, emotions, comfortability, etc., which make development more complicated. A well-designed GUI (Graphical User Interface) is one of the most important aspects to help subjects focus on the game [20]. In [21], the authors built a whack-a-mole game for tablets (Android-based). The game was divided into different speeds, and the time was used to record the subject's score and response time. The authors proved that this game can be used to assess some executive functions, especially those related to inhibition, in their recent study [22]. They also suggested that this game can be developed for the elderly to assess other executive functions [22,23].

In this present study, two serious games were designed to meet the standards of play for the elderly. The purpose of our PC-based games was to measure response performance (reaction time and accuracy rate). Psychologists and clinicians were continuously consulted during system development to obtain a better understanding about the complexity of the external appearance of cognitive functions and the reactions of the elderly. Based on [22], first, we built a similar whack-a-mole game without distractors (the objects in addition to the mole) to focus only on reaction time and accuracy rate when playing the game, as the game's target is to collect information on the reaction time and accuracy rate of the subjects. Then, we designed the second game, hit-the-ball (with a distractor), also to assess judgment ability and to observe how the subjects distinguish between objects. Another issue, as explained in [24], is that elderly people may think that computers are not friendly for them, making these games uncomfortable to play. Therefore, our games were designed to be as simple as possible and easy to play, considering that the subjects are old and that most of them have never experienced playing PC-based games before. It was found that the traditional whack-a-mole machine game was a famous game in the past for Taiwanese people. We designed a special board-button to allow the subjects to be more familiar and comfortable with the game. In our discussion, we analyze and explain the response time and the accuracy rate as the dependent variables. We used the MMSE score (normal group, MCI group, and moderate-to-severe dementia group) and game level (slow, medium, and fast) as the independent variables. We also analyzed judgment ability for the hit-the-ball game. All results were calculated using statistical methods (Kruskal–Wallis Test and Friedman Test) for accuracy rate and one-way ANOVA for reaction time. We found that there are significant differences between these three categories of subjects.

2. Methods and Experimental Design

2.1. Game Design

2.1.1. Whack-a-Mole

The typical whack-a-mole machine was historically very popular at playgrounds in Taiwan. The PC-based whack-a-mole game was designed to simulate the gameplay of a real whack-a-mole game machine. Based on the work in [22], we built the game with only three holes and hidden moles that pop up randomly. The players need to hit the correct button on the button array immediately next to the hole when the mole pops up randomly. Unlike the authors in [22], we did not use another object as a distractor, such as a similar mole with a hat or another object to assess inhibition ability, as our main concern here was the differences in reaction times and accuracy rates between our subjects. We designed the game with 3 holes, as shown in Figure 1, and Table 1 shows the three levels of speed: (1) slow, (2) medium, and (3) fast.

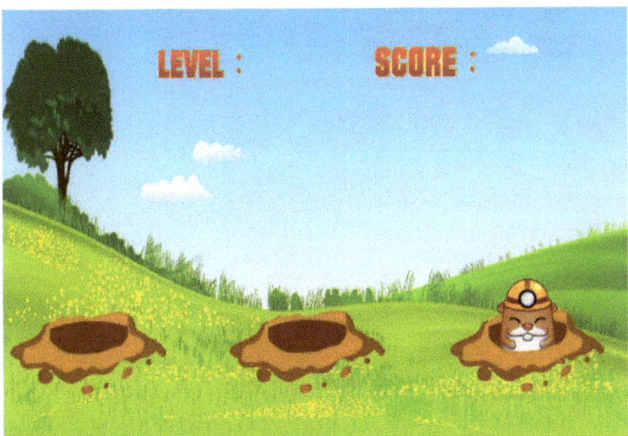

Figure 1. Screenshot demonstration of the whack-a-mole game.

Table 1. Time difference based on the speed level of the whack-a-mole game (in seconds).

Speed-Level	Time Duration	Time Interval between the Mole Appearing
Slow	3	1
Medium	2	1
Fast	1	1

2.1.2. Hit-the-Ball

Based on the whack-a-mole game, we built a second game called *hit-the-ball*. This game has almost the same purpose as that of the whack-a-mole game but with differences to assess judgment ability. We also designed it in a 3D environment. We designed this game considering the participant's mood since they played the games in sequence, which we assumed would be a relatively long time for an elder. This game has three fairways. Every fairway has three segments for evaluating reaction time. Balls are launched far from the end of the fairway and roll toward the player. In this case, the subject has time to think about and anticipate the right ball. The player needs to hit the balls that roll into the red zone of the fairway, while some metal meteors that should not be hit are used to distract the player's judgement. We used a judgment analysis to determine if the subjects had any difficulty in differentiating between the objects. The number of balls and metal meteors are the same and appear randomly. Figure 2 shows the design of the hit-the-ball game, and Table 2 shows the three levels of speed for the *hit-the-ball* game. Three modes with different rolling speeds (from slow to fast) were designed to test reactive ability. A screen demonstration is shown in Figure 3. For further investigations, we included a time-unlimited mode, where we recorded the time when the subject pressed the button even after the ball disappeared.

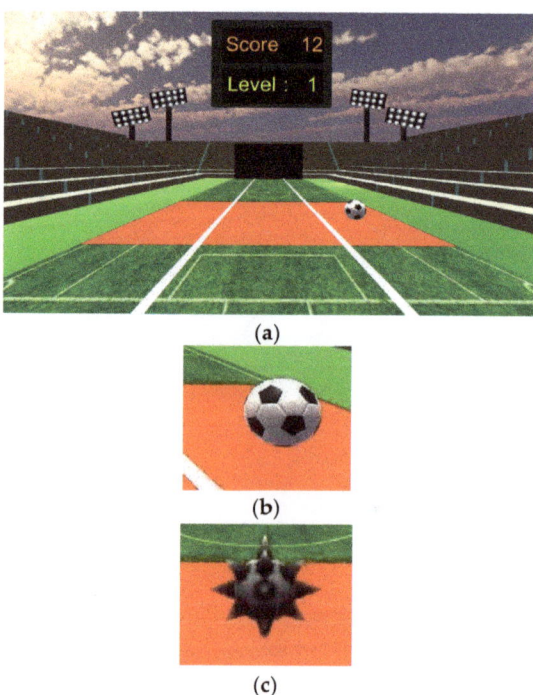

Figure 2. Screen shots of the first stage of the hit-the-ball game: (**a**) the scene, (**b**) the ball, and (**c**) the metal meteor.

Table 2. Time difference based on the speed of the hit-the-ball game (in seconds).

Speed-Level	Time Duration	Time Interval between the Balls	Time on the Redzone
Slow	3.7	5	1.6
Medium	2.8	4	1
Fast	1.8	4	0.5

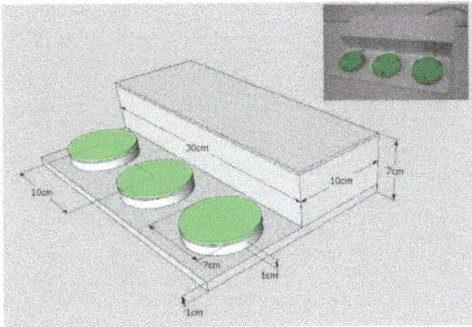

Figure 3. A designed board-button.

2.2. Experimental Design

These games were designed using Unity 2018 and the C# platform with Microsoft Visual Studio 2016. Statistical analyses were performed using the SPSS 25 software package (IBM Corporation, Armonk, NY, USA). The designed board-button was made with an Arduino UNO R3 with FSR sensor as the input. We designed the board-buttons for both of the games since we were concerned about the comfort of the patients (some of them have never played PC-based games with a keyboard or mouse). We considered also the size and distance between the button, which should be as large as when they played the game in an amusement park. The width for each button was 7 cm, with the distance between the centers being 10 cm. For detailed information, Figure 3 shows the specification of the designed board-button. Figure 4 shows the subject playing in front of the screen using the designed board-button.

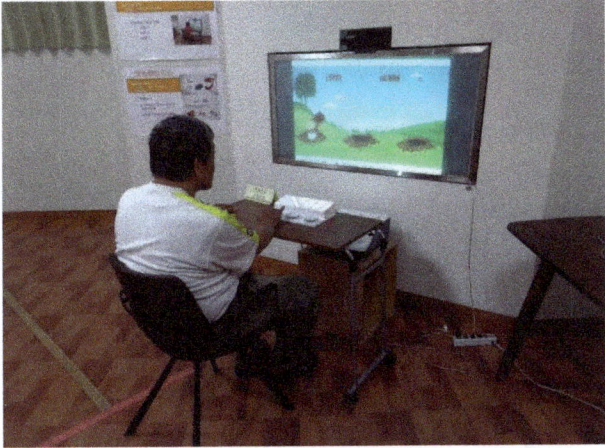

Figure 4. A subject playing a PC serious game in our experimental room using a designed board-button.

This study was approved by the ethics committee of Taichung Veterans General Hospital in Taiwan and conducted in accordance with good clinical practice procedures and the current revision of the Declaration of Helsinki. There were a total of 37 subjects enrolled in this study, including 16 males and 24 females between the ages of 70 and 90 years, with a mean of 75.38 ± 11.41 SD (16 normal subjects, 10 mild cognitive impairment subjects, and 11 moderate-to-severe dementia subjects). Table 3 shows the demographics of the subjects with the clinical questionnaire MMSE scores.

Table 3. Demographic of the subjects with the clinical questionnaire MMSE (Mini Mental State Examination) scores.

Subjects		People (Percentage)	Mean and Standard Deviations
Age		37	75.38 ± 11.41
Sex			
	Male	13 (35%)	
	Female	24 (65%)	
MMSE			
	Normal	16 (43%)	27.81 ± 1.97
	MCI (Mild Cognitive Impairment)	10 (27%)	20.50 ± 1.51
	Moderate	10 (27%)	14.30 ± 1.49
	Severe	1 (3%)	6 ± 0

2.2.1. Clinical Evaluation: MMSE (Mini Mental State Examination)

We used the clinical questionnaire MMSE (Mini Mental State Examination) to categorize our subjects into three different groups: the normal group, the MCI group, and the dementia (moderate-to-severe) group. The MMSE questionnaires were examined by a psychologist along with a doctor specialized in healthcare for the elderly.

2.2.2. Procedure and Consent

The participants signed their consent to ensure they knew all the regulations and the consequences related to the experiments. All participants were instructed before playing to familiarize them with the PC-based games. They also had practice time. In the practice mode, they played in the slow-speed mode for each game and were assisted by the instructor to ensure that they knew how to play the games. They only played both games once, and all data were recorded for analysis. Recorded data during practice were not included.

2.2.3. Modes

In these two games, we separated the measurements into the time-limited mode and time-unlimited mode. The time-limited mode features a limited time to respond when the ball/mole appears, while the time-unlimited mode gives the patients more time to react after the ball/mole disappears. We divided the games this way because we assumed that some of the subjects would be slow to respond to the correct ball and the mole even if they recognized the ball/mole. We believe that the subjects had awareness, even though they reacted slowly. This was proven when they hit the button after the ball had passed the fairway.

2.2.4. Parameters

- Independent Variable To easily observe performance in the hit-the-ball game, the subjects were divided into three groups for observation according to the total score of the subject's MMSE scale: the normal group (MMSE $\geq$ 24), MCI group (18 $\leq$ MMSE $\leq$ 23), and moderate-to-severe group (MMSE $\leq$ 17).
- Dependent Variable
- The hit-the-ball game

- Accuracy rate of the ball In the hit-the-ball game, the accuracy rate considered only correct balls hit by our subjects. Every speed level has 5 balls, and the accuracy rate was calculated for the time-limited and time-unlimited modes in each group of subjects. Time-limited here means the time when the subjects pressed the button while the ball was within the red zone. Time-unlimited is considered the time when the ball appeared until the time the next ball appeared.
- Response time This variable includes all response times when the subject presses the button for the three different speed levels. Here, we consider the time-limited and time-unlimited modes to observe the differences between the three different groups.
- Accuracy rate of the ball and metal meteor (Judgement) In this variable, we consider the balls and the metal meteors to observe the judgement of the subjects. There are 5 balls and 5 meteors balls for every speed level. Every subject has to hit the correct ball and not hit the metal meteors to obtain a point. If the subject presses the metal meteors, he or she misses one point.
- The Whack-A-Mole game
- Accuracy rate of the mole In the whack-a-mole game, the accuracy rate was calculated by all the correct answers when the subjects responded to the mole. There are ten moles for every speed level in this game.
- Response Time The response time for the time-limited mode is the time when the subjects press the button when the mole appears, and for the time unlimited mode, the response time is when the mole appears and disappears before the next mole is launched.

2.3. Statistical Methods

A normality test of the data was performed to determine the use of parametric or nonparametric statistical methods. In the hit-the-ball and whack-a-mole games, the Kruskal–Wallis test was used to compare the accuracy rates among the normal (n_1 = 16), MCI (n_2 = 10), and moderate-to-severe dementia (n_3 = 11) groups. A comparison of the two groups using a Mann–Whitney test was performed after the null hypothesis in the Kruskal–Wallis test was rejected. The median difference among the repeated measures of the 3 speed levels in the game for each group was compared using a Friedman test. A Wilcoxon signed-rank test was used to test the null hypothesis that the median difference between two speed levels is equal to 0. The average response time of the 3 groups was compared by a one-way ANOVA. A post hoc analysis for comparison of the two groups was performed after the null hypothesis in the one-way ANOVA was rejected. The significance level for the statistical analysis was 0.05.

3. Results and Discussion
3.1. Whack-a-Mole
3.1.1. Accuracy Rate Analysis

Table 4 shows the accuracy rate and the results of the Kruskal–Wallis test for comparisons of the three groups at different speed levels for accuracy-rate analysis. In the time-limited mode, the Kruskal–Wallis test was used to observe whether the performance of the three groups was different for the three game speed modes. The results show that the three groups had significant differences at medium speed (X^2 = 17.147, $p < 0.05$) and fast speed (X^2 = 10.187, $p < 0.05$). The results of the posterior comparison with a Mann–Whitney U test indicated that there was a significant difference between the moderate-to-severe and normal groups ($p < 0.05$) as well as a significant difference between the MCI and moderate-to-severe groups ($p < 0.05$) at medium speed. Further, when the speed was fast, the normal and moderate-to-severe groups showed significant differences ($p < 0.05$), and there was also a significant difference between the MCI group and the moderate-to-severe group ($p < 0.05$).

Table 4. Posterior comparisons of the different groups by test scores using Kruskal–Wallis.

	Game Level	MMSE			Kruskal–Wallis	
		Normal (1)	MCI (2)	Moderate-to-Severe (3)	X^2	p-Value
		Mean ± SD [a]	Mean ± SD [a]	Mean ± SD [a]		
Time-limited	Slow	0.98 ± 0.05	0.98 ± 0.04	0.97 ± 0.06	0.229	0.892
	Medium	0.99 ± 0.03	0.99 ± 0.03	0.88 ± 0.10	17.147	0.000 *
	Fast	0.41 ± 0.33	0.11 ± 0.16	0.06 ± 0.09	10.187	0.006 *
Time unlimited	Slow	0.99 ± 0.03	0.99 ± 0.03	0.97 ± 0.06	1.057	0.590
	Medium	1.00 ± 0.00	1.00 ± 0.00	0.95 ± 0.10	4.859	0.088
	Fast	0.97 ± 0.06	0.86 ± 0.19	0.80 ± 0.20	6.247	0.044 *

[a] SD indicates standard deviation. * $p < 0.05$. The null hypothesis that the medians of the three populations are equal is rejected.

In the time-unlimited mode, the Kruskal–Wallis test was used to observe whether the three groups were different at the three game speed levels. The results showed that the three groups were significantly different in the fast speed mode ($p < 0.05$). The Mann–Whitney U test was then used to perform posterior comparisons, and the results showed that, when the speed was fast, there was a significant difference between the moderate-to-severe group and the *normal* group ($p < 0.05$). This means that the time-unlimited mode was relatively easy for the normal group but difficult for the moderate-to-severe group. Some subjects in the MCI group performed well, while others performed poorly.

Table 5 presents posterior comparisons of the impacts of the different game speeds on test scores using a Friedman Test for the time-limited mode to observe whether game speed was different for the three groups. The results show that the differences of all three groups are significant ($p < 0.05$). A Wilcoxon signed-rank test was used to perform the posterior comparison, and the results showed that the performance in the moderate-to-severe group was significantly different between the medium to fast, slow to fast, and medium to slow speeds ($p < 0.05$). The normal group, on the other hand, showed a significant difference ($p < 0.05$) in performance under the medium to fast and slow to fast speeds but no significant difference in slow to medium speeds; the MCI group also had a similar performance. This means that, for the subjects in the moderate-to-severe group, the three speeds provide three different levels of difficulty. For the normal group, there was no difference in performance between the slow and medium speeds. The MCI group presented a similar performance.

Table 5. Posterior comparisons of different speeds based on test scores using a Friedman Test.

	MMSE	Game Level			Friedman	
		Slow(A)	Medium(B)	Fast(C)	X^2	p-Value
		Mean ± SD [a]	Mean ± SD [a]	Mean ± SD [a]		
Time-limited	Normal	0.98 ± 0.05	0.99 ± 0.03	0.41 ± 0.33	28.167	0.000 *
	MCI	0.98 ± 0.04	0.99 ± 0.03	0.11 ± 0.16	19.419	0.000 *
	Moderate-to-Severe	0.97 ± 0.06	0.88 ± 0.10	0.06 ± 0.09	20.600	0.000 *
Time-unlimited	Normal	0.99 ± 0.03	1.00 ± 0.00	0.97 ± 0.06	6.500	0.039 *
	MCI	0.99 ± 0.00	1.00 ± 0.00	0.86 ± 0.19	7.000	0.030 *
	Moderate-to-Severe	0.97 ± 0.06	0.95 ± 0.10	0.80 ± 0.20	11.217	0.004 *

[a] SD indicates standard deviation. * $p < 0.05$. The null hypothesis that the medians of the three populations are equal is rejected.

In the case of the time-unlimited group, a Friedman test was performed to check if the game speeds of every group of MMSE were significantly different. The results showed that, among the three groups, the normal group and the moderate-to-severe groups had significant speed performance differences ($p < 0.05$). A Wilcoxon signed-rank test was used to perform the posterior comparison, and the results showed that the performance under slow-to-fast and medium-to-fast speeds in the moderate-to-severe group was significantly different ($p < 0.05$). This result indicates that, for the subjects in the moderate-to-severe group, each speed is significantly different from the other two speeds.

3.1.2. Reaction-Time Analysis

Table 6 shows the response time(s) of each group of MMSE in the time-limited mode at different game speeds. The table shows that the reaction time decreases as the game speed increases. For the fast speed level, the time taken by the MCI and dementia groups is shorter than that of the normal group. We assume that this occurred because the subjects did not pay attention to which hole the mole appeared in instead of simply pressing the button randomly (which can be observed by the accuracy rate explained in Table 4). For the time-limited mode, after the null hypothesis of the one-way ANOVA was rejected, a post hoc analysis for comparison of two groups was performed and showed differences between the normal group and the moderate-to-severe group, with a T-score = -0.24238 for the slow speed and -0.24998 for medium speed. For the normal group and the MCI group, the T-score was -0.18751 for medium speed. Significance levels were 0.05 for all analyses.

Table 6. Time-limited mode: the response time(s) of each group of MMSE at different game speeds.

Game Level	MMSE			One-Way ANOVA	
	Normal (1)	MCI (2)	Moderate-to-Severe (3)	F	p-Value
	Mean ± SD [a]	Mean ± SD [a]	Mean ± SD [a]		
slow	1.10 ± 0.18	1.27 ± 0.19	1.34 ± 0.21	5.675	0.007 *
medium	1.07 ± 0.19	1.26 ± 0.12	1.32 ± 0.18	7.865	0.002 *
fast	0.71 ± 0.36	0.40 ± 0.46	0.68 ± 0.41	3.581	0.039 *

[a] SD indicates standard deviation. * $p < 0.05$.

Table 7 shows the response time(s) of different MMSE groups at different game speeds in the time-unlimited mode. In the case of the time-unlimited mode, the response time of the normal group was usually shorter than that of the MCI group and the response time of the MCI group was also shorter than that of the moderate-to-severe group at all three speed levels.

Table 7. Time-unlimited mode: posterior comparison of each group of MMSE at different game speeds.

Game Level	MMSE			One-Way ANOVA	
	Normal (1)	MCI (2)	Moderate-to-Severe (3)	F	p-Value
	Mean ± SD [a]	Mean ± SD [a]	Mean ± SD [a]		
slow	1.13 ± 0.19	1.29 ± 0.24	1.34 ± 0.21	3.637	0.037 *
medium	1.08 ± 0.20	1.28 ± 0.15	1.38 ± 0.19	8.792	0.001 *
fast	1.05 ± 0.17	1.23 ± 0.16	1.31 ± 0.16	9.114	0.001 *

[a] SD indicates standard deviation. * $p < 0.05$.

For the time unlimited mode, after rejecting the null hypothesis in one-way ANOVA, a post hoc analysis for a comparison of the two groups was performed and showed differences between the normal group and the moderate-to-severe group only, with a T-score = -0.20988 for slow speed, -0.29224 for medium speed, and -0.9224 for fast speed. The results for the normal group with the MCI group presented a T-score = -0.20037 for medium speed and -0.18090 for fast speed. The significance level was 0.05 for all analyses.

3.2. Hit-the-Ball

3.2.1. Accuracy-Rate Analysis

Table 8 shows the accuracy rate and the results of the Kruskal–Wallis test for comparisons of the three groups at different speed levels for accuracy-rate analysis. In the three groups grouped by MMSE in the time-limited case, the Kruskal–Wallis test was used to observe whether the three groups were different at the three speed levels of the hit-the-ball game. After the posterior test with the Mann–Whitney U test, the results showed that, when the speed is fast, there is a significant difference between the moderate-to-severe group and the normal group ($p < 0.05$) but there is no significant difference between the moderate-to-severe group and the MCI group ($p > 0.05$) as well as no significant difference between the normal group and MCI group ($p > 0.05$). In the time-limited mode, when the game speed is fast, the normal group and the moderate-to-severe group can be distinguished but the normal and MCI groups cannot be distinguished. In Table 8, we can observe that, when the game speed is fast, the performance of those in the normal group and the MCI group is much better than that of those in the moderate-to-severe group.

Table 8. The accuracy rate and the results of the Kruskal–Wallis test for comparisons of the three groups under different speed levels.

Speed Levels of Game		Groups			Kruskal–Wallis Test	
		Normal Mean ± SD [a]	MCI Mean ± SD [a]	Moderate-to-Severe Mean ± SD [a]	X^2	p-Value
Time-limited	Slow	0.86 ± 0.17	0.68 ± 0.38	0.58 ± 0.29	6.587	0.037 *
	Medium	0.83 ± 0.24	0.68 ± 0.40	0.60 ± 0.37	3.096	0.213
	Fast	0.50 ± 0.43	0.16 ± 0.26	0.02 ± 0.06	9.972	0.007 *
Time-unlimited	Slow	1.00 ± 0.00	0.96 ± 0.13	0.78 ± 0.28	12.675	0.002 *
	Medium	1.00 ± 0.00	0.98 ± 0.06	0.78 ± 0.34	7.637	0.022 *
	Fast	0.98 ± 0.07	0.88 ± 0.21	0.56 ± 0.25	19.073	0.000 *
Judgment	Slow	0.98 ± 0.05	0.95 ± 0.16	0.76 ± 0.16	16.826	0.000 *
	Medium	0.99 ± 0.05	0.96 ± 0.10	0.80 ± 0.20	9.778	0.008 *
	Fast	0.96 ± 0.10	0.89 ± 0.12	0.71 ± 0.19	17.175	0.000 *

[a] SD indicates standard deviation. * $p < 0.05$. The null hypothesis that the medians of the three populations are equal is rejected.

In the time-unlimited mode, the Kruskal–Wallis test was used to observe whether the three groups were different under the three game speed modes. The results showed that the performance of the three groups under the three game speeds was significantly different ($p < 0.05$). After a posterior comparison with the Mann–Whitney U test, the results show that, when the speed is slow and fast, there is a significant difference between the moderate-to-severe group and the normal group ($p < 0.05$) as well as a significant difference between the MCI and moderate-to-severe group ($p < 0.05$); when the speed is medium, there is a significant difference between the normal group and the moderate-to-severe group ($p < 0.05$). This means that time-unlimited play is relatively simple for the normal group and the MCI group while the moderate-to-severe group will have some difficulties.

To determine the judgment abilities of the three groups divided by MMSE, by using the Kruskal–Wallis test to observe whether the three groups are different under the three game speeds, the results showed that there were significant differences in performance ($p < 0.05$) between the three groups. After posterior comparison with the Mann–Whitney U test, the results showed a significant difference between the moderate-to-severe group and the normal group ($p < 0.05$) in all three speed modes. There were also significant differences between the MCI and moderate-to-severe groups ($p < 0.05$). This means that it is relatively easy to judge the ball type for the normal and MCI groups, while this same task will be difficult for the moderate-to-severe group.

In the case of the time-limited mode, the performance of the three groups at the three game speeds was analyzed based on Friedman's two-factor level variation. The results show that the groups have significant performance differences at different speeds ($p < 0.05$). In addition, a Wilcoxon signed-rank test was used to perform a posterior comparison and the results showed that the speed score was significant ($p < 0.05$) for the medium vs. fast modes in every group as well as the slow vs. fast modes ($p < 0.05$). This might indicate that the speed was too fast for all subjects, which is why they performed poorly.

For the three game speeds under the time-unlimited mode, the Friedman test was used to observe whether the game speeds produced significant differences between the three groups. The results showed that only the moderate-to-severe groups had significant differences ($p < 0.05$). In addition, the Wilcoxon signed-rank test was used to perform the posterior comparison, and the results showed that there were significant differences ($p < 0.05$) between the speeds of the medium vs. fast and slow vs. fast modes in the moderate-to-severe group. Therefore, for the subjects in the moderate-to-severe group, there will be a large difference in the accuracy rates under high speed compared to other speeds.

For the three groups, judgment ability was discriminated by the different speeds. The analysis was based on the Friedman test, and the MCI group presented significant ($p < 0.05$) results at the different speeds. However, the results showed no significant difference ($p > 0.05$) using the comparison with the Wilcoxon signed-rank test. Therefore, for the subjects in the moderate-to-severe group, there is a slight difference in judging the ball compared to the other two groups, but there is no large difference. The time-limited mode can, therefore, better classify the performance of the three groups than the time-unlimited mode. Table 9 shows the posterior comparisons of the results of different game speeds by test scores using the Friedman Test.

Table 9. Posterior comparisons of the results of different game speeds by test scores using the Friedman Test.

	MMSE	Game Level			Friedman	
		Slow(A)	Medium(B)	Fast(C)	X^2	p-Value
		Mean ± SD [a]	Mean ± SD [a]	Mean ± SD [a]		
Time-limited	Normal	0.86 ± 0.17	0.83 ± 0.24	0.50 ± 0.43	13.378	0.001 *
	MCI	0.68 ± 0.38	0.68 ± 0.40	0.16 ± 0.26	12.000	0.002 *
	Moderate-to-Severe	0.58 ± 0.29	0.60 ± 0.37	0.02 ± 0.06	13.650	0.001 *
Time-unlimited	Normal	1.00 ± 0.00	1.00 ± 0.00	0.98 ± 0.07	4.000	0.135
	MCI	0.96 ± 0.13	0.98 ± 0.06	0.88 ± 0.21	2.923	0.232
	Moderate-to-Severe	0.78 ± 0.28	0.78 ± 0.34	0.56 ± 0.25	7.032	0.030 *
Judgement	Normal	0.98 ± 0.05	0.99 ± 0.05	0.96 ± 0.10	6.500	0.039 *
	MCI	0.95 ± 0.16	0.96 ± 0.10	0.89 ± 0.12	6.421	0.040 *
	Moderate-to-Severe	0.76 ± 0.16	0.80 ± 0.20	0.71 ± 0.19	4.171	0.124

[a] SD indicates standard deviation. * $p < 0.05$. The null hypothesis that the medians of the three populations are equal is rejected.

3.2.2. Reaction-Time Analysis

The response time here is the time from the ball appearing at the start point to the subject pressing the button. Every group uses the response time of each person as an individual datum for analysis. Without considering individual differences, some people may have responded slightly slower and were only able to react when the ball entered the red zone. Reaction time is used to indicate reaction ability in this evaluation. As the game speed increases, the response time gradually decreased in all groups. The response times under different game speeds are shown in Table 10.

Table 10. Response times of subjects at different game level(s) (time-limited).

Game Level	MMSE			One-Way Anova	
	Normal (1)	MCI (2)	Moderate-to-Severe (3)	F	p-Value
	Mean ± SD [a]	Mean ± SD [a]	Mean ± SD [a]		
slow	0.29 ± 0.21	0.32 ± 0.26	0.37 ± 0.27	0.950	0.391
medium	0.22 ± 0.13	0.25 ± 0.15	0.25 ± 0.13	0.587	0.558
fast	0.14 ± 0.07	0.12 ± 0.07	0.15 ± 0.00	0.163	0.850

[a] SD indicates standard deviation. $p < 0.05$.

Like in the whack-a-mole game, at medium and fast speed levels, the MCI group has a shorter reaction time than the normal group, but the accuracy rate is very low (see Table 8). Because the three groups of data were used for the normality analysis and found to be normal, a one-way ANOVA was used to test whether the groups were different, and then a post hoc analysis was performed to compare the differences between the groups.

For the time-limited mode, after the null hypothesis was rejected in the one-way ANOVA, a post hoc analysis for comparison of the two groups was performed, and the results showed differences between the normal group and the MCI group, with a T-score = -0.27715 for medium speed; between the normal group and the MCI group, with a T-score = -0.12272 for fast speed; and between the normal group and the moderate-to-severe group, with a T-score = -0.14359 for fast speed. All significance levels were 0.05 for the analyses.

However, when individual differences are considered, the reaction time in the time-unlimited mode did not increase with an increase in the game speed. However, in the three groups, we found that moderate-to-severe subjects needed a longer response time than the normal and MCI groups (as shown in Table 11), which may also indirectly lead to a lower accuracy rate when game speed is faster.

Table 11. Response times of subjects at different game level(s) (time-unlimited).

Game Level	MMSE			One-Way ANOVA	
	Normal (1) Mean ± SD [a]	MCI (2) Mean ± SD [a]	Moderate-to-Severe (3) Mean ± SD [a]	F	p-Value
slow	0.17 ± 0.38	0.11 ± 0.55	0.28 0.51	1.213	0.301
medium	0.22 ± 0.47	0.49 ± 0.47	0.34 ± 0.22	9.342	0.000 *
fast	0.34 ± 0.23	0.46 ± 0.27	0.48 ± 0.16	6.261	0.002 *

[a] SD indicates standard deviation. * $p < 0.05$.

4. Conclusions

In this study, we found that the response performance of subjects with mild cognitive impairment and dementia were poor compared to normal subjects comprehensively evaluated by reaction time and accuracy rate. Although in the reaction-time analysis, the performance times of the MCI and dementia groups seemed to be shorter than those of the normal group for the same speed level, the accuracy-rate analysis showed poor performance for both the MCI and dementia groups. We observed that these groups reacted randomly by pressing the button when the speed was increased, without considering the accuracy of the object in both the whack-a-mole and hit-the-ball games. Our results, along with those in [6,7], show that those subjects had significantly poorer performance when measured by simple reaction time and accuracy rate. Moreover, we successfully differentiated these three categories of subjects using our serious games. For the reaction-time analysis, we established that the time-unlimited mode in our experiment is a better method to explain the results.

We also found that, even though the two games were designed together to evaluate the reaction performance of the subjects, there were some observable differences in the results of each game. Most subjects had better results with the whack-a-mole game than with the hit-the-ball game. The first reason for this result may be because the hit-the-ball game provides some time for the subject to wait before the ball is on the fairway, which might be related to other cognitive abilities. Further related investigations could be explored in the future. The second reason is because the subjects had to choose between the ball or the meteor ball, which might be related to inhibition ability mentioned by [23], which affect reaction time. This result could also be because the subjects played a similar game (like a whack-a-mole machine at an amusement park (especially in Taiwan)) in the past. This result could, thus, indicate muscle memory that was trained several years ago.

Finally, we concluded that the reaction time and accuracy rates can be evaluated using our two serious games while distinguishing between the three different subjects. However, participation of more subjects will be an important factor for future research. We also believe that these research results could be developed to investigate cognitive function for healthy subjects and patients because such results are associated with neural functioning [5,7]. Therefore, we will also observe potential neural cognitive dysfunction using noninvasive methods such as EEG, MRI, and FMRI with our PC-based serious game. We will also conduct intraindividual variability analysis in future studies to observe the behavior of these subjects. Our hope is that these serious games will be used in the daily life lives of elders to evaluate their performance, followed by and to be followed-up by clinical treatment in the future.

Author Contributions: Y.-T.C., C.-J.H., M.-W.H., and Y.-Y.W. planned and supervised the study, and S.-B.H. designed the study. Analyses were performed by N.D. All authors have read and agreed to the published version of the manuscript.

Funding: The authors acknowledge the financial support for this research from the Ministry of Science and Technology Taiwan (grant No. MOST 107-2218-E-367-001 and MOST 108-2634-F-367-001) and the Higher Education Sprout Project of the Ministry of Education (grant No. 13001090182-EDU).

Institutional Review Board Statement: The study was conducted according to the guidelines of the Declaration of Helsinki and approved by the Institutional Review Board (or Ethics Committee) of Taichung Veteran General Hospital (protocol code SF18297A and 16 January 2019).

Informed Consent Statement: Informed consent was obtained from all subjects involved in the study.

Data Availability Statement: Data available on request due to restrictions eg privacy or ethical. The data presented in this study are available on request from the corresponding author. The data are not publicly available due to [Privacy of the Subjects].

Conflicts of Interest: The authors declare no conflict of interest.

References

1. World Health Organization (WHO). Available online: https://www.who.int/news-room/fact-sheets/detail/dementia (accessed on 12 December 2019).
2. Bruce, W.; Rafik, G.; Frank, K.; Mihaela, P.; Alex, M. Design of Games for Measurement of Cognitive Impairment. In Proceedings of the IEEE-EMBS International Conference on Biomedical and Health Informatics (BHI), Valencia, Spain, 1–4 June 2014. [CrossRef]
3. Alzheimer's Disease International. *World Alzheimer Report 2019: Attitude to Dementia*; Alzheimer's Disease International: London, UK, 2019.
4. Lu, M.-H.; Lin, W.; Yueh, H.-P. Development and Evaluation of a Cognitive Training Game for Older People: A Design-based Approach. *Front. Psychol.* **2017**, *8*, 1837. [CrossRef] [PubMed]
5. Jakobsen, L.H.; Sorensen, J.M.; Rask, I.K.; Jensen, B.S.; Kondrup, J. Validation of reaction time as a measure of cognitive function and quality of life in healthy subjects and patients. *Nutrition* **2011**, *27*, 561–570. [CrossRef] [PubMed]
6. Christ, B.U.; Combrinck, M.I.; Thomas, K.G.F. Thomas Both Reaction Time and Accuracy Measures of Intraindividual Variability Predict Cognitive Performance in Alzheimer's Disease. *Front. Hum. Neurosci.* **2018**, *12*, 124. [CrossRef] [PubMed]
7. Chen, K.; Weng, C.; Hsiao, S.; Tsao, W.; Koo, M. Cognitive decline and slower reaction time in elderly individuals with mild cognitive impairment. *Jpn. Psychogeriatr. Soc.* **2017**, *17*, 364–370. [CrossRef] [PubMed]
8. Phillips, M.; Rogers, P.; Haworth, J.; Bayer, A.; Tales, A. Intra-Individual Reaction Time Variability in Mild Cognitive Impairment and Alzheimer's Disease: Gender, Processing Load and Speed Factors. *PLoS ONE* **2013**, *8*, e65712. [CrossRef] [PubMed]
9. Juan, M.F.M.; Vasileios, A. *Diagnosis of Alzheimer's Disease Based on Virtual Environments*; Information, Intelligence, Systems and Applications (IISA): Sandton, South Africa, 2015.
10. Valladares-Rodríguez, S.; Perez-Rodriguez, R.; Facal, D.; Fernández-Iglesias, M.J.; Anido-Rifon, L.; Mouriño-Garcia, M. Design process and preliminary psychometric study of a video game to detect cognitive impairment in senior adults. *PeerJ* **2017**, *5*, e3508. [CrossRef] [PubMed]
11. McCallum, S.; Boletsis, C. Dementia Games: A Literature Review of Dementia-Related Serious Games. In Proceedings of the 4th International Conference on Serious Games Development and Applications (SGDA 2013), Trondheim, Norway, 25–27 September 2013.
12. Regal, P.; Carter, A. Instrumental Activities of Daily Living Questionnaire for Dementia and Mild Cognitive Impairment. *J. Neurol. Res.* **2015**, *5*, 153–159. [CrossRef]

13. Costas, B.; Simon, M. Smartkuber: A Serious Game for Cognitive Health Screening of Elderly Players. *Games Health J.* **2016**, *5*, 241–251.
14. Costas, B.; Simon, M. Evaluating a Gaming System for Cognitive Screening and Sleep Duration Assessment of Elderly Players: A Pilot Study. In *Games and Learning Alliance. GALA 2016*; Lecture Notes in Computer Science; Springer: Berlin/Heidelberg, Germany, 2016; Volume 10056, pp. 107–119.
15. Costas, B.; Simon, M. Augmented Reality Cube Game for Cognitive Training: An Interaction Study. *Stud. Health Technol. Inform.* **2014**, *200*, 81–87. [CrossRef]
16. Fountoulakis, K.N.; Tsolaki, M.; Chantzi, H.; Kazis, A. Mini mental state examination (MMSE): A validation study in Greece. *Am. J. Alzheimer's Dis. Other Dementiasr.* **2000**, *15*, 342–345. [CrossRef]
17. Chi, H.; Agama, E.; Prodanoff, Z.G. Developing serious games to promote cognitive abilities for the elderly. In Proceedings of the 2017 IEEE 5th International Conference on Serious Games and Applications for Health (SeGAH), Perth, Australia, 2–4 April 2017.
18. Allain, P.; Foloppe, D.; Besnard, J.; Yamaguchi, T.; Etcharry-Bouyx, F.; Le Gall, D.; Nolin, P.; Richard, P. Detecting Everyday Action Deficits in Alzheimer's Disease Using a Nonimmersive Virtual Reality Kitchen. *J. Int. Neuropsychol. Soc.* **2014**, *20*, 468–477. [CrossRef] [PubMed]
19. Fontana, E.; Gregorio, R.; Lucia, E.; Carolina, A. TrainBrain: A Serious Game for Attention Training. *Int. J. Comput. Appl.* **2017**, *160*, 1–6. [CrossRef]
20. Fotis, L.; Kurt, D.; Athanasios, V.; Panagiotis, P.; Alina, E. Comparing interaction techniques for serious games through brain-computer interfaces: A user perception evaluation study. *Entertain. Comput.* **2014**, *5*, 391–399.
21. Tong, T.; Chignell, M.; Tierney, M.C.; Lee, J. Developing a Serious Game for Cognitive Assessment:2014 Choosing Settings and Measuring Performance. *JMIR Serious Games* **2016**, *4*, e7. [CrossRef] [PubMed]
22. Tong, T.; Chignell, M.; DeGuzman, C.A. Using a serious game to measure executive functioning: Response inhibition ability. *Appl. Neuropsychol. Adult* **2019**, 1–12. [CrossRef] [PubMed]
23. Tong, T.; Chignell, M.; Tierney, M.C.; Lee, J.S. Test Retest Reliability of a Serious Game for Delirium Screening in the Emergency Department. *Front. Aging Neurosci.* **2016**, *8*, 258. [CrossRef] [PubMed]
24. Shamsuddin, S.N.W.; Ugail, H.; Lesk, V.; Walters, E. VREAD: A Virtual Simulation to Investigate Cognitive Function in the Elderly. In Proceedings of the 2012 International Conference on Cyberworlds, Darmstadt, Germany, 25–27 September 2012.

Article

A Multivariate Randomized Controlled Experiment about the Effects of Mindfulness Priming on EEG Neurofeedback Self-Regulation Serious Games

Nuno M. C. da Costa [1,2,3,4,*], Estela Bicho [2], Flora Ferreira [5], Estela Vilhena [4] and Nuno S. Dias [4,6,*]

1. MIT Portugal Program, University of Minho, 4804-533 Guimarães, Portugal
2. ALGORITMI Center, School of Engineering, University of Minho, 4800-058 Guimarães, Portugal; estela.bicho@dei.uminho.pt
3. Life and Health Sciences Research Institute (ICVS), School of Medicine, University of Minho, 4710-057 Braga, Portugal
4. 2Ai-School of Technology, IPCA, 4750-810, Barcelos, Portugal; evilhena@ipca.pt
5. Center of Mathematics, School of Sciences, University of Minho, 4800-058 Guimarães, Portugal; fjferreira@math.uminho.pt
6. MindProberlabs, 4470-605 Maia, Portugal
* Correspondence: id6814@alunos.uminho.pt (N.M.C.d.C.); ndias@ipca.pt (N.S.D.)

Citation: da Costa, N.M.C.; Bicho, E.; Ferreira, F.; Vilhena, E.; Dias, N.S. A Multivariate Randomized Controlled Experiment about the Effects of Mindfulness Priming on EEG Neurofeedback Self-Regulation Serious Games. *Appl. Sci.* **2021**, *11*, 7725. https://doi.org/10.3390/app11167725

Academic Editor: Marco Gesi

Received: 1 August 2021
Accepted: 20 August 2021
Published: 22 August 2021

Publisher's Note: MDPI stays neutral with regard to jurisdictional claims in published maps and institutional affiliations.

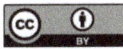

Copyright: © 2021 by the authors. Licensee MDPI, Basel, Switzerland. This article is an open access article distributed under the terms and conditions of the Creative Commons Attribution (CC BY) license (https://creativecommons.org/licenses/by/4.0/).

Featured Application: A mental and emotional state priming BCI to assist Neurofeedback self-regulation serious games.

Abstract: Neurofeedback training (NFT) is a technique often proposed to train brain activity SR with promising results. However, some criticism has been raised due to the lack of evaluation, reliability, and validation of its learning effects. The current work evaluates the hypothesis that SR learning may be improved by priming the subject before NFT with guided mindfulness meditation (MM). The proposed framework was tested in a two-way parallel-group randomized controlled intervention with a single session alpha NFT, in a simplistic serious game design. Sixty-two healthy naïve subjects, aged between 18 and 43 years, were divided into MM priming and no-priming groups. Although both the EG and CG successfully attained the up-regulation of alpha rhythms ($F(1,59) = 20.67$, $p < 0.001$, $\eta_p^2 = 0.26$), the EG showed a significantly enhanced ability ($t(29) = 4.38$, $p < 0.001$) to control brain activity, compared to the CG ($t(29) = 1.18$, $p > 0.1$). Furthermore, EG superior performance on NFT seems to be explained by the subject's lack of awareness at pre-intervention, less vigour at post-intervention, increased task engagement, and a relaxed non-judgemental attitude towards the NFT tasks. This study is a preliminary validation of the proposed assisted priming framework, advancing some implicit and explicit metrics about its efficacy on NFT performance, and a promising tool for improving naïve "users" self-regulation ability.

Keywords: self-regulation; assisted Neurofeedback; neurostimulation; mindfulness; randomized; serious games BCI

1. Introduction

Techniques for self-regulation (SR) of mental states are widely used in clinical, professional, athletic, and the game industry, whether for therapeutic, performance, or entertainment reasons. They include imagery training, music regulation, breathing, meditation, amongst others [1–6]. Many therapeutic implementations of SR have been using serious games to increase user engagement and motivation for anxiety disorders [7], epilepsy [8], attention-deficit/hyperactivity disorder [9], and cognitive training in elders [10]. However, the combined use of SR and serious games is not a mature methodology. Some criticism has been raised, pointing to the need for gradual stimulation, extra personalization of the methodology, and more rigorous validation of its efficacy [7,9].

With the advancement of SR technologies, mechanistic approaches are increasing, such as brain-computer interfaces (BCI) that utilize our ability to learn how to self-regulate brain states when provided with corrective feedback training (in this field SR is also known as self-control) [11–14]. This type of training is defined as neurofeedback training (NFT). Put simply, a neurofeedback (NF) interface works as a virtual "mirror" for neuronal oscillations occurring within the brain, empowering a person to modify them [6–8] explicitly. In this way, NFT acts as a technique to train brain activity SR (in EEG, train brainwave SR). In generic terms, SR is a vital adaptation process to environmental and social challenges. Moreover, SR deficits are linked with diverse behavioural problems and mental disorders such as depression, rumination, distraction, anxiety, stress, and attention control [1,3]. In neurophysiological terms, the adaptation process depends critically on the brain's ability to carefully control the time within—and transitions among—different states [15]. Moreover, NFT promising results attracted the attention and scrutiny of the scientific and medical community, and the technique of NF received criticism concerning the insufficient evaluation, reliability, and validation of its training effects [16]. With the current protocols, the benefits from NFT significantly differ between subjects, with a high percentage of inefficacy (this percentage varies up to ≈50% of non-responders/non-learners, and depending on the protocol, it can be higher). Leading to the frustration of potential users, economic costs, and discredit in NFT and its professionals [5,12,13,17–22].

Multiple mechanisms drive NF SR learning and experimental outcome [14,16]. Nonetheless, it has been hypothesized that an "optimal" self-regulation state is necessary to achieve significant performance in voluntary modulating brainwaves. In this state, the learner should be more engaged, focused (mental focus), undistracted, and mindful of the experiment without judgement of present tasks. Conversely, the learner should avoid self-related thinking (self-monitoring), ruminating, distracting and task-unrelated thoughts, irrelevant associations between internal states and external reward (doubts, questioning, evaluation of progress), and mind-wandering [23–26], suggesting a correlation to focused attention forms of mindfulness meditation (MM). Indeed, during MM, an individual is trained to more efficiently sustain his/her attention toward an intended object (in the current experiment, bodily breathing sensations, BM, and internal imagery of a calm place, IM) and away from external (e.g., external stimulus like sounds, visual cues) or internal sources of distraction (e.g., mind-wandering thoughts) [26–28]. From a dynamical system perspective, the subject needs to "walk" (transition between states) in a trying-sensing continuum until it reaches the "optimal" sensing state [11,15,26]. Therefore, brainwaves SR practice seems closely related to MM, and they both seem to depend upon three core mechanisms: attention control, self-awareness, and emotional regulation [4,25,29,30]. In addition, current "big data" fMRI research investigates the influence of pre-training/priming mechanisms associated with brain structures and NF success [31] and activation levels on NF success [32] to find possible predictors of NFT performance. Moreover, the same group investigated a wide range of different subject- and study-specific factors on real-time fMRI NF success [33], linking the significant positive effect of pre-training to the familiarization of the participants with the NF setup and mental imagery task before NFT runs. Other EEG studies focused on finding predictors from the resting state baseline [22,34–36], psychological factors [23,24,34,37–46], and neurophysiological factors [35,36,47–55].

Additionally, current EEG literature relates these states with up-regulation (synchronization) of alpha rhythm or/and sensory-motor rhythm (SMR), but also with desynchronization (downregulation) of surrounding bands [5,17,18,30,56–61]. The most replicated electro-neurophysiological correlates of MM include phasic increases in the amplitude of EEG alpha oscillations during MM practice and increased resting EEG alpha amplitude. MM and EEG alpha NF have been shown to improve attentional performance and increase full 8–12-Hz EEG alpha amplitude, as shown in the past two decades [4,27,28,30,60,62–67]. As such, EEG alpha rhythm was selected as the feedback signal of interest in the current study.

Based on these previous studies, we hypothesized that it would be possible to develop a "Neurofeedback assisted self-regulation machine" combining the technical, behavioural, psychological, emotional, and electrophysiological components of EEG BCIs, NFT, MM, and SR in a single framework. The current work intends to shed light on the specific question of "how" priming intervention right before NFT (pre-NFT) affects NFT performance (of alpha brainwave) and the emotional state—acquired using qualitative emotional state self-reports and the quantitative emotional state biomarkers of galvanic skin response (GSR) and heart rate variability (HRV). This framework could potentially improve the efficacy of SR serious games targeting therapeutic, performance, or entertainment applications. The current work belongs to a broader three-part study, in which the contributions were: (1) the definition of the foundations of the framework and its design for priming subjects to self-regulate their NF; (2) the development of NeuroPrime [68], an open-source version of the framework in Python for utility, expandability, and reusability; (3) the testing and validation of the framework in different experiments, one previously published [69], that enabled the grasping of the requirements for validation, and the one described in this paper. These preliminary steps aimed to answer what can be gained by developing this framework. Specifically, the fundamental question is, *does priming with external stimulation affect the SR of NF?* Questioning the targets, *which target states (from EEG, GSR, HRV, and self-reports) can be "optimal" for learning SR of brain activity (up-regulation of alpha)?* Regarding the stimulus, *are mindfulness stimuli a good starting primer baseline to arrive at the "optimal" target, compared to, for example, the standard rest baseline tasks?* Measurement-wise, *how can we measure each individual's target performance (learning and behavioural outcomes)?* Regarding the experimental temporal design, *what is the best temporal design to implement the framework?* Regarding the software, *is it possible to develop software to implement this framework?*

This paper focuses on the significance of the current experiment on answering the fundamental question, precisely, which physiological (implicit) and declarative measurements can provide information about the MM priming effects on NFT performance and the emotional state of experimental participants. Hence, following the current NFT experimental checklist [16], we present a randomized controlled intervention with multidimensional signals processing and multivariate statistical analysis.

2. Materials and Methods

2.1. Participants

Criteria. The participants eligible for this study were Portuguese-speaking healthy subjects aged 18–43 years, with normal or corrected-to-normal vision. At study entry, they needed to be naïve or did not perform, at least, in the last year any NFT session. Exclusion criteria were a history of psychiatric or neurological disorders and the taking of psychotropic medications or addictive drugs. In addition, they were requested to give voluntary written informed consent.

Groups sample. Initially, 121 participants were eligible for inclusion. Only 83 were assessed for eligibility, and 62 participants were eventually randomized over two interventions: the experimental priming group (EG, $n = 31$) and the control no-priming group (CG, $n = 31$). Moreover, the priming stimuli (PRIME) and the eyes sequence (ES) of open (EO) and closed (EC) eyes were randomized. The randomization criteria were to balance the groups in sample and gender. Sixty-two participants completed the study; there were no participant dropouts, and no adverse events were recorded. EEG power spectra during the different task conditions were available for 60 participants ($n = 30$ EG, $n = 30$ CG). EEG missing data were due to technical reasons ($n = 1$) and outliers at baseline tasks ($n = 1$). Auxiliary measures like the battery of self-reports and GSR measures were available for the 62 participants, while the HRV was missing data due to technical reasons ($n = 3$). As such, we selected the 60 participants from EEG for the study of this paper. The consort flow diagram of this single session randomized controlled experiment is presented in Figure 1.

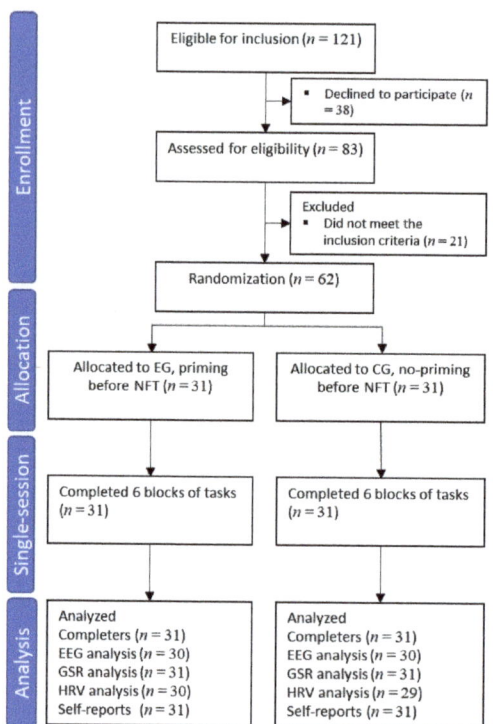

Figure 1. Consort flow diagram of the randomized controlled intervention. Of the 121 participants eligible for inclusion, 38 declined to participate, and 21 did not meet the inclusion criteria. Sixty-two participants were randomized and allocated to the priming and no-priming group. There were no dropouts, and all the subjects completed the tasks. During analysis, missing data from subjects in EEG and HRV were detected, and one CG subject with outlier EEG data was removed.

Procedure. All the protocols were in accordance with the Declaration of Helsinki, and the reported study was approved by an Internal Review Board (IRB), the local Research Ethics Committee of the University of Minho (Subcommission of Life and Health Sciences, SECVS, created under the University of Minho Ethics Commission, CEUM). Written informed consent was obtained before participation. Participants were recruited from the University of Minho student and working community. Intervention measures included questionnaires (psychological traits and states), neuropsychological tasks, EEG, GSR, and HRV.

2.2. Randomizations and Study Blinding

A two-way parallel-group study with balanced randomization in sample and gender was conducted (EG | CG). Randomization was performed using Python "random" package. First, a list of subjects was created with balanced groups (EG | CG, EO | EC, BM | IM) in sample and gender, and then, the list was shuffled using "random.shuffle()" function. From the schedule time slots for experimental acquisition—slot 1 (9:00 a.m. to 11:00 a.m.), slot 2 (11:00 a.m. to 1:00 p.m.), slot 3 (1:00 p.m. to 3:00 p.m.), and slot 4 (3:00 p.m. to 5:00 p.m.)—the participants would choose the slot to be allocated, and they were allocated following the rule first come/first served.

PRIME stimulus (BM | IM) and the ES protocol (EO | EC) were double-blinded, i.e., neither the subject nor the researcher knew the group. The main groups (EG | CG) were single-blinded to the subject.

Power analysis. From a priori analysis, for two dependent groups, a total sample size of 54 (i.e., 27 per group) was calculated (by G*power version 3.1.9 [70]) to be sufficient to detect a medium effect size ($f = 0.25$) in a between moments repeated measure (RM) analysis of variance (ANOVA) with an alpha of 0.05 and a power of 95% (i.e., testing same group intervention on different tasks). While for two independent groups within-moments, a total sample size of 60 (i.e., 30 per group) was only sufficient to detect a large effect size in a one-way ANOVA ($f = 0.47$) and a t-test ($f = 0.86$) with an alpha of 0.05 and a power of 95% (i.e., testing different group interventions on the same task).

2.3. Interventions and Control Condition

Our framework adopts a closed-loop brain state-dependent stimulation (BSDS) design [13] and a simple NFT protocol to test whether mindfulness (focused attention on stimuli) has a role in NF SR. The methodology of a BSDS is to substitute the NFT learner (explicit NF), who is actively engaged and adapting strategies to alter the brain activity in the intended direction, with a stimulator device (implicit NF), which is adapted online to present an experimental stimulus [13]. Hence, our framework for studying brain states and stimuli that complement the NFT for a better self-regulation performance uses the two methodologies for a loop of implicit and explicit training, testing if the implicit priming of the target brain state at pre-NFT (pre-training) can facilitate/scaffold the explicit control of the brain activity towards the target brain state during NFT. Nonetheless, considering that the current experiment represents the first steps within this framework, instead of adapting online the stimulus, we randomized two mindfulness stimuli (BM | IM) to assess the viability of a closed-loop machine learning BSDS framework.

To simplify the analysis of stimulus-response oscillations, PRIME with MM is the target condition, while the resting-state task (REST) is the no-priming control condition.

Priming. The external PRIME stimuli are pure instructional audio manipulations to lead the person from a subjective trying state to a more sensing state before the NFT (pre-training). These transitions can be referred belonging to the trying-sensing continuum discussed by Davelaar and colleagues [26]. During the EO condition, the subject is instructed to "focus on the cross in the centre of the screen and follow the audio-guided instructions", while during the EC condition, the subject is instructed to "close the eyes and follow the audio-guided instructions". The stimuli were adapted from previously published procedures [71], reviewed/transcribed to Portuguese by a specialized mindfulness psychologist, and recorded by a hospital Nurse on macOS using Garageband® software. These meditation instructions are consistent with recent psychological conceptualizations of MM that emphasize the development of attentional abilities combined with a specific, non-judgmental attitude toward the different mental experiences that may arise during MM [4,27–29].

No-priming. The REST task, based on resting-state baseline tasks, is the no-priming control condition. In this type of task, the participant is instructed to "try to relax" for the duration of the task. Moreover, if the task is with EO, the participant is instructed to "focus on the cross in the centre of the screen", while with EC, the participant is instructed to "close the eyes". This choice of control condition was due to the hypothesis that the attentional focus would wander around during the REST control condition when the subject is only instructed to "try to relax".

Additionally, we hypothesize that the MM priming task will promote attentional focus, awareness, and less self-related thinking. Concerning these hypotheses, Davelaar et al. found surprising evidence that the typical instruction, "try to relax and focus on the task", used in NFT and REST tasks, can be detrimental to the learning success [26]. As such, it is expected that the PRIME stimuli, pure implicit instructions guiding the person toward the target subjective experience, can stimulate SR learning performance in short NFT sessions compared to typical REST tasks.

Eyes protocol. To test EO and EC conditions, each subject received a randomized ES intervention. In this study, our distinguishing feature was to use both EO and EC conditions for possible comparisons. Previous single-session studies [42,59,72–74] have tended to use EO conditions for comparisons with the majority of NFT literature in multi-session designs [17,54,60,75,76]. Moreover, the alpha amplitude is generally seen as a function of reduced sensory input from the thalamic nuclei to the cortex [77], and keeping the EO will naturally suppress alpha amplitude relative to an EC condition, providing a lower baseline from which to attempt to increase the alpha amplitude, thereby presumably more amenable to intervention effects via NFT [22,27,78]. Nevertheless, MM is most often practiced with EC in the majority of studies [27,66]. As such, we implemented both conditions, and their resting-state baselines can be used to predict NFT performance [22,35,36,54].

2.4. Experimental Design

The design of the experimental study is represented in the following Figure 2 This study tested 60 participants grouped in 2 interventions: no-priming CG (n = 30) and priming EG (n = 30). Before the intervention, each participant was instructed about the tasks and did the battery of trait self-reports. During the interventions, each participant of CG did a single session of no-priming, while the EG did a single session of priming. The session was divided into six blocks (B), with a total of 14 tasks (T). The first and the last block are equal for the two groups, named block in (Bin) and Block out (Bout). Bin is used to extract the initial baseline threshold from REST EC and EO tasks (T1 and T2 respectably), the first EO NFT, and the first emotional states (using the TMS and POMS). Bout has the same tasks as Bin and serves as the outcome block for comparison. The four blocks between Bin and Bout, B1 to B4, are different for EG and CG. The ES was randomized between two sequences, ES1: EO, EC, EC, EO and ES2: EC, EO, EO, EC. The PRIME stimuli were also randomized between two PRIME sequences (PS), the PS1, BM, IM, BM, IM and PS2: IM, BM, IM, BM. While the CG had a stimuli sequence (SS) of only REST tasks, RS: REST, REST, REST, REST. All participants were randomized between ES1 and ES2 (2 blocks for each condition EO|EC). The CG participants repeated 4 blocks of the REST task (no-priming) followed by the NFT task, while the EG were further randomized between PS1 and PS2 (with two blocks for each condition BM|IM), with each block having the PRIME task followed by the NFT task. After the intervention, participants were tasked to describe the perceived outcome of the experiment and the mental strategy they have used to gain control over the moving bars. The reports were recorded electronically.

NFT Paradigm. The NF system provided audiovisual feedback modality (guided by [13,16]) for increasing alpha power (8–12 Hz). EEG signal was recorded over electrode position Pz. One vertically moving bar, depicting the power of the feedback frequency, was presented on a screen, as shown in Figure 2. The bar in the centre of the screen presented feedback of the alpha power from the Pz channel. Participants were rewarded by getting points, displayed on the feedback screen below the vertical bar and an audible sound cue. Positive feedback was delivered when alpha power increased above an individually calculated threshold. As referred before, at Bin, a 90 s baseline/resting measurement, REST task, was used to define the individual threshold (alpha: mean of alpha power during rest). The thresholds are adapted after each NFT task to prevent the extreme cases of the trained EEG frequency in a single session design due to artefacts [58]: if 90% of epochs are above the threshold, then its value is updated to threshold + 0.1 × threshold and if only 10% of epochs above the threshold then threshold − 0.1 × threshold. The NFT session contained six feedback tasks with four EO NFT runs and two EC NFT runs. Before starting NFT, participants did not receive any specific instruction on how to control the moving bars. They only got the minimal instruction of being physically relaxed, mentally focused, avoiding producing artefacts, and reading the instructions on the screen at the beginning of each block.

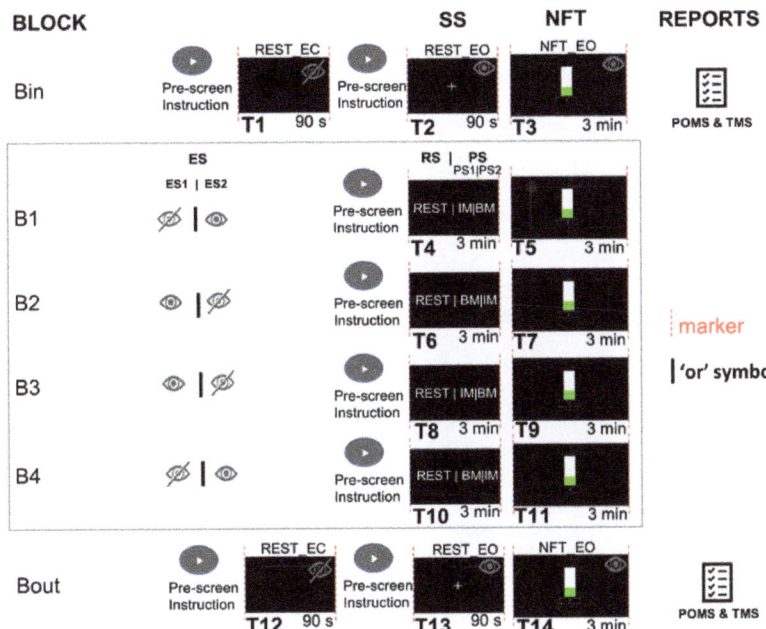

Figure 2. Experiment Block Mockup. Time flows from left to right, top to bottom. In a single session, first, the subject fills the traits self-reports. Then, the training starts. There are 6 blocks and 14 tasks in total. Block in and Block out each begins with rest state with eyes closed then eyes open, followed by alpha NFT. From block 1 to 4, in the EG first is the PRIME, then NFT. In the control group PRIME is substituted by REST. PRIME stimuli are randomized between IM and BM with two PS, PS1 and PS2. Moreover, from blocks 1 to 4, eyes closed and eyes open are randomized between blocks with two ES, ES1, and ES2. In the diagram, the "or" signal is represented by "|". It is used to separate the task for each group or the randomizations of ES (EO | EC) between blocks and the randomizations of PS (BM | IM).

This experimental design enables the study of linear feature changes, within-subjects (i.e., between tasks same group) and between-groups (i.e., same task or combination of tasks in different groups), on the REST, PRIME, and NFT tasks. These feature changes enable to test the main objective: whether the PRIME task before the NFT can facilitate or scaffold the transition to the target brain activity, alpha (see Figure 3).

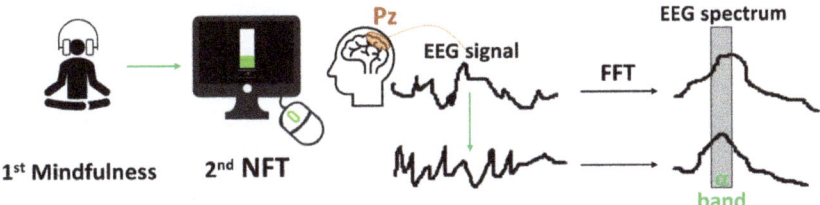

Figure 3. Objective diagram. The external mindfulness stimuli prime the subject to facilitate/scaffold the transition to the target brain activity alpha (α) in the Pz channel during NFT. The EEG spectrum physiological change is also represented.

2.5. Questionnaires

Psychological traits. To investigate different personality traits related to the NF self-regulation performance and for descriptive baseline purposes, participants first completed a sociodemographic questionnaire (SOC), then standard, well-validated Portuguese versions of scales to assess mindfulness, emotional regulation, anxiety, depression, and stress. For mindfulness-related traits, the Five Facet Mindfulness Questionnaire, FFMQ, addressing the traits of *"describe", "observe", "nonjudge", "actaware",* and *"nonreact"* [79,80], was considered. For symptoms of depression, anxiety, and stress, the Depression Anxiety Stress Scale, DASS [81,82], was used. For emotional regulation, the Emotional Regulation Questionnaire, ERQ, measuring *"cognitive reappraisal"* and *"expressive suppression"* [83,84], was applied.

Emotional states. In order to assess the immediate outcomes of the interventions on mood and mindfulness state, participants also completed the Profile of Mood States-Short Form, POMS [85] and the Toronto Mindfulness Scale, TMS [86], which assesses the degree to which participants experience mindful curiosity (e.g., *"I was curious to see what my mind was up to from moment to moment"*) and mindful decentering (e.g., *"I experienced myself as separate from my changing thoughts and feelings"*). Neurofeedback and emotional states results are complementary and offer a way to relate the phenomenological structure of subjective experience with a real-time characterization of large-scale neural operations continuously over the course of the experiment.

For more detail in the trait and states features, go to Appendix A.4.

2.6. Physiological Measures

The EEG, GSR, and HRV signals were continuously acquired to monitor the subjects online during the tasks. The EEG power spectrum, GSR tonic and phasic components of skin conductance level, and HRV photoplethysmography (PPG) signals were collected. The features extracted and analysed from each signal are described in more detail in Appendices A.1–A.3, respectively.

2.7. Recordings

EEG signals were acquired with a 32 channels amplifier ActiCHamp® from Brain Products GmbH. The cap from EASYCAP GmbH has a unified, optimized layout based on an international 10–20 localization system. The ground is located at Fpz position and is a reference-free montage. Any referencing is done post hoc in the software. Before electrode placement, the skin was prepared with a mild skin cleanser, ethanol 70% V/V, to help improve the impedance and conductance of electrodes. Then, electrodes were affixed with a conductive viscose gel, SuperVisc®, high viscosity electrolyte gel for active electrodes, EASYCAP GmbH. Impedances were checked before starting the experiment to be below 30 kOhm and critical channels below 10 KOhm, and the signal was visually inspected to find possible channels with noise. The computer screen was placed 60 cm from the edge of the table. The mouse was only used by the researcher while the keyboard was placed at the edge, close to the participant, so he could use it to interact with the task interface. A cup of water was always present for the subject to drink if needed. Moreover, Bluetooth wireless headphones were used for a lesser impact over the electrodes, consequently less prone to artefacts. A new biosignals device, James One from MindProber Portugal, with a built-in GSR sensor and a PPG sensor that allows HRV measurements [87,88]. The biodevices were placed in the left hand of all the participants, even if they were lefties. GSR sensor was placed in the palm, and the PPG sensor was placed in the index finger. Additionally, a tablet was used to acquire the self-reports answers digitally using Google Forms®.

2.8. Multidimensional Signals Processing

Software. The online experimental paradigm was built from the ground up on Python open-source language, synthesizing and using the best-tested parts of specific BCI and EEG modules. For more detail on NeuroPrime, check [68]. The offline data analysis pipelines were run first in Brain Vision Analyzer (Brain Products GmbH) for visual inspection of noisy channels, noisy epochs, and the processing pipeline's automation planning. Then, NeuroPrime (with Python modules like MNE) was used for advanced signal processing/classification and automation of the pipeline [68].

NFT. During the EEG NFT online loop, the data were updated at an average rate of 200 ms in each iteration. It was concatenated in an epoch buffer of 1 s, meaning that the epoch is made from 800 ms of historical data and 200 ms of new data. There is no real-time loop in the offline analysis, the entire length of each task is analysed instead, and during pre-processing, these data were segmented into epochs of 1 s. Continuous EEG measurements were band-pass filtered with a low cut-off of 1 Hz and a high cut-off value of 40 Hz using a finite impulse response filter (FIR). The original sampling of 1 kHz was not subsampled to maintain a higher resolution on the fast Fourier transform (FFT). Although a common-reference was used for online data analysis, the data are re-referenced to an average-reference previously to offline data processing. Four EEG channels were selected for further processing: Fp1, Fp2, Fz, and Pz. In both online and offline processing pipelines, we excluded epochs with abnormally large amplitudes with a maximum peak-to-peak of over ± 100 µV for online and ± 150 µV for offline and also based on the flatness of the signal with a minimum peak-to-peak acceptance of ± 0.5 µV. Additionally, in offline analysis, epochs contaminated by spurious gross-movement and other non-stereotyped artefacts were also identified by visual inspection and additionally rejected. Afterwards, during processing, the band power values were extracted from the power spectrum of the Pz channel (for theta 4–8 Hz, alpha 8–12 Hz, SMR 12–15 Hz, beta 15–35 Hz). For a list of descriptions of all the EEG features, please go to Appendix A.1.

GSR and HRV. They were continuously monitored for all the participants during the session. Each signal was acquired at a 1 s interval. GSR tonic (skin conductance level—SCL) and phasic components (skin conductance responses—SCR) were extracted offline from each 1 s interval, with an exosomatic direct current sensor [87]. HRV time domain, frequency domain, and non-linear domain features were extracted from the 1 s PPG RR-intervals [88]. For a list of descriptions of all the features, please go to Appendix A.3.

2.9. Data Analysis

Theoretically, an NFT framework implies that any observable measure of brain activity can be extracted and tested for volitional control. Nonetheless, what constitutes successful control, and how to quantify it? In the engineering sense, successful control can be viewed as enhancing the signal-to-noise ratio of a parameter relative to a control condition, a reference condition (e.g., resting-state, sham, or sensory stimulation without control), which could be administered sequentially or interspersed randomly in the experiment [11].

EEG measure. In the current work, the EEG band measure assessing NFT successful control is based on the suggested measures from Dempster and Vernon [89] that can be used to assess feature changes of brain activity during NF. We choose to study changes in absolute values of the alpha amplitude of the Pz channel, reflecting brief and temporally unstable increases over time from the learner. Then, this power spectra measure was $\log_{10}$-transformed to obtain normally distributed data.

Group domains. Apart from the intervention groups (EG, CG) and EEG measures, the additional multivariate data are grouped in four domains, two belonging to qualitative data while the other two are quantitative. Qualitative data are the subject traits groups domain (TG = FFMQ, DASS, ERQ) and emotional states group domain (SG = TMS, POMS). Quantitative emotional states are divided into the skin response (GSR) and heart rate variability (HRV) domains. Each one of these domains and its respective features is detailed in Appendix A.

Statistical Analysis. Statistical analysis was performed using the R language. Significance was assumed if $p < 0.05$ (two-tailed). Demographic data at pre-intervention (T0, referring to the moment right before starting the training session) were compared between groups with one-way ANOVA or χ^2 test with Fisher exact correction. Significant group effects at Bin EC and EO baseline tasks were further explored to locate group differences in band profile using one-way ANOVA. RM ANOVAs were calculated for each condition (REST EC, REST EO, and NFT EO) and frequency band (theta, alpha, SMR, beta) with time (Bin versus Bout) as within-subject factors, and the intervention group (EG vs. CG) as between-subject factor. Only time effects, group main effects, and interactions with a group are reported. For the main outcomes, mean difference and 95% confidence interval [95% CI] are reported. Effect sizes are reported as partial eta-squared (η_p^2), with effects interpreted as small (0.01), medium (0.06), or large (0.14). Afterwards, to perform single session analysis, individual NFT performance was quantified by regression slopes of the trained alpha feedback frequency across the intervention blocks B1 to B4 (regression slopes have a mathematical component of within and between tasks). For that, B1 to B4 were further break down in EO only tasks and EC only tasks, culminating in 3 tasks per subject: "*restBin*", the baseline REST task to get the initial threshold at Bin; "*nft1*", the first NFT task preceded by priming (in the EG) or no-priming (in the CG) and "*nft2*", the second block of NFT preceded by priming or no-priming. Regression slopes were estimated individually (predictor variable = feedback task number; dependent variable = z-transformed power of alpha) and subsequently averaged per group domain (based on [30]). Additionally, to verify group domain effects on NF learning apart from priming (EG) and no-priming (CG), the same alpha regression analysis was performed on two subgroups of participants according to the features in each domain. Each feature (qualitative or quantitative variable) was converted into a dichotomous variable: high value (HV) and low value (LV), representing the groups above and below the best central measure, respectively. We found that the best central measure was mean = (maximum + minimum)/2 for the quantitative regression slopes and the qualitative data of the 60 participants. As such, the statistical hypothesis testing was centred on comparing the regression slopes from each group of HV with LV, HV with zero, and LV with zero. When considering the grouped frequency distribution of HV in the different domains (represent how frequent each HV value occurred within each domain), we selected features with similar HV frequencies in both EG and CG and with nine or more subjects (at least ≈ 1/3 of the EG and CG sample) for balanced comparisons because we are not only comparing with zero slopes but also HV versus LV. One-sample *t*-tests were calculated for each group to test whether the regression slope is different from zero and between groups to test whether the two regression slopes are different. Only features with significant time effects, group main effects, and interactions with groups are reported.

3. Results

3.1. Group Characteristics

At pre-intervention before the training session starts, T0, there were no differences between the intervention groups (EG, CG) in age, gender, and education, see Table 1. There were no baseline differences between groups at Bin in alpha and SMR power during EO and EC tasks in the Pz electrode (using the $\log_{10}$ transformation). However, there were some baseline differences between groups in theta EC ($p < 0.05$) and beta EC ($p < 0.01$) and EO ($p < 0.05$). The number of artefact-free segments was always above 40% of the total task segments.

3.2. EEG Power Spectrum at Pre and Post Priming Intervention

RM ANOVA results for each condition and frequency band are shown in Table 2. $\log_{10}$-transformed EEG power spectra of theta, alpha, SMR, and beta frequency bands at pre- (Bin) and post- (Bout) priming intervention are shown in Figure 4.

Looking at Table 2, the main findings in all the population were a significant decrease between Bin and Bout for the REST EC condition in alpha and beta and an increase in SMR, while for the REST EO a significant increase in theta, alpha, SMR, and beta. As for the NFT EO, a significant increase in theta and alpha was observed. A significant interaction $T \times G$ (time × group) was found for theta value on the REST EC task, while the value of theta in CG group decreases from Bin to Bout. In the EG group, this value is slightly increased. This last result can be confirmed in Figure 4, as well as the similar behaviour of the EG and CG between Bin and Bout.

Table 1. Group characteristics at preintervention (T0) (for $n = 60$).

	EG ($n = 30$)		CG ($n = 30$)		p-Value	
	M	SD	M	SD	F	p
Demographic						
Age (years)	28.87	7.40	27.50	6.38	0.587	ns
Gender (F/M)	18/12		19/11		0.00 [a]	ns
Education (9/12/15/17/21)	0/3/10/12/5		0/8/8/11/3		5.01 [b]	ns
Conditions						
ES (ES1/ES2)	16/14		15/15		0.0 [a]	ns
SS (RS/PS1/PS2)	0/15/15		30/0/0		_[c]	_[c]
Baseline Bands						
theta (EC/EO)	−0.02/−0.16	0.28/0.2	0.27/−0.05	0.42/0.24	9.75/3.92	**/ns
alpha (EC/EO)	0.52/−0.015	0.61/0.47	0.82/0.19	0.56/0.45	3.90/3.04	ns/ns
SMR (EC/EO)	−0.15/−0.35	0.55/0.40	−0.07/−0.28	0.55/0.38	0.23/0.53	ns/ns
beta (EC/EO)	−0.75/−0.94	0.27/0.23	−0.56/−0.79	0.28/0.22	7.31/6.30	**/*

EG, experimental group; CG, control group; M, mean; SD, standard deviation; EC, eyes closed; EO, eyes open; F, female; M, Male; ES, eyes sequence; ES1 and ES2, eyes sequence 1 and 2; SS, stimuli sequence; RS, REST sequence; PS1 and PS2, PRIME sequence 1 and 2. Education level values refer to the number of participants (n) reporting the number of years completed in one of the following five-category: (1) $n \geq 9$, ninth grade; (2) $n \geq 12$, Secondary; (3) $n \geq 15$, Bachelor's degree; (4) $n \geq 17$, Master's degree; (5) $n \geq 21$, Ph.D. Significant tests are marked with asterisks (* $p < 0.05$, ** $p < 0.01$). [a] χ^2 ($df = 1$); [b] χ^2 ($df = 5$). Stimuli sequence (SS) is intended to be different for the CG and the EG.

Table 2. RM ANOVA of pre-(Bin) and postintervention (Bout) power spectra for three conditions.

Task		T			T × G	
		F	η_p^2	Bout-Bin	F	η_p^2
REST EC	theta	3.98	0.06	−0.050	4.86 *	0.08
	alpha	5.04 *	0.08	−0.061	0.01	<0.001
	SMR	4.67 *	0.09	0.054	<0.001	<0.001
	beta	4.45 *	0.07	−0.033	2.13	0.04
REST EO	theta	8.89 **	0.13	0.056	0.64	0.01
	alpha	18.17 ***	0.24	0.096	0.07	0.001
	SMR	33.62 ***	0.38	0.015	0.61	0.01
	beta	5.21 *	0.08	0.033	0.01	<0.001
NFT EO	theta	4.41 *	0.07	0.039	0.77	0.01
	alpha	20.67 ***	0.26	0.109	0.65	0.01
	SMR	0.02	<0.001	0.015	0.02	<0.001
	beta	0.79	0.01	0.012	0.17	0.003

REST, the rest task; NFT, the alpha neurofeedback training; EC, eyes closed, EO, eyes open; T, time; G, group. Bout-Bin, the difference between $\log_{10}$ means from the 60 subjects. Significant tests are marked with asterisks (* $p < 0.05$, ** $p < 0.01$, *** $p < 0.001$).

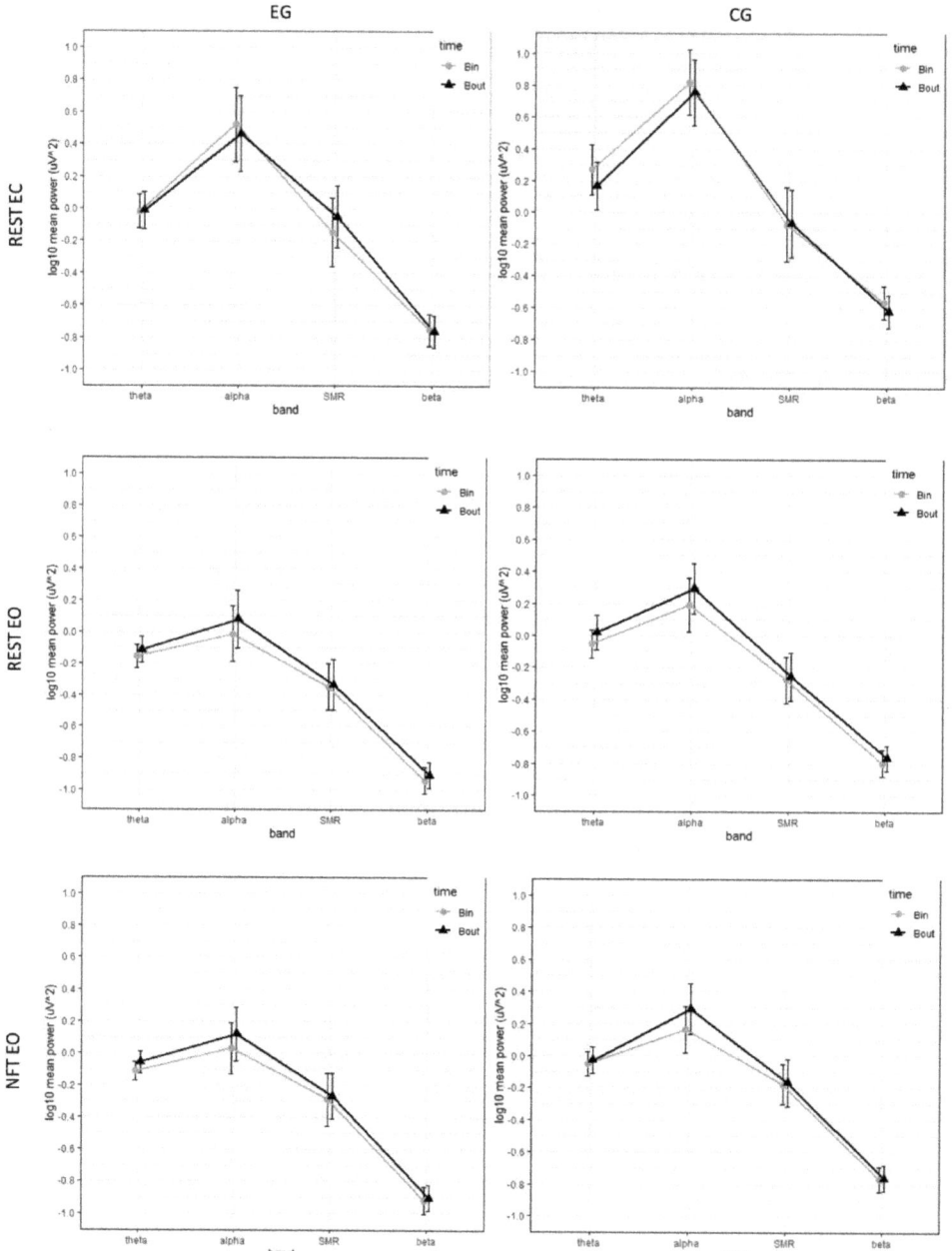

Figure 4. EEG power spectra at Bin and Bout. Estimated marginal means are log-transformed absolute power (μV^2) with 95% confidence intervals. During REST EC, both groups show reductions in alpha, CG also has reductions in theta, while EG increases SMR. While for the REST EO, both groups show up-regulation of alpha, similarly to the NFT EO task.

3.3. NFT Performance in Different Group Domains at Intervention Blocks

As demonstrated in the previous section, results from EO tasks require a different analysis from EC tasks. Therefore, the tasks were analysed separately, as described in Section 2.9.

Regarding the analysis of no-priming (CG) and the priming (EG) results, both groups increased their alpha during EO (voluntarily) and decreased during EC after one session of NFT (Figure 5). These changes were reflected by linear increase and decrease of the power, respectively, matching the results discussed in the previous section at pre- and post-intervention (Figure 4)

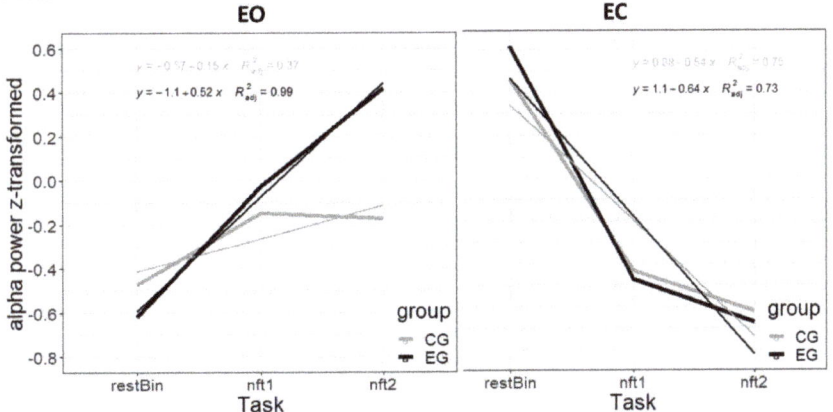

Figure 5. Z-transformed EEG power at intervention blocks. Alpha z-transformed power over the baseline (restBin) and NFT tasks for EO condition and EC at intervention blocks (nft1 and nft2). Three regression slopes are presented separately for CG and EG. Additionally, the regression equations are depicted as well as the regression lines for each group are indicated by thinner lines. The regression slopes at intervention blocks show a significant alpha increase for the EG in the EO condition. In contrast, the EC condition shows a similar downregulation of alpha in both groups.

When individual alpha was regressed on EO NFT tasks, 24 out of 30 EG (80%) participants and 17 out of 30 CG (57%) participants were able to linearly increase their alpha, as suggested by positive individual regression slopes. Checking further, considering half of the maximal slope as the threshold (0.80 = 45.83°) instead of a zero slope, 12 out of 24 (50%) EG participants and 6 out of 17 CG (35%) were able to increase above this slope. One sample t-tests revealed that regression slopes in the EG ($t(29) = 4.38$, $p < 0.001$) were significantly larger than zero, while the CG were not ($t(29) = 1.18$, $p > 0.1$). We also directly compared the slopes between groups. A t-test revealed a significant difference between the slopes of the EG and CG ($t(58) = -2.10$, $p < 0.05$). We have similar results for the EC NFT tasks, as 24 out of 30 EG participants and 24 out of 30 CG participants had negative regression slopes. From these, 17 out of 24 EG and 16 out of 24 CG (~70%) participants had greater negative slopes than half the minimal slope ($-0.72 = -41.14°$). One sample t-tests revealed that regression slopes in the EG ($t(29) = -5.53$, $p < 0.000001$) and CG ($t(29) = -4.50$, $p < 0.001$) were significantly smaller than zero. A t-test revealed no difference between the negative slopes of the EG and CG ($t(58) = 0.62$, $p > 0.05$). As such, we decided to only verify in EO condition the existence of group domain effects on NF learning apart from the EG and CG.

To verify the group domain effects, the first column of Table 3 depicts the HV frequency distribution of each significant domain feature (according to the methodology described in Section 2.9). The subsequent columns represent the average alpha power slope for the HV and LV groups and their t-test's. Considering the alpha regression slope, in the TG domain, the EG with LV of *"actware"* (those acting with less awareness) at T0 (pre-intervention) were the most effective on increasing alpha power in the EO condition. For the SG domain, LV of reported *"vigour"* at Bout in the EG led to the most significant EO NFT performance in this domain, followed by HV of *"decentering"* at Bin and HV of *"tension"* changes (as the difference Bout-Bin). While for the CG, LV of *"fatigue"* changes (as the difference Bout-Bin) led to the most significant EO NFT performance, followed by LV *"confusion"* changes. Considering the GSR regression slopes at intervention blocks, the EG participants with LV of *"scl std"* (standard deviation of the tonic baseline skin conductance level), as well as those with LV of *"scr sumResp"* slope (sum of the amplitudes of phasic event skin conductance responses) had better efficacy on increasing alpha power during EO NFT performance. While for the CG participants, those with HV of *"scl mean"* (mean of the tonic baseline skin conductance level) led to significant alpha slopes during EO NFT. Considering the HRV domain, the alpha power slopes (55 subjects because of missing HRV values) during the EO NFT performance were most significant for the EG participants with LV of *"rmssd"* (it reflects high-frequency influences on HRV—fast or parasympathetic, those influencing larger changes from one beat to the next). In contrast, the CG participants with HV of *"sdnn"* significantly decreased alpha during EO NFT performance.

Table 3. Table by domain at intervention blocks. Alpha z-transformed power over the baseline (restBin) and NFT tasks for EO condition at intervention blocks (nft1 and nft2).

Domain	Feature	HV Frequencies (EG/CG)	EO EG [HV^{p1}/LV^{p2}]^{p3}	EO CG [HV^{p1}/LV^{p2}]^{p3}
TG	FFMQ actaware	13/16	[0.16/0.79 ***] ++	[0.35/−0.08]
SG	TMS decentering (Bin)	18/19	[0.69 ***/0.27]	[0.07/0.29]
	POMS Vigour (Bout)	13/15	[0.2/0.76 ***] +	[0.22/0.09]
	POMS confusion (Bout-Bin)	12/13	[0.64 **/0.44 *]	[−0.23/0.44 *] ++
	POMS fatigue (Bout-Bin)	18/21	[0.48 **/0.58 *]	[−0.06/0.63 *] +
	POMS tension (Bout_Bin)	17/20	[0.69 ***/0.3]	[0.04/0.38]
GSR	GSR scl_mean	19/15	[0.39 */0.74 **]	[0.46 **/−0.15] +
	GSR scl_std	15/17	[0.36/0.68 ***]	[0.1/0.22]
	GSR scr_sumResp	11/10	[0.4/0.59 ***]	[0.24/0.11]
HRV	HRV sdnn	15/15	[0.48 */0.56 *]	[0.44 */−0.12] +
	HRV rmssd	14/9	[0.35/0.69 ***]	[0.23/0.17]

HV, high value; LV, low value; All, EG and CG subjects; EO, eyes open, EC, eyes closed; EG, experimental priming group; CG, control no-priming group. HV frequencies (the frequency distribution) represent how frequently each HV value occurred within each EG and CG domain. Total sample = 60; EG = 30; CG = 30; Total HV = EG HV + CG HV; Total LV = 60—Total HV; EG LV = 30—EG HV; CG LV = 30—CG HV. Note for HRV data: Total = 55, EG = 28 and CG = 27. Statistically significant non-zero regression slopes, $p1$ and $p2$, marked with an asterisk (* $p < 0.05$, ** $p < 0.01$, *** $p < 0.001$). Statistically significant differences between the two regression slopes from HV and LV, $p3$, groups are marked with a cross (+ $p < 0.05$, ++ $p < 0.01$, +++ $p < 0.001$). Green represents the significant results.

4. Discussion

We investigated the ability to gain control over one's brain with the assistance of priming MM techniques right before NFT runs, compared to the no-priming REST tasks.

In this single session design, as initially predicted, the behaviours at pre- and post-priming intervention are similar between the EG and CG. Nonetheless, the EG during the EO intervention blocks showed an improved ability to control their brain activity compared to the CG. While for the EC blocks, a downregulation on both groups was evident. As such, in EC condition, we need further analysis to separate intervention feature changes from the possible downregulation reflex occurring in the Pz channel after closing the eyes, as physiologically expected. Alpha activity in the EEG is dominant during an eyes-closed resting condition and is suppressed during visual stimulation [22,78]. Additionally, the profile of theta power is always lower than alpha (see Figure 4). This result is generally the case in adults during normal wakefulness and, in this case, focus on tasks [90].

Furthermore, within the EG, the most significant subjects on increasing alpha power during NFT had low values of the awareness trait (at pre-intervention) and reported more signs of built-up tension and less *"vigour"* at the end of the experiment protocol (Bout). As such, subjects with a low capacity to act with awareness benefited more from priming, and the demand for focused attention on internal sensations through guiding audio increased the subject's emotional state of tension and lack of vigour. In contrast, the CG participants didn't express these emotional states, as they were not guided and were only required to stare at the screen. Another distinctive EG feature is the higher decentering at Bin, which is connected to the learner's "optimal" state. It reflects higher situational self-awareness (self-regulated awareness of thoughts and feelings), i.e., a capacity of non-judgement by avoiding distractive task-unrelated thoughts—"awareness of one's experience with some distance and disidentification rather than being carried away by one's thoughts and feelings" [86].

Concerning the GSR biomarkers, the EG participants with low changes of SCL standard deviation from the baseline (an almost zero slope between *"baseline"*, *"nft1"* and *"nft2"*) and low changes of SCR sum seem to perform the best. This finding seems to be in line with the literature, since lower values of SCL standard deviation and SCR sum during task performance usually reflect less arousal (diminished stimulation of the sympathetic nervous system) and perhaps, explaining a less stressful, relaxed, and non-judgement attitude (towards stimuli, thoughts or feelings) during task performance [91,92]. Concerning the HRV metrics, the EG participants with low changes of HRV *"rmssd"* values from the baseline (low high-frequency variations of vagal parasympathetic components) performed better, and it might show a more effective task engagement of the subject during the NFT task [93,94]. In contrast, the CG performers had an increase of SCL mean and an increase of HRV *"sdnn"*. In the case of HRV, the literature suggests that a higher baseline HRV is related to concomitants of better self-control and higher vagal withdrawal scores to better attention control and emotional regulation [94–96]. As such, the biomarker results seem to suggest that mindfulness priming stimulates engagement and a relaxed and non-judgement attitude in alpha NFT performers. Nonetheless, these claims must be interpreted with caution, as there is still observable publication bias.

General Discussion and Future Proposals

This work demonstrates a significant effect in priming versus no-priming on NFT performance. In future priming designs, the priming stimuli sequence can be adjusted to the subject's performance in real-time instead of the current protocol's random mindfulness priming sequence. While priming protocols lack some consistency and are not yet ready to be implemented on final products like SR serious games, they potentially provide an essential layer of personalization and mutual game-player adaptation. Actually, a review of attention-deficit hyperactivity disorder (ADHD) randomized control trials indicated that the long-term effects of personalized NF interventions were superior to non-personalized NF [97]. To optimize self-regulation learning, future work will also address the use of neural networks to learn the sequence of stimuli that leads the subject towards their personalized "optimal" state (e.g., using reinforcement learning, deep learning for time series forecasting with long short-term memory networks, multilayer perceptron's, convolutional neural networks, between others). The framework should adapt to the user pace (even slow down user pace if needed) and regulate/control the user's brain state according to the target.

Mindfulness priming seems to facilitate learning in the current single session context, while REST tasks do not. Thus, REST tasks do not seem to be the best primer for this type of protocol. We find it imperative for baseline primer tasks to be discussed and improved since the instruction "try to relax" and even "focus on the cross" does not seem sufficient to diminish self-related mental processes and target a relaxed or/and attentive state (also discussed by Davelaar et al. [26])—leading to uncertain brain states. Although the baseline REST task is often used as a predictor of NFT performance [22,35], the difficulty in monitoring its effects on the brain and emotional states is still meaningful. Therefore, the assumption that a guided instructional approach based on mindfulness techniques can better target a relaxed and focused attention state seems valid. Thus, it is a step further for a more consistent NF operant protocol.

In summary, we addressed the proposed questions in the present work. Regarding the fundamental question, *"Does priming with external stimulation affect the self-regulation of NF?"*, we were able to find significance in priming with MM external neurostimulation. Priming increases the number of subjects with better NFT performance during intervention blocks. As such, some implicit factors in priming were affecting the explicit control of NFT, especially in subjects with a low self-awareness trait. Concerning the mental target state, the hypothesized "optimal" target state seems to correspond to the actual state needed for the learner to self-regulate brain activity, i.e., situational self-awareness (*"decentering"*, a non-judgement attitude towards stimuli, thoughts, or feelings) and task engagement. Following this answer and regarding the stimuli, it seems that MM stimuli are a significant primer to arrive at the "optimal" target. Indeed, the best performers from the EG showed distinct emotional state from the best performers of the CG, as qualitatively analysed by the self-reports' dimensions (*"decentering"*,*" vigour"*, *"tension"*) and quantitively by the GSR (SCL SD, SCR sum) and HRV (*"rmsdd"*) domains. Measurement-wise, the EEG $\log_{10}$ transformed amplitudes, and z-transformed regression slopes seem suitable to track session changes. Nevertheless, future publications will consider other measurements, e.g., the percent time spent in the desired brain state by Vernon and Dempster [77], because it reflects different aspects of brain activity. The percent of time reflects slight differences within the training that are temporally stable, while amplitude reflects brief and unstable increases over time. In the trait self-reports, the *"actware"* of FFMQ predicts that low self-awareness users will significantly benefit from priming. Regarding the subjective experience, it seems essential to target the *"decentering"* dimension of the TMS scale, and the POMS scores seem to quantify the moods relative to the intervention correctly. Moreover, HRV and GSR features seem to correctly separate some emotional states between the EG best performers and the CG best performers. As such, MM priming seems to target mechanisms that scaffold the subject into a superior NF operant. In the future, such mechanisms still need to be discriminated from NF-specific (related to training a target neurophysiological variable), NF non-specific (dependent on the NF context, but independent from the act of controlling a particular brain signal), or general-non-specific mechanisms (including the common benefits of cognitive training as well as psychosocial influences) [16].

We should also not forget that this framework will not substitute other self-regulation mind-body techniques, such as physical exercise, musical training, and meditation, among others. We consider this framework a mechanistic approach to SR techniques, a researching tool for priming the capacity to self-regulate on SR serious games for therapy, performance, and entertainment.

5. Conclusions

This study developed a human-computer framework to assist the SR of NF, aiming to decrease the number of unsuccessful practitioners (non-responders/non-learners) of SR tasks. The assistance was done by priming the subject with mindfulness guided instructions right before the explicit NFT. This intervention was the first step to demonstrate that priming with external stimulation assists NF SR in serious games design and potentially turns NFT non-responders into responders. The main results showed that priming with mindfulness stimuli enables higher significance of EEG target self-regulation during the EO priming intervention blocks in a single session design. Additionally, from the self-reports and biomarkers, the most significant priming performers had low values of the awareness trait at pre-intervention, showed a higher *"decentering"* (situational awareness) at the end of the first block (Bin), and reported signs of built-up tension and less *"vigour"* at the end of the experiment protocol (Bout). As such, especially on subjects with a low capacity to act with awareness, the demand for focused attention on internal sensations through guiding audio seems likely to implicitly support the subject's emotional regulation capacity. In turn, it should increase NFT task engagement and target situational awareness.

Nonetheless, there are remaining questions to be solved that should be addressed in further experiments. In the future, we should be able to: experiment the priming effects in a multi-session design and check if they are only crucial for the first session of the NFT or if they support the subject throughout the multi-session; test different temporal designs to find the best design for this type of framework; find the "optimal" mechanisms that should be primed and validate stimuli able to prime them; test if MM audio-guided is the "optimal" stimuli at priming NF SR mechanisms or if other categories of stimuli or stimuli personalization have better efficacy in leading the subject into the "optimal" learning state; evaluate the hypothesis that non-responders/non-learners depend on the priming protocol personalization, i.e., that non-responders/non-learners can be turned into a responders/learners. In this way, we are trying to answer that brain activity self-regulation can be scaffolded by implicitly priming the "optimal" state at pre-NFT, limiting the number of non-optimal mechanisms, and potentiating optimal mechanisms that affect NF SR performance.

Scaling up this priming assistance research, we envision a machine controller that uses neural networks to classify and select the required neurostimulation to arrive at the desired target—this way, outsourcing the difficulty of sensing the correct mental strategies. Moreover, the machine controller should assist the participant to gravitate/walk towards the desired mental state by implicit neurostimulation, which can affect explicit self-neuromodulation.

In conclusion, we took the first steps towards a better NF operant. Showing that priming with mindfulness stimuli enables higher significance of EEG target self-regulation in a single session. In this way, we find appropriate further research of priming right before NFT for a more precise methodology in this field.

Author Contributions: Conceptualization, N.M.C.d.C. and N.S.D.; Data curation, N.M.C.d.C., F.F. and E.V.; Formal analysis, F.F. and E.V.; Funding acquisition, N.S.D.; Investigation, N.M.C.d.C.; Methodology, N.M.C.d.C., E.B. and N.S.D.; Project administration, E.B. and N.S.D.; Resources, N.S.D.; Software, N.M.C.d.C.; Supervision, E.B. and N.S.D.; Writing—original draft, N.M.C.d.C.; Writing—review & editing, E.B., F.F., E.V. and N.S.D. All authors have read and agreed to the published version of the manuscript.

Funding: This work is co-financed by the ERDF—European Regional Development Fund through the Operational Program for Competitiveness and Internationalisation—COMPETE 2020 (ref.: POCI-01-0145-FEDER-007043; ref: POCI-01-0145-FEDER-007038), the North Portugal Regional Operational Program—NORTE 2020 (ref.: NORTE-01-0145-FEDER-000045) and by the Portuguese Foundation for Science and Technology – FCT under MIT Portugal (author Ph.D. grant ref.: PD/BD/114033/2015) and within the R&D Units Project Scope (ref.: UIDB/00319/2020).

Institutional Review Board Statement: The study was conducted according to the guidelines of the Declaration of Helsinki and approved by the Institutional Review Board (or Ethics Committee) of Subcommission of Life and Health Sciences, SECVS, created under the University of Minho Ethics Commission, CEUM (protocol code: SECVS 011/2018, date: 8 of May 2018, Braga).

Informed Consent Statement: Informed consent was obtained from all subjects involved in the study. Participants were recruited from the University of Minho student and working community. Intervention measures included questionnaires (psychological traits and states), neuropsychological tasks, EEG, GSR, and HRV.

Acknowledgments: Materials and conditions for experimental development were provided by ICVS, University of Minho, Portugal, by ALGORITMI, University do Minho, Portugal, by 2Ai, Polytechnic Institute of Cávado and Ave, Portugal and by MindProber Labs, Porto, Portugal.

Conflicts of Interest: The authors declare no conflict of interest.

Appendix A

Appendix A.1. EEG Features

Sample rate: 1000 Hz.
Feature region of interest (ROI): Pz.
Features extracted per subject:

- [theta, alpha, SMR, beta]: list of bands extracted.
- epoch_a: epochs array of each task = [[band mean, standard deviation] ... , [n-epoch]]. Bands power spectrum density (PSD) is calculated from 1000 samples per second.

The measure used to detect brain activity changes due to neurofeedback [89]:

- Mean: changes in absolute values of frequency band mean amplitude (power spectra measures were log_{10}-transformed to obtain normally distributed data), reflecting brief and temporally unstable increases over time from the learner.

Appendix A.2. GSR Features

Sample rate: 100 Hz.
Features extracted per subject:

- epoch_a: epochs array of each task = [[TIMESTAMP, SAMPLE_COUNTER, GSR_VALUE,], ... , [n-epoch]]. Each epoch is 1 sample of GSR value, calculated from the 100 samples per second.

Tonic GSR Features, skin conductance level (SCL) [91,92]:

- scl_mean: GSR mean per task.
- scl_std: GSR standard deviation per task.

Phasic GSR Feature, skin conductance responses (SCR) [91,92]:

- scr_sumResp: sum of response amplitude per task.

Appendix A.3. HRV Features

Sample rate: 100 Hz.
Features extracted per subject:

- epoch_a: epochs array of each task = [[TIMESTAMP, SAMPLE_COUNTER, BPM_VALUE, RR_VALUE], ... , [n-epoch]]. Each epoch is 1 sample of RR value, calculated from the 100 samples per second.

Time Domain Features [93,98]:

Mainly used on long-term recordings (24 h), but some studies use some of these statistical features on short term recordings such as in our case, from 1 to 5 min window.

- sdnn: The standard deviation of the time interval between successive normal heart beats (i.e., the RR-intervals).
- rmssd: The square root of the mean of the sum of the squares of differences between adjacent NN-intervals. Reflects high frequency (fast or parasympathetic) influences on HRV (i.e., those influencing larger changes from one beat to the next).

Appendix A.4. Self-Reports Features

The reader can check out the digital forms at the following links:

- First questionnaire at T0 (pre-intervention): https://forms.gle/2uT7f7oH3pd4c9FD9 (accessed on 21 August 2021).
- Second questionnaire at Bin: https://forms.gle/nQNRQkBWEVtbKySo8 (accessed on 21 August 2021).
- Third questionnaire at Bout: https://forms.gle/k1zVwzwVacu7hBYRA (accessed on 21 August 2021).

Appendix A.4.1. Traits (TG)

See the form online (1st questionnaire).

FFMQ

Five dimensions were obtained by summing the items: [describe, observe, nonjudge, actaware, nonreact].

(R) = reverse item.

- Observe. "I notice the smells and aromas of things."
- Describe. "I am good at finding words to describe my feelings."
- Actaware (acting with awareness). "I find myself doing things without paying awareness attention" (R).
- Nonjudge (nonjudging of inner emotions). "I think some of my emotions are bad or experience inappropriate and I should not feel them"(R).
- Nonreact (nonreactivity to inner emotions). "I perceive my feelings and emotions experience without having to react to them."

ERQ

Two dimensions were obtained by summing the items: [cognitive reappraisal, expressive suppression].

- Cognitive reappraisal. Where a person attempts to change how he or she thinks about a situation in order to change its emotional impact.
- Expressive suppression. "I keep my emotions to myself"—where a person attempts to inhibit the behavioural expression of his or her emotions.

DASS

Three dimensions were obtained by summing the items: [stress, anxiety, depression].

Appendix A.4.2. Sates (SG)

TMS

Two dimensions obtained by summing the items: [curiosity, decentering].

Decentering: awareness of one's experience with some distance and disidentification rather than being carried away by one's thoughts and feelings.

Curiosity: reflect awareness of present moment experience with a quality of curiosity.

POMS

Four dimensions obtained by summing the items: [tension, fatigue, vigour, confusion].

- Tension: state of preoccupation and muscle tension.
- Fatigue: state of tiredness, inertia, boredom.
- Confusion: state of confusion.
- Vigour: state of energy and physical and psychological vigour.

References

1. Damasio, A.R. *Self Comes to Mind: Constructing the Conscious Brain*; Pantheon Books: New York, NY, USA, 2010; ISBN 9780307378750.
2. Gruzelier, J. Differential effects on mood of 12–15 (SMR) and 15–18 (beta1) Hz neurofeedback. *Int. J. Psychophysiol.* **2014**, *93*, 112–115. [CrossRef]
3. Heatherton, T.F. Neuroscience of Self and Self-Regulation. *Annu. Rev. Psychol* **2011**, *62*, 363–390. [CrossRef]
4. Tang, Y.-Y.; Hölzel, B.K.; Posner, M.I. The neuroscience of mindfulness meditation. *Nat. Rev. Neurosci.* **2015**, *16*, 213–225. [CrossRef]
5. Gruzelier, J. EEG-neurofeedback for optimising performance. II: Creativity, the performing arts and ecological validity. *Neurosci. Biobehav. Rev.* **2013**, *44*, 142–158. [CrossRef]

6. Jin, J.; Xiao, R.; Daly, I.; Miao, Y.; Wang, X.; Cichocki, A. Internal Feature Selection Method of CSP Based on L1-Norm and Dempster-Shafer Theory. *IEEE Trans. Neural Netw. Learn. Syst.* **2020**, 1–12. [CrossRef]
7. Pinheiro, J.; de Almeida, S.R.; Marques, A. Emotional self-regulation, virtual reality and neurofeedback. *Comput. Hum. Behav. Rep.* **2021**, *4*, 100101. [CrossRef]
8. Ninaus, M.; Witte, M.; Kober, S.E.; Friedrich, E.V.C.; Kurzmann, J.; Hartsuiker, E.; Neuper, C.; Wood, G. Neurofeedback and serious games. *Psychol. Pedagog. Assess. Serious Games* **2013**, 82–109. [CrossRef]
9. Coenen, F.; Scheepers, F.E.; Palmen, S.J.M.; de Jonge, M.V.; Oranje, B. Serious Games as Potential Therapies: A Validation Study of a Neurofeedback Game. *Clin. EEG Neurosci.* **2020**, *51*, 87–93. [CrossRef]
10. Israsena, P.; Jirayucharoensak, S.; Hemrungrojn, S.; Pan-Ngum, S. Brain Exercising Games with Consumer-Grade Single-Channel Electroencephalogram Neurofeedback: Pre-Post Intervention Study. *JMIR Serious Games* **2021**, *9*, e26872. [CrossRef]
11. Ros, T.; Baars, B.; Lanius, R.R.A.; Vuilleumier, P.; Baars, B.J.; Lanius, R.R.A.; Vuilleumier, P. Tuning pathological brain oscillations with neurofeedback: A systems neuroscience framework. *Front. Hum. Neurosci.* **2014**, *8*, 1008. [CrossRef]
12. Sitaram, R.; Ros, T.; Stoeckel, L.; Haller, S.; Scharnowski, F.; Lewis-Peacock, J.; Weiskopf, N.; Blefari, M.L.; Rana, M.; Oblak, E.; et al. Closed-loop brain training: The science of neurofeedback. *Nat. Rev. Neurosci.* **2016**, *18*, 86–100. [CrossRef]
13. Enriquez-Geppert, S.; Huster, R. EEG-neurofeedback as a tool to modulate cognition and behavior: A review tutorial. *Front. Hum.* **2017**, *11*, 51. [CrossRef]
14. Davelaar, E. Mechanisms of neurofeedback: A computation-theoretic approach. *Neuroscience* **2017**, *378*, 175–188. [CrossRef] [PubMed]
15. Gu, S.; Cieslak, M.; Baird, B.; Muldoon, S.F.; Grafton, S.T.; Pasqualetti, F.; Bassett, D.S. The Energy Landscape of Neurophysiological Activity Implicit in Brain Network Structure. *Sci. Rep.* **2018**, *8*, 2507. [CrossRef] [PubMed]
16. Ros, T.; Enriquez-Geppert, S.; Zotev, V.; Young, K.D.; Wood, G.; Whitfield-Gabrieli, S.; Wan, F.; Vuilleumier, P.; Vialatte, F.; Van De Ville, D.; et al. Consensus on the reporting and experimental design of clinical and cognitive-behavioural neurofeedback studies (CRED-nf checklist). *Brain* **2020**, *143*, 1674–1685. [CrossRef] [PubMed]
17. Zoefel, B.; Huster, R.J.; Herrmann, C.S. Neurofeedback training of the upper alpha frequency band in EEG improves cognitive performance. *NeuroImage* **2010**, *54*, 1427–1431. [CrossRef]
18. Gruzelier, J. EEG-neurofeedback for optimising performance. I: A review of cognitive and affective outcome in healthy participants. *Neurosci. Biobehav. Rev.* **2013**, *44*, 124–141. [CrossRef]
19. Thibault, R.; Veissière, S.; Olson, J.; Raz, A. Treating ADHD with suggestion: Neurofeedback and placebo therapeutics. *J. Atten. Disord.* **2018**, *22*, 707–711. [CrossRef]
20. Zuberer, A.; Brandeis, D. Are treatment effects of neurofeedback training in children with ADHD related to the successful regulation of brain activity? A review on the learning of regulation of brain activity and a contribution to the discussion on specificity. *Front. Hum.* **2015**, *9*, 135. [CrossRef]
21. Alkoby, O.; Abu-Rmileh, A.; Shriki, O.; Todder, D. Can We Predict Who Will Respond to Neurofeedback? A Review of the Inefficacy Problem and Existing Predictors for Successful EEG Neurofeedback Learning. *Neuroscience* **2018**, *378*, 155–164. [CrossRef] [PubMed]
22. Nan, W.; Wan, F.; Tang, Q.; Wong, C.M.; Wang, B.; Rosa, A. Eyes-Closed Resting EEG Predicts the Learning of Alpha Down-Regulation in Neurofeedback Training. *Front. Psychol.* **2018**, *9*, 1607. [CrossRef] [PubMed]
23. Witte, M.; Kober, S.E.S.; Ninaus, M.; Neuper, C.; Wood, G. Control beliefs can predict the ability to up-regulate sensorimotor rhythm during neurofeedback training. *Front. Hum. Neurosci.* **2013**, *7*, 478. [CrossRef]
24. Ninaus, M.; Kober, S.E.; Witte, M.; Koschutnig, K.; Stangl, M.; Neuper, C.; Wood, G. Neural substrates of cognitive control under the belief of getting neurofeedback training. *Front. Hum. Neurosci.* **2013**, *7*, 914. [CrossRef]
25. Wood, G.; Kober, S.; Witte, M. On the need to better specify the concept of "control" in brain-computer-interfaces/neurofeedback research. *Front. Syst.* **2014**, *8*, 171. [CrossRef]
26. Davelaar, E.J.; Barnby, J.M.; Almasi, S.; Eatough, V. Differential Subjective Experiences in Learners and Non-learners in Frontal Alpha Neurofeedback: Piloting a Mixed-Method Approach. *Front. Hum. Neurosci.* **2018**, *12*, 402. [CrossRef]
27. Chow, T.; Javan, T.; Ros, T.; Frewen, P. EEG Dynamics of Mindfulness Meditation Versus Alpha Neurofeedback: A Sham-Controlled Study. *Mindfulness* **2017**, *8*, 572–584. [CrossRef]
28. Tang, Y. *The Neuroscience of Mindfulness Meditation: How the Body and Mind Work Together to Change Our Behaviour*; Palgrave Macmillan: London, UK, 2017. [CrossRef]
29. Lutz, A.; Slagter, H.A.; Dunne, J.D.; Davidson, R.J. Attention regulation and monitoring in meditation. *Trends Cogn. Sci.* **2008**, *12*, 163–169. [CrossRef]
30. Kober, S.; Witte, M.; Ninaus, M. Ability to Gain Control Over One's Own Brain Activity and its Relation to Spiritual Practice: A Multimodal Imaging Study. *Front. Hum.* **2017**, *11*, 271. [CrossRef]
31. Zhao, Z.; Yao, S.; Zweerings, J.; Zhou, X.; Zhou, F.; Kendrick, K.M.; Chen, H.; Mathiak, K.; Becker, B. Putamen volume predicts real-time fMRI neurofeedback learning success across paradigms and neurofeedback target regions. *Hum. Brain Mapp.* **2021**, *42*, 1879–1887. [CrossRef]
32. Haugg, A.; Sladky, R.; Skouras, S.; McDonald, A.; Craddock, C.; Kirschner, M.; Herdener, M.; Koush, Y.; Papoutsi, M.; Keynan, J.N.; et al. Can we predict real-time fMRI neurofeedback learning success from pre-training brain activity? *Hum. Brain Mapp.* **2020**, *41*, 3839–3854. [CrossRef]

33. Haugg, A.; Renz, F.M.; Nicholson, A.A.; Lor, C.; Götzendorfer, S.J.; Sladky, R.; Skouras, S.; McDonald, A.; Craddock, C.; Hellrung, L.; et al. Predictors of real-time fMRI neurofeedback performance and improvement—A machine learning mega-analysis. *Neuroimage* **2021**, *237*, 118207. [CrossRef] [PubMed]
34. Diaz Hernandez, L.; Rieger, K.; Koenig, T. Low Motivational Incongruence Predicts Successful EEG Resting-state Neurofeedback Performance in Healthy Adults. *Neuroscience* **2018**, *378*, 146–154. [CrossRef] [PubMed]
35. Reichert, J.L.; Kober, S.E.; Neuper, C.; Wood, G. Resting-state sensorimotor rhythm (SMR) power predicts the ability to up-regulate SMR in an EEG-instrumental conditioning paradigm. *Clin. Neurophysiol.* **2015**, *126*, 2068–2077. [CrossRef] [PubMed]
36. Wan, F.; Nan, W.; Vai, M.; Rosa, A. Resting alpha activity predicts learning ability in alpha neurofeedback. *Front. Hum.* **2014**, *8*, 500 [CrossRef] [PubMed]
37. Hardman, E.; Gruzelier, J.; Cheesman, K.; Jones, C. Frontal interhemispheric asymmetry: Self regulation and individual differences in humans. *Neuroscience* **1997**, *221*, 117–120. [CrossRef]
38. Egner, T.; Gruzelier, J. Learned self-regulation of EEG frequency components affects attention and event-related brain potentials in humans. *NeuroReport* **2001**, *12*, 4155–4159. [CrossRef]
39. Nijboer, F.; Sellers, E.; Mellinger, J.; Jordan, M. A P300-based brain–computer interface for people with amyotrophic lateral sclerosis. *Clinical* **2008**, *119*, 1909–1916. [CrossRef]
40. Dickhaus, T.; Sannelli, C.; Müller, K.R.; Curio, G.; Blankertz, B. Predicting BCI performance to study BCI illiteracy. *BMC Neurosci* **2009**, *10*, P84. [CrossRef]
41. Kleih, S.; Nijboer, F.; Halder, S.; Kübler, A. Motivation modulates the P300 amplitude during brain–computer interface use. *Clin. Neurophysiol.* **2010**, *121*, 1023–1031. [CrossRef]
42. Hammer, E.M.; Halder, S.; Blankertz, B.; Sannelli, C.; Dickhaus, T.; Kleih, S.; Müller, K.R.; Kübler, A. Psychological predictors of SMR-BCI performance. *Biol. Psychol.* **2012**, *89*, 80–86. [CrossRef] [PubMed]
43. Kober, S.E.S.; Witte, M.; Ninaus, M.; Neuper, C.; Wood, G. Learning to modulate one's own brain activity: The effect of spontaneous mental strategies. *Front. Hum. Neurosci.* **2013**, *7*, 695. [CrossRef] [PubMed]
44. Enriquez-Geppert, S.; Huster, R.J.; Herrmann, C.S. Boosting brain functions: Improving executive functions with behavioral training, neurostimulation, and neurofeedback. *Int. J. Psychophysiol.* **2013**, *88*, 1–16. [CrossRef]
45. Ruiz, S.; Buyukturkoglu, K.; Rana, M.; Birbaumer, N.; Sitaram, R. Real-time fMRI brain computer interfaces: Self-regulation of single brain regions to networks. *Biol. Psychol.* **2014**, *95*, 4–20. [CrossRef] [PubMed]
46. Hammer, E.; Kaufmann, T.; Kleih, S. Visuo-motor coordination ability predicts performance with brain-computer interfaces controlled by modulation of sensorimotor rhythms (SMR). *Front. Hum.* **2014**, *8*, 574. [CrossRef]
47. Kotchoubey, B.; Strehl, U.; Holzapfel, S. Negative potential shifts and the prediction of the outcome of neurofeedback therapy in epilepsy. *Clinical* **1999**, *110*, 683–686. [CrossRef]
48. Neumann, N.; Birbaumer, N. Predictors of successful self control during brain-computer communication. *J. Neurol. Neurosurg.* **2003**, *74*, 1117–1121. [CrossRef] [PubMed]
49. Blankertz, B.; Sannelli, C.; Halder, S.; Hammer, E.M.; Kübler, A.; Müller, K.R.; Curio, G.; Dickhaus, T. Neurophysiological predictor of SMR-based BCI performance. *NeuroImage* **2010**, *51*, 1303–1309. [CrossRef]
50. Weber, E.; Köberl, A.; Frank, S.; Doppelmayr, M. Predicting successful learning of SMR neurofeedback in healthy participants: Methodological considerations. *Appl. Psychophysiol. Biofeedback* **2011**, *36*, 37–45. [CrossRef]
51. Nan, W.; Rodrigues, J.P.; Ma, J.; Qu, X.; Wan, F.; Mak, P.-I.; Mak, P.U.; Vai, M.I.; Rosa, A. Individual alpha neurofeedback training effect on short term memory. *Int. J. Psychophysiol.* **2012**, *86*, 83–87. [CrossRef]
52. Halder, S.; Varkuti, B.; Bogdan, M.; Kübler, A.; Rosenstiel, W.; Sitaram, R.; Birbaumer, N. Prediction of brain-computer interface aptitude from individual brain structure. *Front. Hum. Neurosci.* **2013**, *7*, 105. [CrossRef]
53. Enriquez-Geppert, S.; Huster, R.; Scharfenort, R. The morphology of midcingulate cortex predicts frontal-midline theta neurofeedback success. *Front. Hum. Neurosci.* **2013**, *7*, 453. [CrossRef] [PubMed]
54. Nan, W.; Wan, F.; Vai, M.I.; Da Rosa, A.C. Resting and Initial Beta Amplitudes Predict Learning Ability in Beta/Theta Ratio Neurofeedback Training in Healthy Young Adults. *Front. Hum. Neurosci.* **2015**, *9*, 677. [CrossRef] [PubMed]
55. Weber, L.A.; Ethofer, T.; Ehlis, A.C. Predictors of neurofeedback training outcome: A systematic review. *NeuroImage Clin.* **2020**, *27*, 102301. [CrossRef] [PubMed]
56. Klimesch, W.; Sauseng, P.; Hanslmayr, S. EEG alpha oscillations: The inhibition-timing hypothesis. *Brain Res. Rev.* **2007**, *53*, 63–88. [CrossRef]
57. Gruzelier, J.; Thompson, T.; Redding, E.; Brandt, R. Application of alpha/theta neurofeedback and heart rate variability training to young contemporary dancers: State anxiety and creativity. *Int. J. Psychophysiol.* **2014**, *93*, 105–111. [CrossRef]
58. Kober, S.E.; Schweiger, D.; Witte, M.; Reichert, J.L.; Grieshofer, P.; Neuper, C.; Wood, G. Specific effects of EEG based neurofeedback training on memory functions in post-stroke victims. *J. Neuroeng. Rehabil.* **2015**, *12*, 107. [CrossRef] [PubMed]
59. Hanslmayr, S.; Sauseng, P.; Doppelmayr, M.; Schabus, M.; Klimesch, W. Increasing individual upper alpha power by neurofeedback improves cognitive performance in human subjects. *Appl. Psychophysiol. Biofeedback* **2005**, *30*, 1–10. [CrossRef]
60. Gruzelier, J.; Inoue, A.; Smart, R.; Steed, A.; Steffert, T. Acting performance and flow state enhanced with sensory-motor rhythm neurofeedback comparing ecologically valid immersive VR and training screen scenarios. *Neurosci. Lett.* **2010**, *480*, 112–116. [CrossRef]

61. Van Lutterveld, R.; Houlihan, S.; Pal, P.; Sacchet, M.; McFarlane-Blake, C.; Patel, P.R.; Sullivan, J.S.; Ossadtchi, A.; Druker, S.; Bauer, C.; et al. Source-space EEG neurofeedback links subjective experience with brain activity during effortless awareness meditation. *NeuroImage* **2016**, *151*, 117–127. [CrossRef]
62. Aftanas, L.; Golosheikin, S. Changes in cortical activity in altered states of consciousness: The study of meditation by high-resolution EEG. *Hum. Physiol.* **2003**, *29*, 143–151. [CrossRef]
63. Cahn, B.R.; Polich, J. Meditation states and traits: EEG, ERP, and neuroimaging studies. *Psychol. Bull.* **2006**, *132*, 180–211. [CrossRef]
64. Lagopoulos, J.; Xu, J.; Rasmussen, I.; Vik, A.; Malhi, G.S.; Eliassen, C.F.; Arntsen, I.E.; Sæther, J.G.; Hollup, S.; Holen, A.; et al. Increased theta and alpha EEG activity during nondirective meditation. *J. Altern. Complement. Med.* **2009**, *15*, 1187–1192. [CrossRef]
65. Chiesa, A.; Serretti, A. A systematic review of neurobiological and clinical features of mindfulness meditations. *Psychol. Med.* **2010**, *40*, 1239–1252. [CrossRef] [PubMed]
66. Lomas, T.; Ivtzan, I.; Fu, C.H.Y. A systematic review of the neurophysiology of mindfulness on EEG oscillations. *Neurosci. Biobehav. Rev.* **2015**, *57*, 401–410. [CrossRef] [PubMed]
67. Navarro Gil, M.; Escolano Marco, C.; Montero-Marín, J.; Minguez Zafra, J.; Shonin, E.; García Campayo, J. Efficacy of Neurofeedback on the Increase of Mindfulness-Related Capacities in Healthy Individuals: A Controlled Trial. *Mindfulness* **2018**, *9*, 303–311. [CrossRef]
68. Da Costa, N.M.C. Nmc-Costa/Neuroprime: A Framework for Real-Time HCI/BCI. Specifically Developed for Advanced Human-Computer Assisted Self-Regulation of Neurofeedback. Available online: https://github.com/nmc-costa/neuroprime (accessed on 19 April 2020).
69. Da Costa, N.M.C.; Bicho, E.G.; Dias, N.S. Priming with mindfulness affects our capacity to self-regulate brain activity? In Proceedings of the 2020 IEEE 8th International Conference on Serious Games and Applications for Health (SeGAH), Online, 12–14 August 2020; pp. 1–8. [CrossRef]
70. Faul, F.; Erdfelder, E.; Lang, A.G.; Buchner, A. G*Power 3: A flexible statistical power analysis program for the social, behavioral, and biomedical sciences. In *Proceedings of the Behavior Research Methods*; Psychonomic Society Inc.: Chicago, IL, USA, 2007; Volume 39, pp. 175–191. Available online: https://link.springer.com/content/pdf/10.3758/BF03193146.pdf (accessed on 21 August 2021).
71. Frewen, P.A.; Unholzer, F.; Logie-Hagan, K.R.J.; MacKinley, J.D. Meditation Breath Attention Scores (MBAS): Test-Retest Reliability and Sensitivity to Repeated Practice. *Mindfulness* **2014**, *5*, 161–169. [CrossRef]
72. Ros, T.; Théberge, J.; Frewen, P.A.; Kluetsch, R.; Densmore, M.; Calhoun, V.D.; Lanius, R.A. Mind over chatter: Plastic up-regulation of the fMRI salience network directly after EEG neurofeedback. *NeuroImage* **2013**, *65*, 324–335. [CrossRef]
73. Peeters, F.; Ronner, J.; Bodar, L.; van Os, J.; Lousberg, R. Validation of a neurofeedback paradigm: Manipulating frontal EEG alpha-activity and its impact on mood. *Int. J. Psychophysiol.* **2013**, *93*, 116–120. [CrossRef] [PubMed]
74. Wells, R.; Outhred, T.; Heathers, J.A.J.; Quintana, D.S.; Kemp, A.H. Matter over mind: A randomised-controlled trial of single-session biofeedback training on performance anxiety and heart rate variability in musicians. *PLoS ONE* **2012**, *7*, e46597. [CrossRef] [PubMed]
75. Angelakis, E.; Stathopoulou, S.; Frymiare, J.L.; Green, D.L.; Lubar, J.F.; Kounios, J. EEG neurofeedback: A brief overview and an example of peak alpha frequency training for cognitive enhancement in the elderly. *Clin. Neuropsychol.* **2007**, *21*, 110–129. [CrossRef]
76. Van Boxtel, G.J.M.; Denissen, A.J.M.; Jäger, M.; Vernon, D.; Dekker, M.K.J.; Mihajlović, V.; Sitskoorn, M.M. A novel self-guided approach to alpha activity training. *Int. J. Psychophysiol.* **2012**, *83*, 282–294. [CrossRef]
77. Vernon, D.; Dempster, T.; Bazanova, O.; Rutterford, N.; Pasqualini, M.; Andersen, S. Alpha Neurofeedback Training for Performance Enhancement: Reviewing the Methodology. *J. Neurother.* **2009**, *13*, 214–227. [CrossRef]
78. Barry, R.J.; Clarke, A.R.; Johnstone, S.J.; Magee, C.A.; Rushby, J.A. EEG differences between eyes-closed and eyes-open resting conditions. *Clin. Neurophysiol.* **2007**, *118*, 2765–2773. [CrossRef]
79. Baer, R.A.; Smith, G.T.; Lykins, E.; Button, D.; Krietemeyer, J.; Sauer, S.; Walsh, E.; Duggan, D.; Williams, J.M.G. Construct validity of the five facet mindfulness questionnaire in meditating and nonmeditating samples. *Assessment* **2008**, *15*, 329–342. [CrossRef]
80. Gregório, S.; Gouveia, J.P. Facetas de mindfulness: Características psicométricas de um instrumento de avaliação. *Psychologica* **2011**, 259–279. [CrossRef]
81. Crawford, J.R.; Henry, J.D. The Depression Anxiety Stress Scales (DASS): Normative data and latent structure in a large non-clinical sample. *Br. J. Clin. Psychol.* **2003**, *42*, 111–131. [CrossRef] [PubMed]
82. Pais-Ribeiro, J.L.; Honrado, A.; Leal, I. Contribuição para o Estudo da Adaptação Portuguesa das Escalas de Ansiedade, Depressão e Stress (EADS) de 21 itens de Lovibond e Lovibond. *Psicol. Saúde Doenças* **2004**, *5*, 229–239.
83. Lovibond, P.; Lovibond, S. The structure of negative emotional states: Comparison of the Depression Anxiety Stress Scales (DASS) with the Beck Depression and Anxiety Inventories. *Behav. Res. Ther.* **1995**, *33*, 335–343. [CrossRef]
84. Vaz, F.; Martins, C.; Martins, E.C. Diferenciação emocional e regulação emocional em adultos portugueses. *Psicologia* **2008**, *22*, 123. [CrossRef]
85. Viana, M.; Almeida, P.; Santos, R. Adaptação Portuguesa da Versão Reduzida do Perfil de Estados de Humor: POMS. *Aná. Psicol.* **2001**, *19*, 77–92. [CrossRef]

86. Lau, M.A.; Bishop, S.R.; Segal, Z.V.; Buis, T.; Anderson, N.D.; Carlson, L.; Shapiro, S.; Carmody, J.; Abbey, S.; Devins, G. The toronto mindfulness scale: Development and validation. *J. Clin. Psychol.* **2006**, *62*, 1445–1467. [CrossRef]
87. Moreira, P.S.; Chaves, P.; Dias, R.; Dias, N.; Almeida, P.R. Validation of wireless sensors for psychophysiological studies. *Sensors* **2019**, *19*, 4824. [CrossRef] [PubMed]
88. Correia, B.; Dias, N.; Costa, P.; Pêgo, J.M. Validation of a Wireless Bluetooth Photoplethysmography Sensor Used on the Earlobe for Monitoring Heart Rate Variability Features during a Stress-Inducing Mental Task in Healthy Individuals. *Sensors* **2020**, *20*, 3905. [CrossRef] [PubMed]
89. Dempster, T.; Vernon, D. Identifying indices of learning for alpha neurofeedback training. *Appl. Psychophysiol. Biofeedback* **2009**, *34*, 309–318. [CrossRef] [PubMed]
90. Louis, E.K.S.; Frey, L.C.; Britton, J.W.; Frey, L.C.; Hopp, J.L.; Korb, P.; Koubeissi, M.Z.; Lievens, W.E.; Pestana-Knight, E.M.; Louis, E.K.S. The Normal EEG. 2016. Available online: https://www.ncbi.nlm.nih.gov/books/NBK390343/ (accessed on 21 August 2021).
91. Boucsein, W.; Fowles, D.C.; Grimnes, S.; Ben-Shakhar, G.; Roth, W.T.; Dawson, M.E.; Filion, D.L. Publication recommendations for electrodermal measurements. *Psychophysiology* **2012**, *49*, 1017–1034. [CrossRef]
92. Posada-Quintero, H.F.; Chon, K.H. Innovations in Electrodermal Activity Data Collection and Signal Processing: A Systematic Review. *Sensors* **2020**, *20*, 479. [CrossRef]
93. Malik, M.; John Camm, A.; Thomas Bigger, J.; Breithardt, G.; Cerutti, S.; Cohen, R.J.; Coumel, P.; Fallen, E.L.; Kennedy, H.L.; Kleiger, R.E.; et al. Heart rate variability: Standards of measurement, physiological interpretation, and clinical use. *Circulation* **1996**, *93*, 1043–1065. [CrossRef]
94. Zahn, D.; Adams, J.; Krohn, J.; Wenzel, M.; Mann, C.G.; Gomille, L.K.; Jacobi-Scherbening, V.; Kubiak, T. Heart rate variability and self-control—A meta-analysis. *Biol. Psychol.* **2016**, *115*, 9–26. [CrossRef]
95. Beauchaine, T. Vagal tone, development, and Gray's motivational theory: Toward an integrated model of autonomic nervous system functioning in psychopathology. *Dev. Psychopathol.* **2001**, *13*, 183–214. [CrossRef]
96. Graziano, P.; Derefinko, K. Cardiac vagal control and children's adaptive functioning: A meta-analysis. *Biol. Psychol.* **2013**, *94*, 22–37. [CrossRef]
97. Pimenta, M.G.; Brown, T.; Arns, M.; Enriquez-Geppert, S. Treatment Efficacy and Clinical Effectiveness of EEG Neurofeedback as a Personalized and Multimodal Treatment in ADHD: A Critical Review. *Neuropsychiatr. Dis. Treat.* **2021**, *17*, 637. [CrossRef] [PubMed]
98. Champseix, R. Aura-Healthcare/Hrv-Analysis: Package for Heart Rate Variability Analysis in Python. Available online: https://github.com/Aura-healthcare/hrv-analysis (accessed on 12 May 2021).

Article

Hybrid Spine Simulator Prototype for X-ray Free Pedicle Screws Fixation Training

Sara Condino [1,*], Giuseppe Turini [2], Virginia Mamone [1], Paolo Domenico Parchi [3] and Vincenzo Ferrari [1]

1. Information Engineering Department, University of Pisa, 56126 Pisa, Italy; virginia.mamone@unipi.it (V.M.); vincenzo.ferrari@unipi.it (V.F.)
2. Department of Computer Science, Kettering University, Flint, MI 48504, USA; gturini@kettering.edu
3. 1st Orthopaedic and Traumatology Division, Department of Translational Research and of New Surgical and Medical Technologies, University of Pisa, 56124 Pisa, Italy; paolo.parchi@unipi.it
* Correspondence: sara.condino@unipi.it

Abstract: Simulation for surgical training is increasingly being considered a valuable addition to traditional teaching methods. 3D-printed physical simulators can be used for preoperative planning and rehearsal in spine surgery to improve surgical workflows and postoperative patient outcomes. This paper proposes an innovative strategy to build a hybrid simulation platform for training of pedicle screws fixation: the proposed method combines 3D-printed patient-specific spine models with augmented reality functionalities and virtual X-ray visualization, thus avoiding any exposure to harmful radiation during the simulation. Software functionalities are implemented by using a low-cost tracking strategy based on fiducial marker detection. Quantitative tests demonstrate the accuracy of the method to track the vertebral model and surgical tools, and to coherently visualize them in either the augmented reality or virtual fluoroscopic modalities. The obtained results encourage further research and clinical validation towards the use of the simulator as an effective tool for training in pedicle screws insertion in lumbar vertebrae.

Keywords: surgical simulation; augmented reality; spine surgery; hybrid simulator; pedicle screws fixation training; unity game engine

1. Introduction

Simulation is becoming an essential part of surgical training as it allows for repetitive practice in a safe controlled environment whose complexity can be tailored to the trainee's expertise level and needs. Currently, there is a consensus among the orthopedic community that the acquisition of trainees' surgical skills should commence in a simulated training environment prior to progression to the surgical room [1] in order to improve surgical outcomes and patient safety.

Pedicle screws fixation, the gold standard among posterior instrumentation techniques to stabilize spine fusion, is a technically demanding procedure which requires long training to avoid catastrophic neurovascular complications due to screw misplacement. The risk of misplacement, which is exacerbated by the complexity of the anatomy (e.g., deformity of the spine together with dysplastic anatomy) can be very high, indeed literature studies report an error rate of 10–40% [2,3].

This leads to the need of enriching traditional educational methods, largely based on the Halstedian model "see one, do one, teach one" [4], with surgical training sessions outside the operating theatre. According to the literature, cadavers are an effective medium for teaching surgical skill outside the operating room due to their realism [5]; however, their availability may be limited and their use has ethical, legal, and cost implications [6].

Since a few years ago, the use of three-dimensional (3D)-printed spine models has been emerging as a low-cost, easy-to-handle, and store alternative which allows the overcoming of ethical issues and/or legal constraints of training on cadavers [7].

Today, 3D printing is playing an emerging role in the domain of orthopedic education, allowing the development of high-fidelity anatomical reproductions which can be fruitfully used to learn and understand the pathological anatomy, but also to plan a surgical procedure, and to simulate surgical steps using real orthopedic instruments [8]. Furthermore, patient specific 3D-printed spine models, obtained starting from computed tomography (CT) images, overcome the intrinsic morphological constraints of cadavers. In fact, a user may wish to rehearse a particular surgical case or anatomical variation, but it is unlikely to find ex-vivo tissues that exhibit the desired pathology. Recent literature studies show that life-size 3D-printed spine models can be an excellent tool for training beginners in the use of free-hand pedicle screw instrumentation [9], enabling the training course administrator to select the surgical case from a digital library of anatomical models, and to tailor the simulation difficulty level to fit the needs of the learner [7].

3D printing of patient-specific models offers great benefits for surgical training and rehearsal, and also overcomes limits of standard commercial mannequins which cover a very limited range of individual differences and pathologies. However, a recent review [10] on orthopedic simulation technologies suggests that *"an ideal simulator should be multimodal, combining haptic, visual and audio technology to create an immersive training environment"*: this highlights the need for further studies to develop "high-tech" simulators.

Virtual reality (VR) has been well-established as a learning and training tool [11]. An interesting example of VR simulators available for spine surgery is the ImmersiveTouch Surgical Simulation Suite for Spine Surgery [12] that provides surgeons the ability to visualize 3D models of real patients, measure the exact dimensions of anatomical irregularities, etc. The effectiveness of this VR simulator was tested by Gasco et al. in [13], who demonstrated that it can effectively improve pedicle screw placement compared to traditional (oral/verbal/visual) teaching. However, the availability of realistic haptic feedback is the bottleneck in developing high fidelity VR simulators, especially in open surgery, and conventional haptic interfaces are limited in the magnitude of the forces being rendered (so they do not enable a realistic simulation of the surgical instruments/bone interaction) [14], thus a hybrid approach based on 3D printing and augmented reality (AR) is promising to overcome current technological limits [14].

Hybrid simulators combine physical anatomical models with virtual reality elements by exploiting AR technologies to enrich the synthetic environment, for example: to visualize hidden anatomical structures, and/or additional information to guide the surgical tasks and to help the trainee [15,16].

For these reasons, in a previous work, we presented a patient-specific hybrid simulator for orthopedic open surgery featuring wearable AR functionalities [14]. That simulator, which uses the Microsoft HoloLens (1st gen) head-mounted display (HMD) [17] for an interactive and immersive simulation experience for hip arthroplasty training, received positive feedback from medical staff involved in the study to evaluate visual/audio perceptions, and gesture/voice interactions.

Head-mounted displays are increasingly recognized as the most ergonomic solution for AR applications including manual tasks performed under direct vision like what happens in open surgery; however, literature studies [18] highlight some possible pitfalls to consider when using HMDs not specifically designed for the peripersonal space, to guide manual tasks: the perceptual issue related to vergence-accommodation conflict (VAC) and focal rivalry (FR) which hinder visual performance and cause visual fatigue [19], and the physical burdening of wearing an HMD for a prolonged period of time. Indeed, the HMD weight demands the forceful action of the neck extensors muscles to support and stabilize the neck and maintain the posture [20]. For these reasons the simulation environment should be carefully set up so that the virtual content appears in the optimal/comfort zone for most of the simulation, and so that the head tilt is sustainable.

Furthermore, one should consider that the availability of an HMD during the simulation is a technological addon not coherent with the devices available in a traditional surgical room. Other non-wearable AR-enabling devices deserve consideration to develop hybrid simulators for the training of image-guided surgical procedures, such as spinal fluoroscopic-guided interventions, where the operator is constantly required to switch attention between the patient and a monitor showing real-time fluoroscopic images of the spinal anatomy. For these reasons, a traditional stand-up display appears the best technological choice in terms of realism, since it is consistent with the equipment of a real surgical scenario.

In this work we describe and test an innovative hybrid spine simulator consisting of a torso mannequin with a patient-specific spine, and a PC with a traditional monitor to render the scene generated by a software module. Specifically, this latter provides:

- A "Virtual X-Ray Visualization", simulating X-ray images of the anatomy to train for the uniplanar fluoroscopic targeting of pedicles without any exposure to harmful radiation.
- An "AR Visualization", allowing the observation of the torso with overlaid virtual content to assist in the implantation of the screws at the proper anatomical targets (vertebral peduncles).

Fluoroscopic images simulation has been previously proposed by Bott et al. in [21] to improve the effectiveness of C-arm training for orthopedic and reconstructive surgery. Specifically, the system designed by Bott et al. can generate digitally reconstructed radiographs based on the relative position of a real C-arm and a mannequin representing the patient: a virtual camera is used to simulate the X-ray detector, providing views of a CT volume (selected from a database containing surgical cases) from various perspectives. The mannequin is not patient-specific, and it does not contain a replica of the bony structures corresponding to the CT dataset. Moreover, the trainee can only interact with the mannequin to simulate different positioning of the patient on the surgical bed, without using any surgical instruments.

In this work, the patient specific physical bone replica and virtual information are consistent with each other, the trainee can interact with the spinal anatomy by using real surgical instrumentations, and the simulated fluoroscopic images are updated according to the current pose of the orthopedic tools and the positioning of each single vertebra.

2. Materials and Methods

This section describes both the design and development of the simulator hardware and software components (in Sections 2.1 and 2.2), and its qualitative testing (in Section 2.3).

2.1. Hardware Components

The hardware components of the simulator include (Figure 1a): the spine phantom, the surgical instruments, the camera and markers for tracking, a calibration cube, as well as a desktop computer.

The spine phantom contains patient-specific vertebral synthetic models, generated by processing CT datasets, and manufactured with a fused deposition modeling (FDM) 3D printer (Dimension Elite 3D Printer Stratasys Ltd., Minneapolis, MN, USA and Rehovot, Israel). The CT datasets are processed using a semi-automatic tool, the "EndoCAS Segmentation Pipeline" integrated in the ITK-SNAP 1.5 open-source software [22], to generate the 3D virtual meshes of the patient vertebrae. Then, following the image segmentation, these 3D meshes are refined into printable 3D models, via the open-source software MeshLab [23] by performing a few optimization stages (e.g., removal of non-manifold edges and vertices, holes filling, and finally mesh filtering).

Acrylonitrile butadiene styrene (ABS) is used to manufacture vertebral models via 3D printing: this material is commonly employed for 3D printing in the orthopedic domain to replicate the bone mechanical behavior [24]. Mockups of intersomatic disks are manufactured with a soft room-temperature-vulcanizing silicone (RTV silicone), modeled to replicate the size and to maintain a mobility similar to the in-vivo human spine [25]. The spine mannequin is embedded in a soft synthetic polyurethane foam to simulate paravertebral soft tissues, and a skin-like covering made of RTV silicone is added to allow an accurate simulation of palpation and surgical incision (Figure 1b).

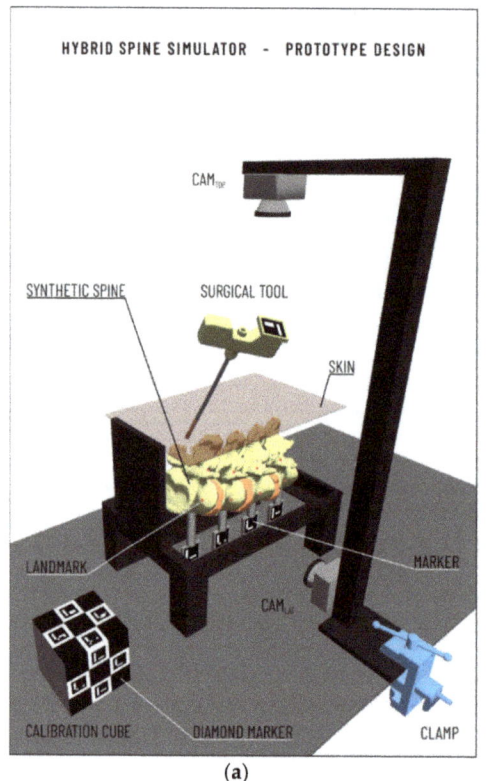 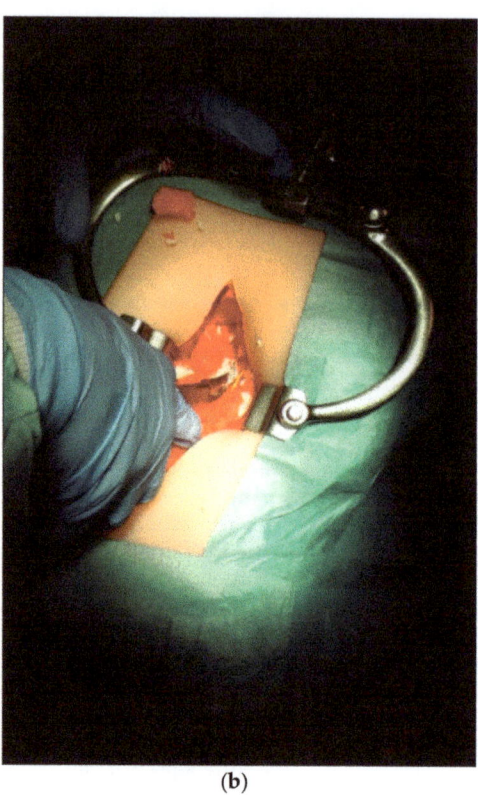

Figure 1. (**a**, **left**) Overview of the final design of the simulator hardware components: a spine phantom, equipped with markers for tracking, surgical tools with markers, two cameras for tracking, and a calibration cube. (**b**, **right**) The final appearance of the 3D printed spine embedded in the soft synthetic foam and covered with a skin-like silicone layer.

Vertebrae tracking is necessary to update the Virtual X-Ray Visualization and the AR Visualization accordingly to any vertebral displacement during the simulated surgical intervention. The selected tracking strategy is based on the using of low-cost cameras to reduce the total cost of the simulator. Cameras and markers' positioning are chosen considering both technical requirements and the consistency with a real surgical scenario. ArUco markers [24], square (2 cm × 2 cm) fiducial markers composed of a binary matrix (white and black) and a black border, are used for real-time tracking of anatomical models and instrumentation.

Ad-hoc supports are designed to apply these planar fiducial markers on each vertebra, allowing us to determine their real-time pose during the entire surgical simulation. Given that the intervention is commonly performed with a posterior access, vertebral supports are designed to emerge from the bottom side of the phantom (Figure 2a), so that they are visible by a lateral camera (Cam_{Lat}) which is used to track in real-time the pose of vertebrae. An additional top camera (Cam_{Top}), opportunely calibrated with Cam_{Lat}, is placed above the phantom to acquire posterior images and then to offer AR views of the simulated torso, to help the trainee in the identification of pedicles and implantation of screws (e.g., vertebra models or virtual targets showing the ideal trajectory for screw insertion). At the same time, this second camera (Cam_{Top}) offers an additional point of view to track the surgical instruments (e.g., pedicle access tool equipped with a trackable fiducial marker), when they are not visible for the Cam_{Lat} camera. The calibration between the reference systems of Cam$_{Lat}$ and Cam$_{Top}$ is performed as described in Section 2.2.2 thanks to the calibration cube.

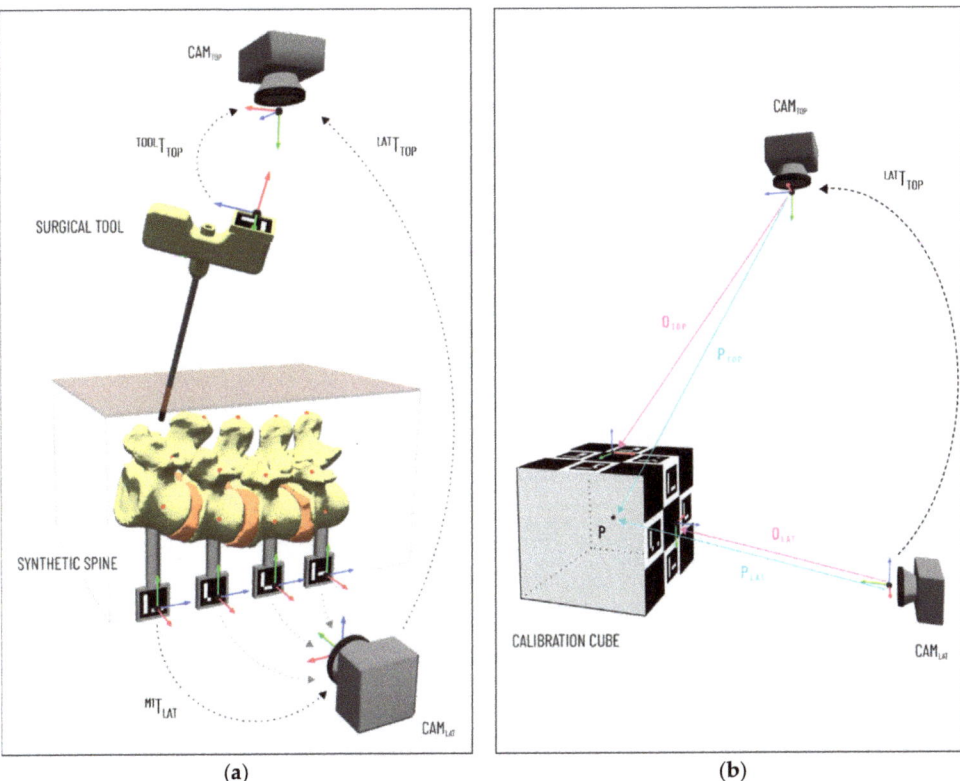

Figure 2. (**a**, **left**) Cameras and fiducial markers setup with schematic representation of transformation matrix involved. (**b**, **right**) Calibration of the lateral and top cameras with the calibration cube.

The cameras selected for the implementation of our application are the UI-164xLE camera from IDS Imaging with a 1/3″ CMOS color sensor (resolution 1280 × 1024 pixels). The UI-164xLE is a compact USB camera with an S-mount adapter allowing the use of small low-cost lenses, and it allows the user to set focus manually.

2.2. Software Architecture

In addition to the hardware components described in the previous paragraph, the architecture of the simulator (represented in Figure 3) also comprises software components. The latter have been developed using the Unity game engine [26], with OpenCV plugin for Unity [27] to perform the video-based tracking necessary for the rendering in both the AR Visualization and Virtual X-Ray Visualization.

As summarized in Figure 3, the software architecture includes the following modules: ArUco 3D Tracking, Camera Calibration, Virtual X-Ray Visualization, AR Visualization, and User Interface. The ArUco 3D Tracking module acquires images from the two cameras and receives input parameters from the Camera Calibration module to model the projection matrix of the two cameras. It runs image-processing steps allowing the Virtual X-Ray Visualization module, and the AR Visualization module to, respectively, perform the proper graphics rendering of the surgical scenario. Finally, the User Interface module allows the user to load the cameras' intrinsics and to control both the visualization modules. Each software module is described in detail in the following sections.

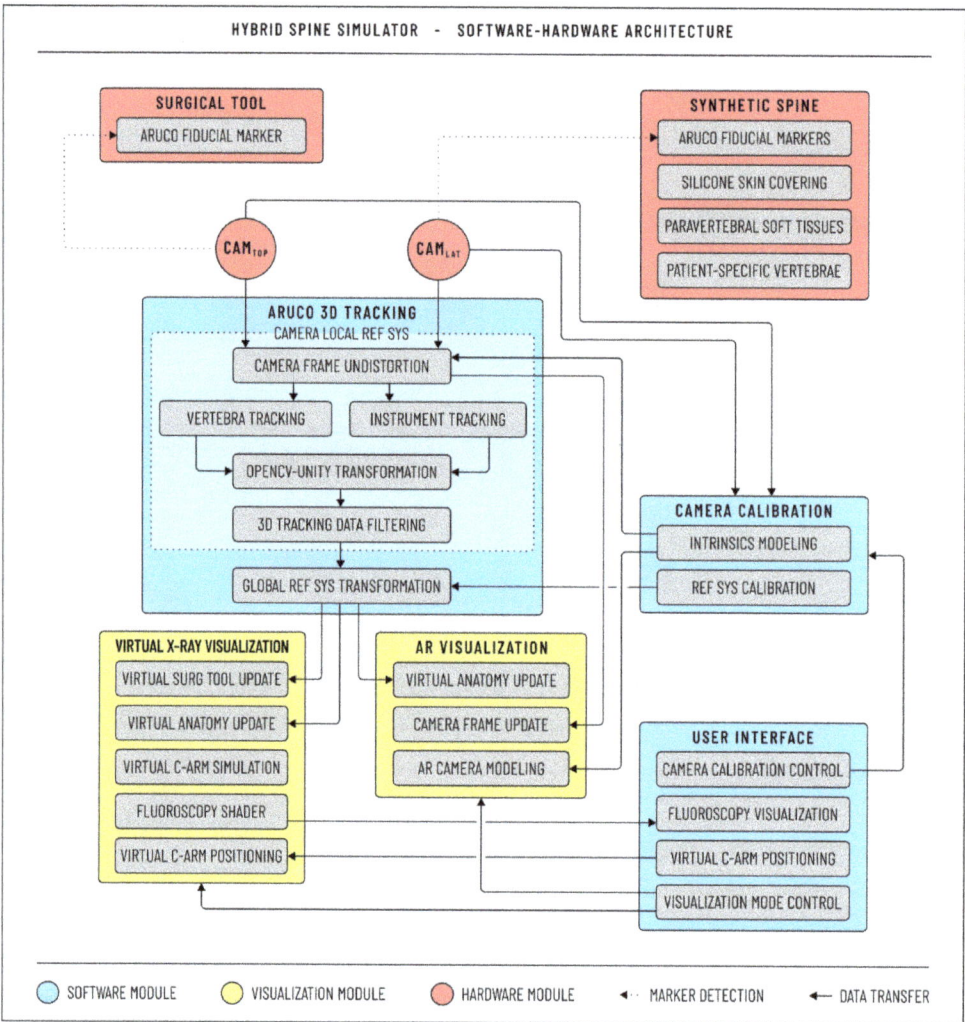

Figure 3. Architecture of the simulator. The Hardware module consists of two cameras, a synthetic spine, and surgical tools with ArUco fiducial markers. The simulator also includes: the Camera Calibration module to model the projection matrix of the two cameras; the ArUco calibration module to track the spine and the surgical instrumentations; the User Interface to load the cameras' intrinsics, to control the virtual C-Arm and the visualization modules, and to visualize the generated images; the Virtual X-Ray and the augmented reality (AR) visualization module to generate and update the fluoroscopic images and the AR view.

2.2.1. ArUco 3D Tracking

The ArUco library [28,29], a popular library for detection of square fiducial marker based on OpenCV, is used for tracking purposes. ArUco marker tracking is based on image segmentation to extract the marker region, contour extraction to extract the polygons in the interior of the marker images, identification of marker codes by the pre-defined dictionary, and finally marker pose computation with the Levenberg–Marguardt algorithm [30].

The OpenCV undistort function is used to transform images acquired by the two cameras (Cam_{Lat} and Cam_{Top}) to compensate for lens distortion (mainly radial) according to the distortion coefficients stored by the Camera Calibration module. Undistorted images are then processed by the ArUco 3D Tracking module to determine the pose of each vertebra and the surgical instrumentation.

The ArUco tracking expresses the pose of each marker according to the right-handed reference system of OpenCV, whereas Unity uses a left-handed convention (the Y-axis is inverted as shown in Figure 4): thus, a change-of-basis transformation is applied to transform the acquired tracking data from OpenCV convention to Unity convention.

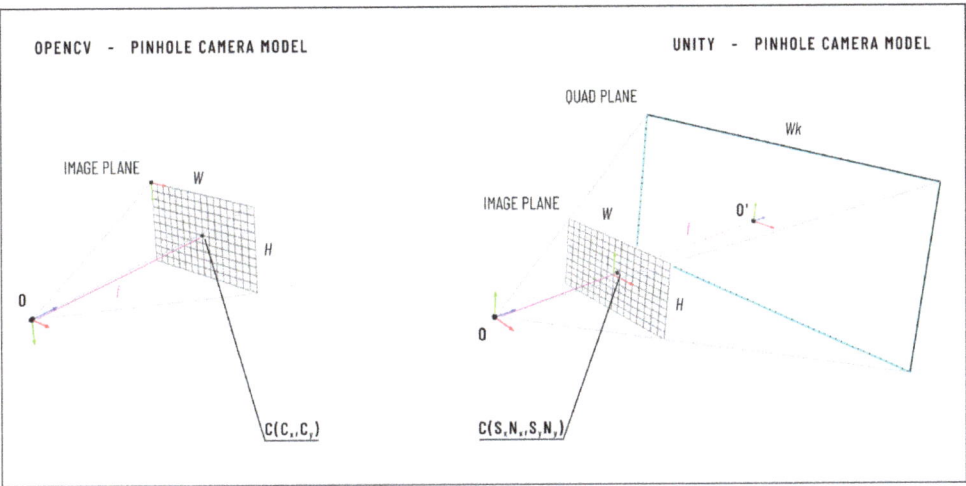

Figure 4. Camera coordinate frame and image coordinate frame of the pinhole camera model in OpenCV and in Unity. Both OpenCV and Unity assume that the camera principal axis is aligned with the positive Z-axis of the camera coordinate system, but the OpenCV coordinate system is right-handed (the Y-axis is oriented downward) while the Unity coordinate system is left-handed (the Y-axis is oriented upward). Moreover, in OpenCV, the origin of the image coordinate system is the center of the upper-left image pixel while in Unity the origin of the image coordinate system is at the image center. This picture also shows the coordinate system of the quad primitive used in Unity.

A moving average filter is then applied to denoise marker tracking: the number of points in the average was empirically set to five to stabilize the marker pose with an acceptable delay for real-time monitoring. Finally, a calibration procedure is performed: indeed, the pose of markers on vertebra replicas and the pose of instrumentations are, respectively, acquired in the Cam_{Lat} and Cam_{Top} local reference system and they should be expressed in the same global coordinate system. In this work, the global reference system corresponds to Cam_{Top} local reference systems (see Figure 2). The roto-translation matrix between the two reference systems is computed by the Camera Calibration module as described in the following paragraph.

2.2.2. Camera Calibration

Cameras are modeled with the well-known pinhole camera model. Figure 4 depicts the camera coordinate frame and image coordinate frame of the pinhole camera model in OpenCV and in Unity.

An asymmetric checkerboard is used to estimate cameras' intrinsic parameters offline using the Camera Calibrator application of the MATLAB Computer Vision Toolbox™ [31] based on the Zhang method [32]. The calibration process involves the detection of the checkerboard from at least 10 different viewpoints, and it is repeated until the reprojection error is less than 0.15 pixels.

Once the calibration is completed, the results are saved in a text file (.txt format), including:

- the horizontal and vertical focal length expressed in pixels (f_x, f_y);
- the coordinates of the principal point in pixels (c_x, c_y);
- two radial distortion coefficients (K_1 and K_2); and
- the input image size in pixels (N_x, N_y).

The Camera Calibration module of our software acquires these data and makes them available to the ArUco 3D Tracking and the AR Visualization modules.

The Virtual X-Ray Visualization and AR Visualization modules require the pose of vertebral models and instruments to be expressed in the same reference system. With this aim, the Camera Calibration module also computes the extrinsic calibration consisting of the roto-translation matrix between the reference systems of Cam_{Lat} and Cam_{Top}. This calibration is performed by acquiring the pose of a calibration cube with two ArUco diamond markers ($Diamond_{Top}$ and $Diamond_{Lat}$) placed, respectively, on two adjacent faces (Figure 2b). ArUco diamond markers are chessboards composed of 3×3 squares with four ArUco fiducial markers, and they can be used for accurate pose computation in all situations when the marker size is not an issue for the application. Each diamond marker is represented by an identifier and four corners: these latter corners correspond to the four chessboard corners and they are derived from the previous detection of the four ArUco markers. The coordinate system of the diamond pose is in the center of the diamond marker with the Z-axis pointing outward, as in a simple ArUco marker [33].

For this application, diamonds markers are printed in a size of 9×9 cm (the four ArUco markers of a diamond marker measure 2×2 cm each). The calibration process includes the following steps:

1. The calibration cube is positioned inside the field of view (FOV) of both cameras, and Cam_{Lat} and Cam_{Top} simultaneously acquire the diamond markers.
2. ArUco libraries are used to estimate the pose of each diamond marker in the reference system of the corresponding tracking camera. We refer to the position vector from the Cam_{Top} reference system to the origin of the $Diamond_{Top}$ reference system as $\vec{O}_{Top}$, while we use $\vec{O}_{Lat}$ to denote the position vector from the origin of the Cam_{Lat} reference system to the origin of the reference system of the $Diamond_{Lat}$ (see Figure 2b).
3. The position of the cube center is estimated in each camera reference system from the position of the two diamond markers ($\vec{O}_{Top}$ and $\vec{O}_{Lat}$), the orientation of their Z-axis ($\hat{z}_{Top}$, $\hat{z}_{Lat}$) expressed in the tracking camera reference system, and the size (l) of the ArUco Diamond marker according to Equations (1) and (2).

$$\vec{P}_{Top} = \vec{O}_{Top} + \frac{l}{2}\hat{z}_{Top} \tag{1}$$

$$\vec{P}_{Lat} = \vec{O}_{Lat} + \frac{l}{2}\hat{z}_{Lat} \tag{2}$$

where $\vec{P}_{Top}$ is the position vector from the origin of the Cam_{Top} reference system to the calibration cube center, and $\vec{P}_{Lat}$ is the position vector from the origin of the Cam_{Lat} reference system to the calibration cube center.

4. Steps 1–2–3 are repeated at least three times moving the cube in the camera FOV to collect two clouds of n-positions ($n \geq 3$).
5. A rigid point cloud registration algorithm based on singular value decomposition (SVD) is used to calculate the transformation matrix ($^{Top}T_{Lat}$ in Figure 2b) between the reference systems of the two cameras from the collected clouds of positions (n-

positions of the center of the calibration cube expressed in the reference systems of the two cameras).

2.2.3. AR Visualization

The visualization of the AR scene requires configuration of the virtual camera using the intrinsic parameters of the corresponding real camera to obtain the same projection model and thus to guarantee the virtual–real matching. To do this in Unity, we used the "Physical Camera" component that can simulate real-world camera attributes: focal length, sensor size, and lens shift.

The lens shift (S_x, S_y) of a Physical Camera in Unity is a dimensionless value which *"offsets the camera's lens from its sensor horizontally and vertically"* [34] and it can be used to model the principal point offset. This lens shift is relative to the sensor size, and it is derived from the principal point coordinates expressed in pixels (c_x, c_y) and the input image size in pixels (N_x, N_y), according to Equations (3) and (4).

$$S_x = \frac{c_x - \frac{N_x}{2}}{N_x} \qquad (3)$$

$$S_y = -\frac{c_y - \frac{N_y}{2}}{N_y} \qquad (4)$$

A quad primitive is used to render the images acquired by the camera after undistortion. The quad size is set as a multiple of the sensor size (W, H) and its position $\vec{O'}$ is determined as in Equation (5), where k is the ratio between the quad size and the sensor size.

$$\vec{O'} = \begin{pmatrix} S_x\, N_x\, k \\ S_y\, N_y\, k \\ fk \end{pmatrix} \qquad (5)$$

2.2.4. Virtual X-ray Visualization

This module generates realistic virtual fluoroscopic images of the current surgical scene that comprises: the surgical tool, the patient-specific vertebrae, a virtual human body, and a C-arm 3D model (the "Virtual C-Arm"). The pose of the vertebrae and the tool are expressed in the same reference system thanks to the Camera Calibration module. The human body (a standard 3D model, with size compatible with the patient-specific virtual spine) is manually registered according to the anatomical correct positioning of the spine The Virtual C-Arm is scaled to a realistic size (the source-to-detector distance, SDD, is 0.120 m as in [35]), and a "virtual isocenter" is placed at a distance of 0.64 m from the source (source-to-isocenter distance, SID, of 0.64 m).

X-ray simulation is obtained through the implementation of a virtual camera (the "X-ray Camera"), positioned at the Virtual C-Arm source. The FOV of the X-ray Camera and its clipping planes are manually tuned according to the size of the Virtual C-Arm.

The X-ray beam projection of a C-arm device is commonly defined using two rotation angles (Figure 5): the left/right anterior oblique (LAO/RAO) angle, α; and the caudal/cranial (CAUD/CRAN) angle, β (in the literature, these are also referred to as the angular and orbital rotation angles, respectively) [36]. A custom Unity script-component was implemented to allow the user to rotate the Virtual C-Arm around its isocenter, adjusting α and β values with keyboard inputs to obtain different image projections. Moreover, this script also implements the Virtual C-Arm translation along the three main axes.

The X-ray Camera uses a custom replacement shader to render the vertebral meshes and the tracked instrumentation: the "X-ray effect" is implemented with a colored, semi-transparent shader, with no backface culling to also render polygons that are facing away from the viewer (Figure 6).

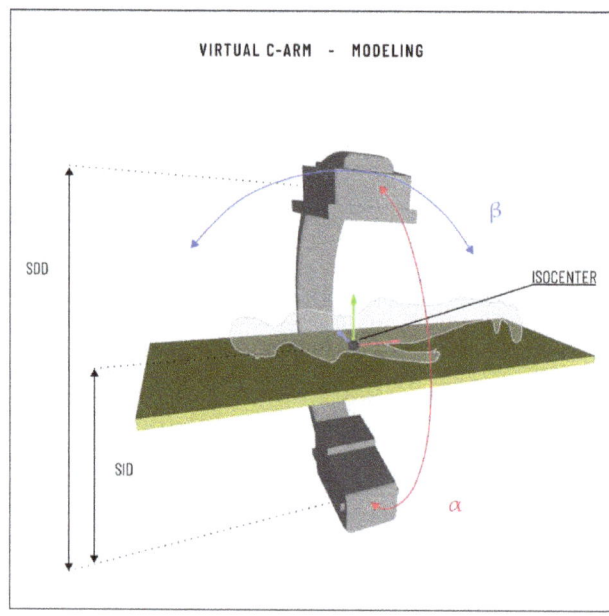

Figure 5. Virtual C-Arm modeling for the Virtual X-Ray Visualization module. The Virtual C-Arm can rotate around its isocenter, adjusting α and β values with keyboard inputs to obtain different image projections.

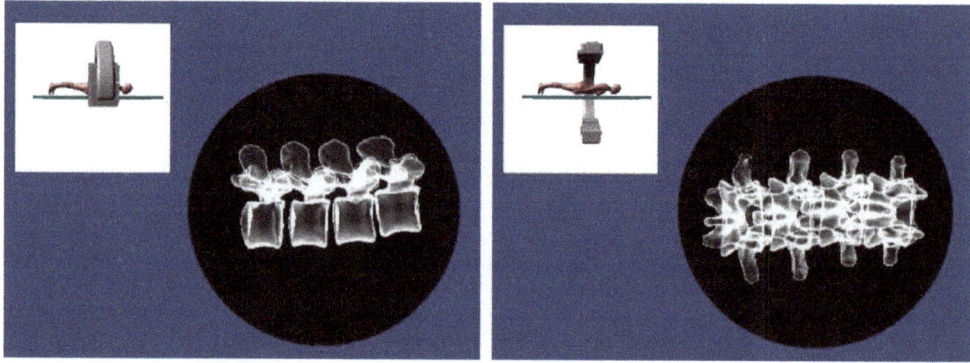

Figure 6. Two screenshots of the User Interface during the simulation in Virtual X-ray Visualization modality. The User Interface shows the relative positioning of the Virtual C-Arm and the patient and the corresponding simulated fluoroscopic image.

2.2.5. User Interface

The User Interface allows the user to load the cameras' intrinsics, to control the Virtual C-Arm, and to visualize the generated images. Moreover, the user can switch between the calibration (Figure 7a) and the simulation application. During the simulation, the user can turn on both the AR Visualization and the Virtual X-ray Visualization modalities at the same time (Figure 7b), or activate the Virtual X-ray Visualization alone (Figure 6). The Virtual X-ray Visualization allows the visualization of the Virtual C-Arm pose and the corresponding simulated fluoroscopic image. The user can move the Virtual C-Arm (by adjusting the angular and orbital rotation angles and translating the Virtual C-Arm with respect to the patient bed) via keyboard input.

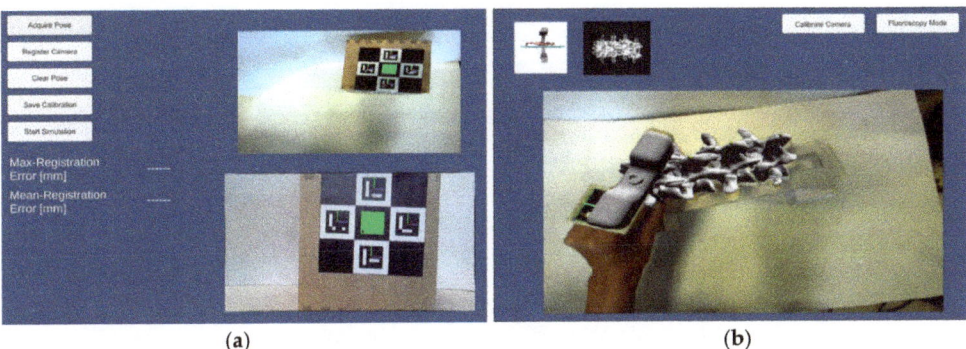

Figure 7. Screenshots of the User Interface: (**a**, **left**) the User Interface during a calibration procedure; (**b**, **right**) the User Interface during a simulation session. This second screenshot shows both the virtual fluoroscopic image (from the selected Virtual C-Arm pose) and the AR view from the top camera (Cam_{Top}).

2.3. Simulator Testing

Quantitative tests were performed to evaluate the accuracy of both the AR Visualization (that in turn gives information about the calibration of the two cameras), and the Virtual X-Ray Visualization. Figure 8 illustrates the testing setup: the two cameras are held in position by an articulated arm, and the vertebral models are assembled and inserted into a support structure.

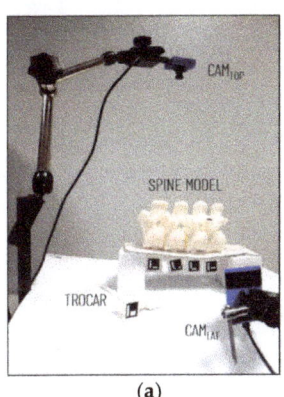
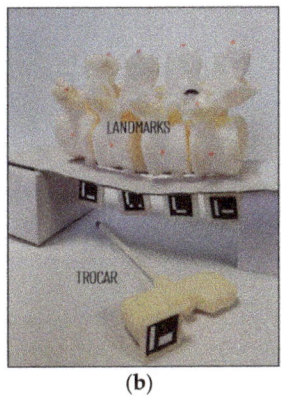

Figure 8. Testing setup: (**a**, **left**) configuration of the two cameras and the spine model; (**b**, **right**) a close-up of the spine model with 3D-printed spherical landmarks, and the trocar mockup.

2.3.1. Evaluation of the Camera Calibration and AR Visualization

Three fiducial spherical landmarks (2 mm in diameter) were added to each vertebra model at known positions to evaluate the cameras' calibration: one was positioned at the vertebral body so that it is visible by the lateral camera (Cam_{Lat}), and the other two at the vertebral peduncle and the spinous process so that are visible by the top camera, Cam_{Top} (Figure 8).

The VR models of landmarks were added to the AR scene for estimating the target visualization error (TVE), thus evaluating the accuracy of the AR overlay (a similar procedure was adopted in [16] to evaluate the accuracy of a hybrid simulator). With this aim, the vertebral models were moved in ten different positions, acquiring each time the AR image of both virtual cameras.

More specifically, for each position, two images were captured from each virtual camera. The first image was acquired with AR switched-off; therefore, this image contains only the scene as viewed by the camera, without AR information. The second image was acquired with AR switched-on, thus it also shows the virtual landmarks. This produced for each camera two sets of corresponding images: we refer to the set with AR switched-off as the "Real Set", and to the set with AR switched-on as the "AR Set". The correspondence between the Real Set and the AR Set guarantees an accurate modeling of the camera projection models and their intrinsic and extrinsic calibration, which is a requirement for the realism and fidelity of both the AR Visualization and the Virtual X-ray Visualization modalities.

The acquired sets were automatically processed to estimate the 2D target visualization error (TVE2D), that is: the offset, expressed in pixels, between the virtual and real objects in the image plane (i.e., the centroids of the virtual landmarks, and the corresponding real 3D-printed landmarks). The Real Set and the AR Set were processed in the hue–saturation-value (HSV) color space that allows a robust segmentation even when the target objects show non-uniformities in illumination, shadows, or shading [37]. The image processing, performed in MATLAB, included the following steps:

1. Transformation from RGB to HSV color space.
2. Detection of the virtual landmarks in the AR Set (Figure 9a).
3. Detection of the 3D-printed landmarks in the Real Set (Figure 9b).

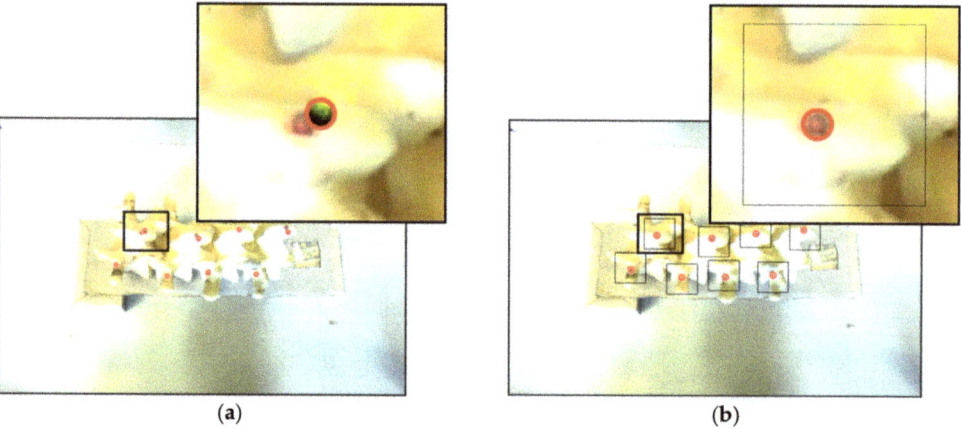

Figure 9. Examples of corresponding images of AR Set and Real Set from the Cam_{Top} view. (**a**, **left**) Image from the AR Set: the eight detected digital markers are circled in red, and a zoomed view of the first top left marker is provided. (**b**, **right**) Image from the Real Set: the detected 3D-printed markers are circled in red with each region of interest (ROI) enclosed by a black-edged square, and a zoomed view of the first top left marker is provided.

Virtual landmarks were detected with the circular Hough transform, using their diameter as an input parameter. The Hough transform sensitivity was adjusted to detect all the landmarks in the image (four markers for Cam_{Lat} and eight for Cam_{Top}): an increase in the sensitivity allows the detection of more circular objects, including weak and partially obscured circles (however higher sensitivity values also increase the risk of false detection) [38].

The knowledge of the virtual markers position derived from step 2 was used to improve the robustness of step 3. Each 3D-printed landmark indeed was searched within a region of interest (ROI) centered on the position of the corresponding virtual landmark.

The ROI was segmented to identify the red areas through filtering on the hue (H) and saturation (S) channels.

Detected 2D positions were used to calculate the TVE2D, and subsequently to derive the TVE3D, a rough estimation of the visualization error in space at a fixed distance, expressed in mm [39]. The TVE3D was estimated by inverting the projection equation as in Equation (6).

$$TVE_{3D} = \frac{TVE_{2D}}{k} \frac{Z_c}{f} \quad (6)$$

In Equation (6): Z_C is the estimated working distance, f is the camera focal length estimated in the calibration stage, and k is the scaling factor of the image sensor (number of pixels per unit of length).

2.3.2. Evaluation of the Total Error

Inaccurate tracking of surgical instrumentation is a source of error that can affect the realism and fidelity of the system, particularly of the Virtual X-ray Visualization that simultaneously shows the tracked vertebra and instruments. For this reason, we performed additional tests, using a mockup of a Jamshidi trocar (a tool for percutaneous pedicle cannulation) equipped with an ArUco marker (Figure 9) to estimate the total error. We pointed the trocar tip at the vertebra landmarks under direct visual control, and we calculated the accuracy as the distance between the tracked tip position and the virtual landmark. Targeting landmarks under direct visualization allowed us to minimize positioning inaccuracy due to the experience level of the experimenter, compared to targeting under Virtual X-ray Visualization.

The error was calculated as the projection of the Euclidean distance on the XZ- and XY- planes that coincide with the simulated anteroposterior and latero–lateral fluoroscope projections, respectively.

3. Results

The target visualization errors (both TVE2D and TVE3D) were estimated for each spine pose for a total of: 40 measurements for the lateral camera, Cam_{Lat} (4 markers detected in each of the 10 images); and 80 measurements for the top camera, Cam_{Top} (8 markers detected in each of the 10 images). Table 1 summarizes mean (μ) and standard deviation (σ) values for each of the 10 images.

Table 1. Mean (μ) and standard deviation (σ) of target visualization errors (TVE)2D and TVE3D values for each of the 10 poses.

		Pos 1	Pos 2	Pos 3	Pos 4	Pos 5	Pos 6	Pos 7	Pos 8	Pos 9	Pos 10	Total
Cam_{Lat}	TVE2D (pixel)	μ= 8.1	9.1	10.1	10	6.5	8.8	7.4	7.5	5.5	6.6	8
		σ= 7.7	7.8	9.9	9.2	5.5	9.2	8.4	8.5	6.1	6.4	4.1
	TVE3D (mm)	0.7	0.9	1	1	0.6	0.9	0.8	0.8	0.6	0.7	0.8
		0.3	0.4	0.4	0.7	0.3	0.4	0.3	0.4	0.3	0.5	0.4
Cam_{Top}	TVE2D (pixel)	5.9	6.5	4.9	4.7	4.5	6.6	6.6	3.9	4.1	6.8	5.5
		2.8	3.8	3.2	3.6	1.2	3.4	3.2	2.2	2.2	3.1	3
	TVE3D [mm]	1.7	1.9	1.5	1.4	1.4	2	2	1.1	1.3	2	1.6
		0.8	1.1	0.9	1.1	0.4	1	1	0.6	0.7	0.9	0.4

The total error was calculated for each vertebra (for a single spine pose), three times for each of the landmarks (landmarks on the vertebral body, pedicle and spinous process) for a total of 36 measurements. Table 2 summarizes mean (μ) and standard deviation (σ) values for each vertebra.

Table 2. Mean (μ) and standard deviation (σ) of the targeting error latero–lateral (LL) and anteroposterior (AP) projections.

		Vertebra 1	Vertebra 2	Vertebra 3	Vertebra 4	Total
Targeting Error	LL (mm)	1.9 0.8	2.2 0.6	2.1 1.1	2.1 1.3	2.1 1.0
	AP (mm)	2.5 0.5	1.7 0.8	1.6 0.4	1.8 1.4	1.9 0.9

The obtained TVE3D and targeting errors confirm the feasibility of the proposed strategy to track the vertebral models/surgical tools, and to coherently visualize them both in AR Visualization mode and in Virtual X-ray Visualization as an aid for the training of pedicle screw implantation in lumbar vertebrae. The errors are indeed lower than half the size of lumbar pedicle radius which, according to [40], is 6.4–6.5 mm for L1 (left and right pedicle, respectively) increases from L1 to L4, and increased sharply at L5 reaching a mean size of 17.5–17.7 mm (left and right pedicle, respectively).

The TVE3D of the Cam_{Top} is an estimation of the error in the registration of vertebral models in the global (Cam_{Top}) reference systems (Vertebra Registration Error). As for the targeting error we should consider the following sources of error: Vertebra Registration Error, error in the localization of the ArUco marker used to track the surgical tool in the global (Cam_{Top}) reference system, inaccuracy of the users in the alignment of the tool tip with the marker, and finally the error in the tool calibration.

The instrument calibration is required to infer the pose of the tool tip from the pose of the detected marker. In this study, we used a built-in marker to track the trocar mockup and we derived the calibration matrix from the CAD (computer-aided design) project; a procedure such as the pivot calibration [41] can be used instead for localizing a real surgical tool using a marker whose relative pose with the respect to the tool tip is unknown a priori. Given the obtained TVE3D and targeting error we can assume that, even using a real surgical tool, the final accuracy of the system would be enough for the proposed application (screw implantation in lumbar vertebrae).

Figure 10 illustrates the simulated lateral (Figure 10a) and anterior–posterior (Figure 10b) fluoroscopic view of the spine during the targeting of one marker with the Jamshidi trocar mockup. The corresponding actual positioning of the trocar is shown by the images captured by the lateral (Cam_{Lat}) and the top camera (Cam_{Top}). For these experiments, the "X-ray" shader was applied only to the vertebral models while a standard opaque material was used for the landmarks and the instrument model for a better visualization of their pose.

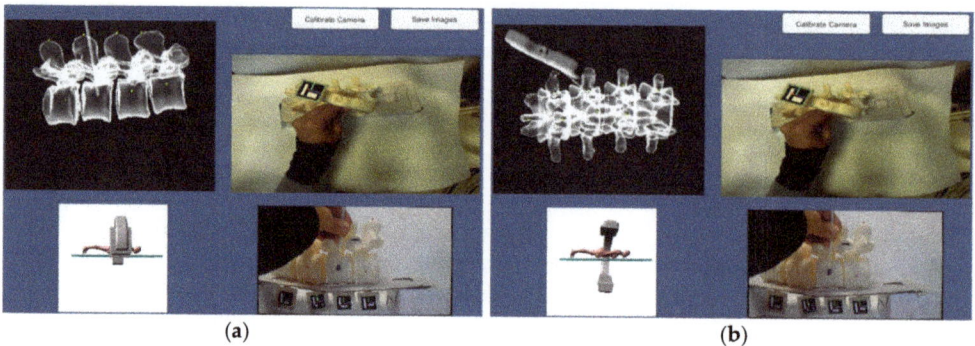

Figure 10. Two screenshots of the User Interface during the targeting of a landmark with a trocar mockup. (**a, left**) The pose of the Virtual C-Arm is adjusted to simulate a lateral fluoroscopic image. (**b, right**) The pose of the Virtual C-Arm is adjusted to simulate an anterior–posterior fluoroscopic image.

4. Discussion and Conclusions

A recent literature review on orthopedic surgery simulation highlights the need for "high-tech" multimodal simulators allowing the trainees to develop visuospatial awareness of the anatomy and a "sense of touch" for surgical procedures. Starting from these considerations, in a previous study we have presented a hybrid simulator for open orthopedic surgery using the Microsoft HoloLens [14]. Although HDMs represent an ideal solution to develop an immersive training environment for open surgery, other non-wearable AR-enabling devices deserve consideration to develop hybrid simulators for training of image-guided surgical procedures such as spinal fluoroscopic guided interventions. For this reason, in this work we present and technically test a prototype of an innovative hybrid spine simulator for pedicle screws fixation, based on the use of a traditional stand-up display, that is consistent with the equipment of a real surgical scenario and thus appears the best technological choice in terms of realism.

The proposed strategy to build the spine simulator takes advantage of:

- patient-specific modeling to improve the realism of the simulated surgical pathology;
- rapid prototyping for the manufacturing of synthetic vertebral models;
- AR to enrich the simulated surgical scenario and help the learner to carry out the procedure;
- VR functionalities for simulating X-ray images of the anatomy to train for the uniplanar fluoroscopic targeting of pedicles without any exposure to harmful radiations.

Fiducial markers are used to track in real-time the position of each vertebra (which can move relative to adjacent vertebrae to simulate the mobility of the human spine) and surgical instrumentation. Two calibrated cameras, arranged in an orthogonal configuration, are proposed to track the vertebral models (lateral camera) and to track the instrumentation and produce an AR view of the simulated torso (top camera). A simulated virtual C-arm is used to generate synthetic fluoroscopic projections, using a simple approach based on shader programming to achieve an "X-ray effect".

Quantitative tests show that the proposed low-cost tracking approach is accurate enough for training in pedicle screws insertion in lumbar vertebrae.

Future studies will improve the robustness of the simulator, involving clinicians to test the system and define the best positioning of the cameras (an ad-hoc support structure will be designed to hold in position the two cameras), fiducial markers, and lights so that the accuracy is maximized and, at the same time, the tracking set-up (camera, markers and lights) does not hinder the surgeon's movements and manipulation of the instruments. To this end, the proposed tracking strategy that is based on the optical tracking of the passive markers, is advantageous compared to other techniques using wired sensors (e.g., electromagnetic sensors). On the other hand, the selected tracking approach can fail due to marker occlusions: in our simulator, this is particularly true for the markers placed on the instruments. However, for our application, continuous instrument tracking is not necessary because, even in the real surgical workflow, fluoroscopic imaging is not continuous but intermittent to minimize the radiation dose to the patient.

In the future, Face Validity, Content Validity, and Construct Validity tests will be performed for a complete assessment of the proposed simulator for training in pedicle screws insertion.

Author Contributions: Conceptualization, S.C., G.T.; methodology, S.C., G.T., V.F. and P.D.P.; software, S.C.; validation, S.C., V.M.; formal analysis, S.C. and V.M.; investigation, S.C.; resources, V.F.; data curation, S.C. and V.M.; writing—original draft preparation, S.C., G.T. and V.M.; writing—review and editing, G.T., P.D.P. and V.F.; visualization, V.F.; project administration, S.C.; funding acquisition, V.F. All authors have read and agreed to the published version of the manuscript.

Funding: This research was partially funded by the CRIO2AR project, Fas Salute 2018—Regione Toscana. This work was also supported by the Italian Ministry of Education and Research (MIUR) in the framework of the CrossLab project (Departments of Excellence) of the University of Pisa, Laboratory of Augmented Reality.

Institutional Review Board Statement: Not applicable.

Informed Consent Statement: Not applicable.

Data Availability Statement: The data presented in this study are available on request from the corresponding author. The data are not publicly available due to its proprietary nature.

Conflicts of Interest: The authors declare no conflict of interest.

References

1. Atesok, K.; Hurwitz, S.; Anderson, D.D.; Satava, R.; Thomas, G.W.; Tufescu, T.; Heffernan, M.J.; Papavassiliou, E.; Theiss, S.; Marsh, J.L. Advancing Simulation-Based Orthopaedic Surgical Skills Training: An Analysis of the Challenges to Implementation. *Adv. Orthop.* **2019**, *2019*, 2586034. [CrossRef]
2. Parchi, P.; Evangelisti, G.; Cervi, V.; Andreani, L.; Carbone, M.; Condino, S.; Ferrari, V.; Lisanti, M. Patient's Specific Template for Spine Surgery. In *Computer-Assisted Musculoskeletal Surgery*; Ritacco, L.E., Milano, F.E., Chao, E., Eds.; Springer International Publishing: Berlin/Heidelberg, Germany, 2016. [CrossRef]
3. Ferrari, V.; Parchi, P.; Condino, S.; Carbone, M.; Baluganti, A.; Ferrari, M.; Mosca, F.; Lisanti, M. An optimal design for patient-specific templates for pedicle spine screws placement. *Int. J. Med. Robot. Comput. Assist. Surg.* **2013**, *9*, 298–304. [CrossRef]
4. Kotsis, S.V.; Chung, K.C. Application of the "see one, do one, teach one" concept in surgical training. *Plast. Reconstr. Surg.* **2013**, *131*, 1194–1201. [CrossRef]
5. Stirling, E.R.; Lewis, T.L.; Ferran, N.A. Surgical skills simulation in trauma and orthopaedic training. *J. Orthop. Surg. Res.* **2014**, *9*, 126. [CrossRef] [PubMed]
6. Yiasemidou, M.; Gkaragkani, E.; Glassman, D.; Biyani, C.S. Cadaveric simulation: A review of reviews. *Ir. J. Med. Sci.* **2018**, *187*, 827–833. [CrossRef] [PubMed]
7. Parchi, P.; Condino, S.; Carbone, M.; Gesi, M.; Ferrari, V.; Ferrari, M.; Lisanti, M. Total hip replacement simulators with virtual planning and physical replica for surgical training and rehearsal. In Proceedings of the 12th IASTED International Conference on Biomedical Engineering, BioMed, Innsbruck, Austria, 15–17 February 2016; pp. 97–101.
8. Anderson, P.A. Chapter 6—3D Printing for Education and Surgical Planning in Orthopedic Surgery. In *3D Printing in Orthopaedic Surgery*; Dipaola, M., Wodajo, F.M., Eds.; Elsevier: Amsterdam, The Netherlands, 2019; pp. 55–63. [CrossRef]
9. Park, H.J.; Wang, C.; Choi, K.H.; Kim, N. Use of a life-size three-dimensional-printed spine model for pedicle screw instrumentation training. *J. Orthop. Surg. Res.* **2018**, *13*, 1–8. [CrossRef] [PubMed]
10. Vaughan, N.; Dubey, V.N.; Wainwright, T.W.; Middleton, R.G. A review of virtual reality based training simulators for orthopaedic surgery. *Med. Eng. Phys.* **2016**, *38*, 59–71. [CrossRef] [PubMed]
11. Pfandler, M.; Lazarovici, M.; Stefan, P.; Wucherer, P.; Weigl, M. Virtual reality-based simulators for spine surgery: A systematic review. *Spine J.* **2017**, *17*, 1352–1363. [CrossRef] [PubMed]
12. Immersive Touch Surgical Simulation Suite for Spine Surgery. Available online: https://www.immersivetouch.com/ivsp-for-spine-surgery (accessed on 11 December 2020).
13. Gasco, J.; Patel, A.; Ortega-Barnett, J.; Branch, D.; Desai, S.; Kuo, Y.F.; Luciano, C.; Rizzi, S.; Kania, P.; Matuyauskas, M.; et al. Virtual reality spine surgery simulation: An empirical study of its usefulness. *Neurol. Res.* **2014**, *36*, 968–973. [CrossRef]
14. Condino, S.; Turini, G.; Parchi, P.D.; Viglialoro, R.M.; Piolanti, N.; Gesi, M.; Ferrari, M.; Ferrari, V. How to Build a Patient-Specific Hybrid Simulator for Orthopaedic Open Surgery: Benefits and Limits of Mixed-Reality Using the Microsoft HoloLens. *J. Healthc. Eng.* **2018**, *2018*. [CrossRef] [PubMed]
15. Viglialoro, R.M.; Condino, S.; Gesi, M.; Ferrari, M.; Ferrari, V. Augmented reality simulator for laparoscopic cholecystectomy training. In *Lecture Notes in Computer Science (Including Subseries Lecture Notes in Artificial Intelligence and Lecture Notes in Bioinformatics)*; Springer: Cham, Switzerland, 2014; Volume 8853, pp. 428–433.
16. Viglialoro, R.M.; Esposito, N.; Condino, S.; Cutolo, F.; Guadagni, S.; Gesi, M.; Ferrari, M.; Ferrari, V. Augmented Reality to Improve Surgical Simulation: Lessons Learned Towards the Design of a Hybrid Laparoscopic Simulator for Cholecystectomy. *IEEE Trans. Biomed. Eng.* **2019**, *66*, 2091–2104. [CrossRef] [PubMed]
17. Microsoft HoloLens (1st Gen). Available online: https://docs.microsoft.com/en-us/hololens/hololens1-hardware (accessed on 12 January 2021).
18. Condino, S.; Carbone, M.; Piazza, R.; Ferrari, M.; Ferrari, V. Perceptual Limits of Optical See-Through Visors for Augmented Reality Guidance of Manual Tasks. *IEEE Trans. BioMed Eng.* **2019**. [CrossRef] [PubMed]
19. Kim, J.; Kane, D.; Banks, M.S. The rate of change of vergence–accommodation conflict affects visual discomfort. *Vis. Res.* **2014**, *105*, 159–165. [CrossRef] [PubMed]
20. Kim, E.; Shin, G. Head Rotation and Muscle Activity When Conducting Document Editing Tasks with a Head-Mounted Display. *Proc. Hum. Factors Ergon. Soc. Annu. Meet.* **2018**, *62*, 952–955. [CrossRef]
21. Bott, O.; Dresing, K.; Wagner, M.; Raab, B.-W.; Teistler, M. Use of a C-Arm Fluoroscopy Simulator to Support Training in Intraoperative Radiography. *Radiographics* **2011**, *31*, E65–E75. [CrossRef]
22. Yushkevich, P.A.; Piven, J.; Hazlett, H.C.; Smith, R.G.; Ho, S.; Gee, J.C.; Gerig, G. User-guided 3D active contour segmentation of anatomical structures: Significantly improved efficiency and reliability. *NeuroImage* **2006**, *31*, 1116–1128. [CrossRef]

23. Cignoni, P.; Callieri, M.; Corsini, M.; Dellepiane, M.; Ganovelli, F.; Ranzuglia, G. MeshLab: An Open-Source Mesh Processing Tool. In Proceedings of the Eurographics Italian Chapter Conference, Salerno, Italy, 2–4 July 2008; Volume 1, pp. 129–136.
24. Parchi, P.D.; Ferrari, V.; Piolanti, N.; Andreani, L.; Condino, S.; Evangelisti, G.; Lisanti, M. Computer tomography prototyping and virtual procedure simulation in difficult cases of hip replacement surgery. *Surg. Technol. Int.* **2013**, *23*, 228–234.
25. Parchi, P.; Carbone, M.; Condino, S.; Stagnari, S.; Rocchi, D.; Colangeli, S.; Ferrari, M.; Scaglione, M.; Ferrari, V. Patients Specific Spine Simulators for Surgical Training and Rehearsal in Pedicule Screws Placement: A New Way for Surgical Education. In Proceedings of the CAOS 2020. The 20th Annual Meeting of the International Society for Computer Assisted Orthopaedic Surgery, Brest, France, 10–13 June 2020; pp. 225–230.
26. Unity3D. 2020. Available online: https://unity.com/ (accessed on 27 October 2020).
27. OpenCV for Unity. Available online: https://enoxsoftware.com/opencvforunity/ (accessed on 27 October 2020).
28. Romero-Ramirez, F.J.; Muñoz-Salinas, R.; Medina-Carnicer, R. Speeded up detection of squared fiducial markers. *Image Vis. Comput.* **2018**, *76*, 38–47. [CrossRef]
29. Garrido-Jurado, S.; Muñoz-Salinas, R.; Madrid-Cuevas, F.; Medina-Carnicer, R. Generation of fiducial marker dictionaries using Mixed Integer Linear Programming. *Pattern Recognit.* **2015**, *51*, 481–491. [CrossRef]
30. Kam, H.C.; Yu, Y.K.; Wong, K.H. An Improvement on ArUco Marker for Pose Tracking Using Kalman Filter. In Proceedings of the 2018 19th IEEE/ACIS International Conference on Software Engineering, Artificial Intelligence, Networking and Parallel/Distributed Computing (SNPD), Busan, Korea, 27–29 June 2018; pp. 65–69.
31. Matlab Computer Vision Toolbox. Available online: https://www.mathworks.com/products/computer-vision.html (accessed on 29 October 2020).
32. Zhang, Z. A flexible new technique for camera calibration. *IEEE Trans. Pattern Anal. Mach. Intell.* **2000**, *22*, 1330–1334. [CrossRef]
33. OpenCV—Detection of Diamond Markers. Available online: https://docs.opencv.org/master/d5/d07/tutorial_charuco_diamond_detection.html (accessed on 15 December 2020).
34. Unity Manual—Using Physical Cameras. Available online: https://docs.unity3d.com/Manual/PhysicalCameras.html (accessed on 11 December 2020).
35. Daly, M.J.; Siewerdsen, J.H.; Cho, Y.B.; Jaffray, D.A.; Irish, J.C. Geometric calibration of a mobile C-arm for intraoperative cone-beam CT. *Med. Phys.* **2008**, *35*, 2124–2136. [CrossRef] [PubMed]
36. Ritschl, L.; Kuntz, J.; Kachelrieß, M. *The Rotate-Plus-Shift C-Arm Trajectory: Complete CT Data with Limited Angular Rotation*; SPIE: Bellingham, WA, USA, 2015; Volume 9412.
37. Mamone, V.; Viglialoro, R.M.; Cutolo, F.; Cavallo, F.; Guadagni, S.; Ferrari, V. Robust Laparoscopic Instruments Tracking Using Colored Strips. In Proceedings of the Augmented Reality, Virtual Reality, and Computer Graphics, Ugento, Italy, 12–15 June 2017; pp. 129–143.
38. Yuen, H.K.; Princen, J.; Illingworth, J.; Kittler, J. Comparative study of Hough Transform methods for circle finding. *Image Vis. Comput.* **1990**, *8*, 71–77. [CrossRef]
39. Ferrari, V.; Viglialoro, R.M.; Nicoli, P.; Cutolo, F.; Condino, S.; Carbone, M.; Siesto, M.; Ferrari, M. Augmented reality visualization of deformable tubular structures for surgical simulation. *Int. J. Med. Robot. Comput. Assist. Surg.* **2016**, *12*, 231–240. [CrossRef] [PubMed]
40. Lien, S.-B.; Liou, N.-H.; Wu, S.-S. Analysis of anatomic morphometry of the pedicles and the safe zone for through-pedicle procedures in the thoracic and lumbar spine. *Eur. Spine J.* **2007**, *16*, 1215–1222. [CrossRef] [PubMed]
41. Yaniv, Z. Which pivot calibration? In *Medical Imaging 2015: Image-Guided Procedures, Robotic Interventions, and Modeling*; SPIE: Bellingham, WA, USA, 2015. [CrossRef]

Review

Augmented Reality, Mixed Reality, and Hybrid Approach in Healthcare Simulation: A Systematic Review

Rosanna Maria Viglialoro [1,*], Sara Condino [1,2,*], Giuseppe Turini [1,3], Marina Carbone [1,2], Vincenzo Ferrari [1,2] and Marco Gesi [4,5]

1. EndoCAS Center, Department of Translational Research and of New Surgical and Medical Technologies, University of Pisa, 56124 Pisa, Italy; gturini@kettering.edu (G.T.); marina.carbone@endocas.unipi.it (M.C.); vincenzo.ferrari@endocas.unipi.it (V.F.)
2. Dipartimento di Ingegneria dell'Informazione, University of Pisa, 56122 Pisa, Italy
3. Computer Science Department, Kettering University, Flint, MI 48504, USA
4. Department of Translational Research and of New Surgical and Medical Technologies, University of Pisa, 56126 Pisa, Italy; marco.gesi@med.unipi.it
5. Center for Rehabilitative Medicine "Sport and Anatomy", University of Pisa, 56121 Pisa, Italy
* Correspondence: rosanna.viglialoro@endocas.org (R.M.V.); sara.condino@endocas.unipi.it (S.C.); Tel.: +39-050-995-689 (R.M.V. & S.C.)

Abstract: Simulation-based medical training is considered an effective tool to acquire/refine technical skills, mitigating the ethical issues of Halsted's model. This review aims at evaluating the literature on medical simulation techniques based on augmented reality (AR), mixed reality (MR), and hybrid approaches. The research identified 23 articles that meet the inclusion criteria: 43% combine two approaches (MR and hybrid), 22% combine all three, 26% employ only the hybrid approach, and 9% apply only the MR approach. Among the studies reviewed, 22% use commercial simulators, whereas 78% describe custom-made simulators. Each simulator is classified according to its target clinical application: training of surgical tasks (e.g., specific tasks for training in neurosurgery, abdominal surgery, orthopedic surgery, dental surgery, otorhinolaryngological surgery, or also generic tasks such as palpation) and education in medicine (e.g., anatomy learning). Additionally, the review assesses the complexity, reusability, and realism of the physical replicas, as well as the portability of the simulators. Finally, we describe whether and how the simulators have been validated. The review highlights that most of the studies do not have a significant sample size and that they include only a feasibility assessment and preliminary validation; thus, further research is needed to validate existing simulators and to verify whether improvements in performance on a simulated scenario translate into improved performance on real patients.

Keywords: healthcare simulation; augmented reality; mixed reality; hybrid; medical training

1. Introduction

Until the 20th century, the apprenticeship model, focused on the educational philosophy of "see one, do one, teach one", was the standard teaching methodology in medical education. This model, developed by Dr. William Halsted in 1890, is based on progressive responsibility culminating in almost-independence [1–3]. In other words, the trainee directly observes a procedure performed by the expert supervisor several times, then (once the apprentice is considered ready) he/she executes the same procedure by imitating the supervisor's skills; possible mistakes are prevented or fixed immediately by the supervisor to protect the patient. This model undoubtedly has strengths thanks to the trainee's early immersion in the clinical environment which allows him/her to acquire practical and applied knowledge. However, it is inefficient because it is characterized by long hours of work with poorly defined goals and random experiences depending on the flow of patients in the operating theatre [4].

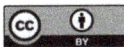

Over the last decades, the rapid introduction of new techniques and surgical approaches, such as the minimally invasive and robotic procedures, combined with the new legislative restrictions on surgeons' working hours have worsened the issues of the apprenticeship model [5–7]. Thus, based on these considerations, the surgical community was forced to reconsider training strategies [8].

Simulation-based training, relying on "see one, simulate many deliberately, do one" principle, has been proposed as an excellent adjunct method to traditional medical education [9,10]. Simulation is defined as "a technique to replace or amplify real experiences with guided experiences, often immersed in nature, that evoke or replicate substantial aspects of the real world in a fully interactive way" [11]. Healthcare simulation provides the opportunity to develop the knowledge, the skills, and the attitude of medical professionals, without any risk to the patient. The trainee can explore, repeat the surgical practice in a setting that "fosters permission to fail", recognize the mistakes and correct them, and try different approaches without jeopardizing patient safety. Thus, simulation-based medical training can be a platform for learning to mitigate ethical tensions and acquire/refine technical skills [12–15]. The main simulation techniques in healthcare include virtual reality (VR) simulation, physical simulation, and hybrid (virtual-physical) simulation.

VR simulation is based on the principles of immersion, interaction, and user involvement at different degrees: learners are immersed in a highly realistic virtual clinical environment (e.g., an operating room or an intensive care unit) and interact in real-time with the environment through virtual interactions/interfaces (e.g., virtual menus, point-and-click, etc.). Two interesting features of VR simulation are the objective evaluation of the trainee's performance, and the flexibility in selecting the virtual scenario. The latter allows the simulation to be adapted to the trainee's learning needs, enabling the learner to gain new cognitive skills, or develop and refine technical skills (e.g., instrumental navigation, clipping, slicing, etc.). However, two major limitations of VR-based simulation are the moderate sense of haptic feedback during interactions and the high costs making it prohibitively expensive for many institutions [16–18].

On the contrary, physical simulation is based on the reproduction of clinical scenarios with various degrees of realism. Low-fidelity scenarios include simple synthetic models (such as tubes or rings) made of plastic, rubber, and latex that are used to train basic clinical skills (such as knot-tying and suturing). High-fidelity scenarios include human organs or mannequins that can be used to perform the physical examination and to complete more complex procedures than just basic clinical tasks, and, unlike VR simulation, they provide the trainee realistic haptic feedback during all tool–tissue interactions [19,20]. However, the main negative aspects of this type of simulation are the need to replace the model in case of a destructive task increasing training costs and the lack of the objective evaluation of trainee's performance.

Hybrid simulators combine VR elements and physical models of the anatomy which can have an active or passive role in the simulation. Hybrid systems retain the natural haptic feedback of the physical simulation and the performance evaluation tools typical of VR simulation.

We present a systematic review of simulation techniques based on augmented reality (AR), mixed reality (MR), and hybrid approaches in the context of healthcare, to investigate the challenges and trends in this discipline. Firstly, we define AR, MR, and hybrid approaches (Section 2.1), then we examine the simulation techniques in terms of the implementation of their virtual and physical components and the accuracy validity of the adopted techniques. Finally, we evaluate the clinical validity of the simulators and their frequency of use.

2. Materials and Methods

2.1. Simulation Approach

In the literature, there is no univocal definition of the terms hybrid simulator, AR simulator, and mixed reality simulator. In performing this review, we have categorized the simulators using the following definitions:

- Augmented reality (AR) simulator: an interactive simulator in which the real-world environment is enhanced by computer-generated content perceived by the user using different senses. In these simulators, the specifically designed physical component could be absent (using only pre-existing elements of the real-world environment, such as the ground, a wall etc.), passive (not actively participating in the simulation), or active (providing/enabling specific functionalities in the simulation).
- Hybrid simulator: an interactive simulator in which the system integrates both a virtual and a physical module. In these simulators the physical parts are always present, but they could play either a passive or active role in the simulation.
- Mixed reality (MR) simulator: an interactive simulator in which real content (physical objects) and virtual information (computer-generated content) are merged so that they can interact with each other in real time. In these simulators the physical parts can interact with the virtual content (and/or vice versa).

Therefore, as an example, a simulation system could have been classified as AR and hybrid but not as MR if the system integrated both virtual content and physical parts but did not enable any virtual physical interaction.

The results of the classification according to these definitions are given in Section 3.10, which reports the associate statistical data collected by answering statistical questions SQ2 ("How many AR simulators are there?"), SQ3 ("How many MR simulators are there?"), and SQ4 ("How many hybrid simulators are there?").

2.2. Literature Search

The literature search was conducted using the following nine electronic databases: Scopus, Google Scholar, PubMed, ProQuest, ScienceDirect, Wiley Online Library, IEEE Xplore, Taylor & Francis Online and SAGE. The searches were limited to studies published between February 2008 and April 2020 inclusive. The review was conducted by four reviewers and the searches in all the databases above returned 262 results.

We have used the following research terms:

- (Augmented Reality OR AR) AND (Simulation OR Simulator) AND (Healthcare OR Medicine OR Surgery OR Surgical)
- (Mixed Reality OR MR) AND (Simulation OR Simulator) AND (Healthcare OR Medicine OR Surgery OR Surgical)
- (Hybrid) AND (Simulation OR Simulator) AND (Healthcare OR Medicine OR Surgery OR Surgical)

The search in the online digital libraries was conducted in April 2020.

2.3. Study Selection

The selection process started with 262 studies collected from online digital libraries. We defined three questions to select and include relevant studies:

Q1: Is the study relevant to healthcare simulation for improving the medical technical and/or non-technical skills?
Q2: Are the simulation techniques based on AR, MR, and/or hybrid approach?
Q3: Does the study concern the development of an ad-hoc simulator or the evaluation of a commercial simulator?

The selection process has been divided into four phases:

1. Removal of duplicates from nine different databases. After removing them, 98 studies remained.

2. Removal of editorials (1), reviews (2), book chapters (1), conference abstracts (8), thesis (9), reports (1), and reflections (4). After removing them, 72 studies remained for the next phase.
3. Removal of studies after reading the title and abstract. The removed articles do not resolve question Q1. After removing them, 35 studies remained.
4. Removal of studies after reading the full text, since some papers are still dubious after step 3. The removed articles do not resolve questions Q2 and Q3. A total of 23 studies remained relevant for our review.

Figure 1 shows the flow chart for the selection of studies according to PRISMA statements [21].

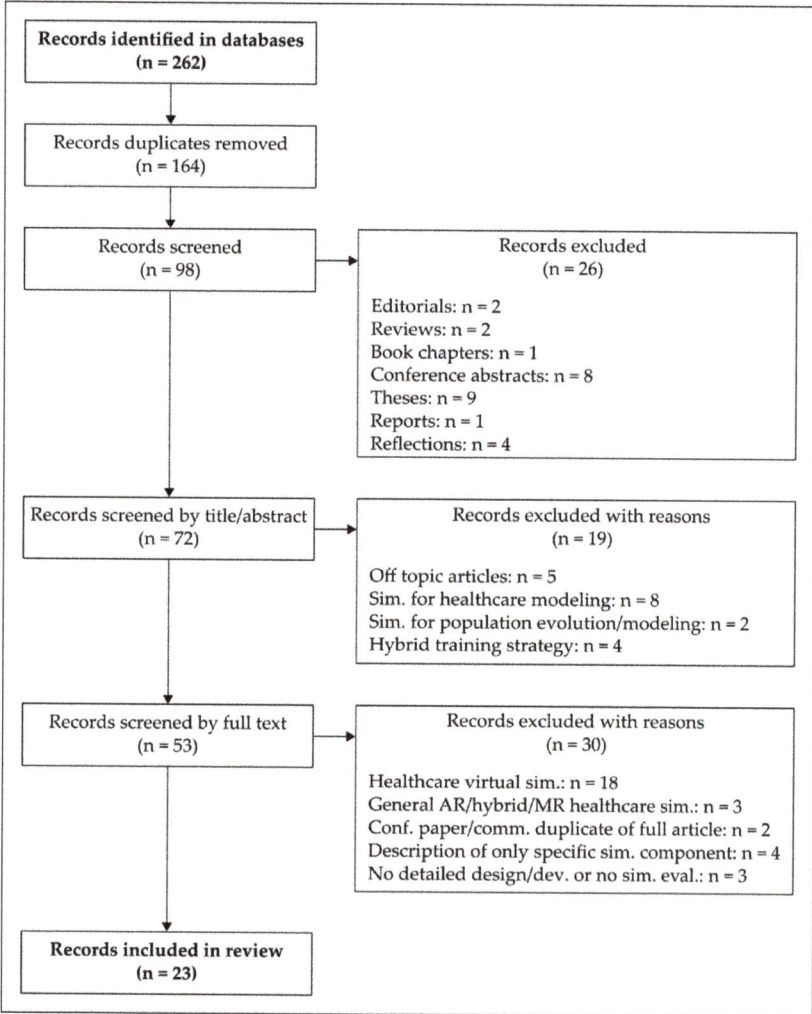

Figure 1. Flow chart illustrating the selection of studies according to PRISMA statements.

2.4. Research Questions

To guide the entire methodology and to help define the purpose of our systematic review, we have defined 23 research questions that have been classified into three categories: General Question (GQ), Focus Question (FQ), and Statistical Question (SQ). All these research questions (GQs, FQs, and SQs) are listed in Table 1.

Table 1. Research questions.

Type/Code		Research Questions
General Questions	GQ1	Which is the target clinical area?
	GQ2	Which skills are addressed by simulator? (technical skills, non-technical skills)
	GQ3	Does the simulator integrate haptic feedback?
	GQ4	What kind of sensors are used?
	GQ5	Is the simulator patient-specific? (patient-specific, not-patient-specific)
	GQ6	Are the simulator components reusable?
	GQ7	Is a clinical performance evaluation performed?
	GQ8	Does the simulator allow the selection of different scenarios based on trainee's needs?
	GQ9	How portable is the simulator? (very portable, portable, not portable)
Focus Questions	FQ1	How invasive is the simulated surgical approach? (non-inv., minimally-inv., inv.)
	FQ2	Which mode is used to convey haptic feedback?
	FQ3	Which tracking approach is used to implement AR? (marker-based or marker-less)
	FQ4	What visualization type is used? (monitor, hand-held display, HMD, projection)
	FQ5	What kind of artificial intelligence technique is implemented?
	FQ6	Which types of phantom are used? (commercial, custom-made)
	FQ7	Which simulator manufacturing technique is used?
	FQ8	Which metric is used for performance evaluation?
	FQ9	Which evaluation method is performed to validate the simulator?
	FQ10	Is a statistical analysis performed?
Statistical Questions	SQ1	How many commercial simulators are used?
	SQ2	How many AR simulators are there?
	SQ3	How many MR simulators are there?
	SQ4	How many hybrid simulators are there?

GQs concern the target clinical area (GQ1), the skills addressed by the simulator (GQ2), the presence of haptic feedback (GQ3), integrated sensor types (GQ4), the presence of patient-specific anatomy (GQ5), the reusability of simulator components (GQ6), the evaluation of clinical performance (GQ7), the possibility to select different scenarios based on the trainee's needs (GQ8), and simulator portability level (GQ9).

FQs refer to specific questions to help answering GQs providing more details on how invasive the simulated surgical approach is (FQ1), the mode used to convey haptic feedback (FQ2), the tracking approach adopted (FQ3), the visualization techniques used (FQ4), the artificial intelligence technique implemented (FQ5), the phantom type used (FQ6), the manufacturing techniques adopted (FQ7), the performance evaluation metric used (FQ8), the evaluation method performed (FQ9), and the presence of statistical analysis (FQ10).

SQs concern the current trends in the choice of simulation approaches in the healthcare sector (SQ2, SQ3, and SQ4) and the types of simulators (commercial or custom-made) used to implement a specific approach or to compare two different approaches (SQ1).

3. Results

A total of 23 studies remained relevant for our review. Table 2 contains basic information on the selected studies: the authors and year of publication and reference number (column Reference) and the publication title (column Title).

Table 2. Selected studies.

Reference	Title of Selected Study
Coelho 2020 [22]	Augmented reality and physical hybrid model simulation for preoperative planning of metopic craniosynostosis surgery.
Condino 2018 [23]	How to build a patient-specific hybrid simulator for orthopedic open surgery: benefits and limits of mixed-reality using the Microsoft HoloLens.
Condino 2011 [24]	How to build patient-specific synthetic abdominal anatomies. An innovative approach from physical toward hybrid surgical simulators.
Feifer 2011 [25]	Randomized controlled trial of virtual reality and hybrid simulation for robotic surgical training.
Ferrari 2016 [26]	Augmented reality visualization of deformable tubular structures for surgical simulation.
Fuerst 2014 [27]	A novel augmented reality simulator for minimally invasive spine surgery.
Fushima 2016 [28]	Mixed-reality simulation for orthognathic surgery.
Halic 2010 [29]	Mixed reality simulation of rasping procedure in artificial cervical disc replacement (ACDR) surgery.
Huang 2018 [30]	The use of augmented reality glasses in central line simulation: "see one, simulate many, do one competently, and teach everyone"
Jain 2019 [31]	Virtual reality based hybrid simulation for functional endoscopic sinus surgery.
Keebler 2014 [32]	Building a simulated medical augmented reality training system.
Lahanas 2015 [33]	A novel augmented reality simulator for skills assessment in minimal invasive surgery.
Lee 2013 [34]	Augmented reality intravenous injection simulator based 3D medical imaging for veterinary medicine.
Lin 2012 [35]	The development of optical see-through display based on augmented reality for oral implant surgery simulation.
Loukas 2013 [36]	An integrated approach to endoscopic instrument tracking for augmented reality applications in surgical simulation training.
Nomura 2015 [37]	Laparoscopic skill improvement after virtual reality simulator training in medical students as assessed by augmented reality simulator.
Onishi 2013 [38]	AR dental surgical simulator using haptic feedback.
Parkes 2009 [39]	A mixed reality simulator for feline abdominal palpation training in veterinary medicine.
Tai 2009 [40]	Augmented-reality-driven medical simulation platform for percutaneous nephrolithotomy with cybersecurity awareness.
Thomas 2014 [41]	The validity and reliability of a hybrid reality simulator for wire navigation in orthopedic surgery.
Tsujita 2018 [42]	Development of a surgical simulator for training retraction of tissue with an encountered-type haptic interface using MR fluid.
Van Duren 2018 [43]	Augmented reality fluoroscopy simulation of the guide-wire. insertion in DHS surgery: a proof of concept study.
Viglialoro 2018 [44]	Augmented reality to improve surgical simulation. Lessons learned towards the design of a hybrid laparoscopic simulator for cholecystectomy.

3.1. Target Clinical Area (GQ1, FQ1)

Simulation-based education is widely incorporated as a means of effective training to learn technical and non-technical skills in almost all areas of healthcare. In the past, it has been mainly used for training medical professionals to reduce errors during surgery. Today, there is a growing trend to use simulation both as a tool for objective skill assessment and as an anatomy learning tool to circumvent the drawbacks associated with conventional anatomy training based on cadaver dissection.

With regard to question GQ1 ("Which is the target clinical area?"), 22 of the 23 studies concern simulators for training of surgical tasks/procedures (such as neurosurgery [22,42], abdominal surgery [24,26,40,44], orthopedic surgery [23,27,29,41,43], dental surgery [28,35,38], otorhinolaryngological surgery [31], laparoscopic basic tasks [25,33,36], abdominal surgery and basic tasks [37], palpation [39], intravenous injection [34], and central venous catheter insertion [30]); eight of them use the simulation also as an assessment tool [25,33,34,37,40,41,43]. One study reports the use of simulation only for didactive purposes to learn anatomy [32].

Surgical Approaches (FQ1)

A surgical procedure can be classified according to the degree of invasiveness in non-invasive surgery, minimally invasive surgery (MIS), or invasive surgery (i.e., open surgery). The non-invasive surgical approach is a conservative treatment that does not require any incision in the skin; such procedures range from simple observation to surgical specialties such as radiosurgery. The MIS approach refers to surgical procedures using small incisions. This approach allows the patient to recover faster with less pain than the open surgery approach characterized by large incisions.

In answering question FQ1 ("What surgical approach is implemented in sim.? (non inv., minimally inv., inv.)"), a total of 15 studies concern the simulation of MIS procedures [24–27,29–31,33,34,36,37,40,41,43,44], six concern the simulation of invasive approaches [22,23,28,35,38,42], and only one concerns the simulation of a non-invasive approach [39].

3.2. Technical and Non-Technical Skills in Surgery (GQ2)

Mastery of both technical and non-technical skills is required to perform a safe procedure. The former are defined as psychomotor actions or related mental faculties acquired through practice and learning, pertaining to a particular craft or profession. The latter are defined as the social (teamwork, leadership, communication), cognitive (situation awareness, decision-making), and personal resource skills (stress, fatigue, and stress management) that complement technical skills, contributing to safe and effective performance [45]. As reported by [46], the technical skills are no longer enough for the delivery of a modern and safe surgical practice; indeed, more frequently the risk to the patient is from failure of non-technical skills [45,46].

Regarding question GQ2 ("Which skills are addressed by simulator? (technical skills, non-technical skills)"), in the largest part of the analyzed studies [22–31,33,34,37,38,40,41,44], the simulators address both the technical and non-technical skills. Only in five studies [35,36,39,42,43] do the simulators address only the technical skills. Indeed, many studies show that simulation-based education is a powerful tool to teach both technical and non-technical skills to individual surgeons and surgical teams without risking patient safety.

3.3. Haptic Feedback (GQ3, FQ2)

Haptic feedback plays a key role in medical simulations because it increases the simulation fidelity with beneficial effects on training. In particular, haptic feedback is an important add-on for virtual reality simulators because it improves the perception of virtual objects giving the user the illusion of touch. Many VR simulators recreate the sense of touch through haptic devices that apply forces, vibrations, or motions to the user during their interaction with the virtual environment.

In particular, haptic technology can be used to simulate the tactile properties of tissues (i.e., the stiffness of a tissue is essential during a palpation procedure) and the manipulation of surgical instrumentation [47].

With regard to question GQ3 ("Does the simulator integrate haptic feedback?"), 22 [22–31,33–44] of the 23 studies integrate haptic feedback. The only system that does not offer such feedback is the simulator presented in [32] designed for the AR visualization of anatomical models for educational purposes.

In more detail, answering question FQ2 ("Which mode is used to convey haptic feedback? (actual interaction with physical components, haptic interface)"), the largest part of the studies analyzed [22–24,26,27,29–31,33,34,36,38,41–44] offer the trainee the possibility to use actual surgical instruments and/or manipulate/palpate physical anatomical replicas.

Two of the reviewed simulators [39,40] incorporate a haptic software module and deliver the simulated haptic experience via commercial haptic interfaces: Phantom Premium devices [39] and Phantom Omni devices [40] (Sensable Technologies, Woburn, MA). The main difference between the two studies is that haptic interfaces are used in [39] to interact with virtual models of organs superimposed on a physical model (a cat toy), whereas in [40] they are used to interact with a purely virtual representation of anatomy to mimic the insertion of a percutaneous needle and to mimic hand palpation.

3.4. Implementation of the Virtual Component of the Simulators (FQ2–5)

In the following paragraphs we report technical details on the implementation of the virtual component of the simulator, including the tracking approach adopted for deriving the spatiotemporal relationship between the real and virtual worlds (FQ3), the display technologies to provide the user with computer-generated information (FQ4), and the implementation of artificial intelligence (AI) techniques (FQ5).

3.4.1. Tracking Approach (FQ3)

The knowledge of the spatiotemporal relationship between the real and virtual worlds is a key aspect in the development of a MR simulator for allowing a proper interaction of virtual elements (e.g., virtual models of the anatomy) with real objects (e.g., surgical tools). Moreover, accurate and fast estimation of the viewing pose relative to the real objects is a crucial challenge for a proper alignment of the virtual content to the real-world in AR/MR application.

Tracking methods commonly employed comprise the following approaches:

1. Vision-based approaches, that can be further categorized into two mutually non-exclusive methods: marker-based and marker-less (i.e., location-based position).

A marker is a distinguishable artificial element that a computer system can detect using image segmentation, pattern recognition, and computer vision techniques. Marker-based methods are fast; however, inherent drawbacks of these approaches lie in the fact that marker detection is very sensitive to marker occlusion and poor ambient lighting (that can make the makers unrecognizable). As for the latter issue, infrared (IR) retro-reflective markers can be used to improve the reliability of tracking, reducing the effects of ambient illumination.

2. Other sensor-based approaches (apart from vision sensors) including electromagnetic tracking, acoustic tracking, and inertial tracking sensors.

3. Hybrid techniques that combine marker-based with marker-less approaches or vision-based and sensor-based techniques.

Our analysis shows that none of the literature simulators employ a marker-less method alone, instead there are several systems based on the use of markers. Explored marker-based solutions mainly use planar printable markers such as Vuforia Image Targets (images that Vuforia Engine can detect and track) [48], square black and white patterns [32–35,42], and colored strips [41]. Only two systems [29,43] employ non-planar markers: retroreflective IR markers tracked by the Vicon system in [29] and two colored (green and yellow) markers in [43].

As for the sensor-based approach, our literature search shows that the most common sensors used for the development of AR/MR simulators are electromagnetic (EM) coils [24,26,31,41,44] that do not require line-of-sight and can be used to track hidden anatomical structures as described in [24,26,44].

Finally, some simulators adopt a hybrid approach. For example, the minimally invasive laparoscopic system described in [33] employs a planar marker to track the box-trainer; an electromagnetic sensor, a rotary encoder, and IR sensors are instead used to provide the laparoscopic tool kinematics (3D pose of the tool in six DOF (degrees of freedom), shaft rotation, and opening angle of the tooltip). The simulator in [34] employs a gyro sensor coupled with a planar marker for an accurate tracking of the instrument (a syringe). Another hybrid approach is presented in [41] for estimating the pose of the surgical instrument with respect to the camera: first, an algorithm creates an adaptive model of a color strip attached to the distal part of the tool, then another program tracks the endoscopic shaft, using a combined Hough–Kalman approach.

3.4.2. Visualization Modality (FQ4)

Available display technologies to provide the user with computer-generated information include: 2D monitors, hand-held displays (mobile phones and tablets), head-mounted displays (HMDs), and spatial projection-based AR displays.

Most of the revised simulators [25–28,33,34,36,38,39,41,43,44] use a traditional 2D display. In these simulators (except for the commercial LapSim® and ProMIS® systems), the virtual information is not designed to interact in real-time with the real content (physical objects). Moreover, most of these simulators are for minimally invasive procedures not performed under direct vision. Indeed, [25,26,36,44] are designed for laparoscopy, for endoscopic surgery [33], and for wire navigation in minimally invasive procedures [41,43]. Finally, in [27] the monitor is used to show simulated fluoroscopic images to guide spine surgery. Among the other simulation systems for procedures involving the direct visualization of the anatomy, a particular solution is presented in [38]. This system uses a traditional monitor in a tilted position coupled with a half mirror placed horizontally between the user's head and his/her hands to visualize the virtual information superimposed onto the anatomical physical replica.

Six papers [23,29,30,34,35,40] report the use of a HMDs. These intrinsically provide the user with an egocentric viewpoint and allow handsfree work; for these reasons, HMDs are deemed the most ergonomic solution for applications including manual tasks performed by the user under direct vision, similar to what happens in open surgery. The devices selected by the AR/MR simulators evaluated are optical see-through HMDs (OST HMDs): these displays offer an instantaneous and unobstructed full resolution view of the real environment allowing a naturalistic experience. In more detail, the simulators in [23,40] are based on Microsoft HoloLens (1st generation), [30] is based on AiRScouter WD-200B, and [35] presents the design of an innovative custom-made OST HMD. Finally, HMDs are also used in [29] (NVIS nVisor ST50) and [31] (HTC VICE MIS) for virtual reality immersive experience.

Only two simulators [22,32] employ a hand-held display: these systems are designed for AR visualization of VR anatomical models for surgical planning [22] or training of medical and anatomy students [32]. None of the simulators employ a spatial projection-based AR display.

3.4.3. Artificial Intelligence Techniques Integrated in the Simulation (FQ5)

The use of AI algorithms is raising in the development of surgical simulators as the AI potential is huge for automatic performance evaluation, metrics extraction, simulation level adaptation to the trainee performance, and realistic force feedback implementation.

Actually, in the literature, AI methods are studied but not yet robustly integrated. Indeed, among all the studies analyzed, only four report the use of AI methods [25,36,37,40]. In [25] and [37], the authors use the commercial ProMIS hybrid laparoscopic simulator in a training program. ProMIS integrates a machine learning algorithm for the tracking of the laparoscopic instrumentation. In particular, the instruments are optically recognized through color-contrasted adhesive labels that are affixed to their distal tips and through a proprietary formula that combines time and path length the simulator manages to record and evaluate the economy of motion, and then generates a numeric score for the execution time. The same approach is used in [36] with the scope to estimate the 3D pose of the surgical instrument with respect to the camera and follow its movements. In this paper the adaptive algorithm developed through the color tracking method is compared with a second algorithm that tracks the endoscopic shaft using a combined Hough–Kalman approach. Here the final aim is to achieve a robust interaction with the virtual world and to improve the realism of the rendering when the virtual scene is occluded by the instrument.

In [40], AI is used to improve the realism of the force feedback provided in the AR simulator. In particular, the authors use a cyber security algorithm to anonymously and safely record actual force feedback from real surgical interventions, then they analyze the data recorded to provide precise muscle memory acquisition during the training procedure.

3.5. Implementation of the Physical Component of the Simulator (GQ4, FQ6–7)

The physical components of the simulators are based mostly on phantoms (plastic structures) simulating parts of the patient body or a full human body. The more complex phantoms are equipped with sensors and computer software that allow an objective performance assessment and the implementation of advanced functionalities such as guidance information to the trainee, simulation of physiological functions, etc. The main advantage of using physical models is that they provide a realistic training environment owing to the real haptic feedback provided and the possibility to use actual surgical tools.

3.5.1. Materials and Fabrication Techniques (FQ6–7)

Simulators can consist of commercial or custom-made physical components. The analysis performed to answer question FQ6 ("Which phantoms are used? (commercial, custom-made)") reveals that most of the simulators analyzed are custom-made; indeed, a total of 13 studies employ custom-made phantoms, and only five studies employ commercial phantoms.

Below, the manufacturing techniques for both of these types of simulators are reported to answer question FQ7 ("Which simulator manufacturing technique is used?"). As for the simulators with custom-made anatomical replicas, only three studies [29,35,38] do not provide details on the manufactured process, while the others provide a description of the manufacturing method useful to reproduce the simulator.

The study in [27] presents a peculiar method for fabricating the anatomical replicas. The phantom includes artificial vertebrae and soft tissue. The synthetic vertebrae are manufactured starting from frozen and formalin-fixed thoracolumbar spines; they are defrosted and dissected, then embedded using a fast curing plastic. In particular, polyurethane foam recipe is used for the inner cancellous core of vertebrae while a resin is used covering a layer of cortical bone. Finally, different mixtures of silicone rubber are used to manufacture the human's erector spinae and the skin, while a thin plastic foil is used to imitate a muscle fascia.

In a large part of the studies [22–24,26,28,29,31,34,44], the authors instead developed phantoms extracting the 3D anatomical models from CT images of real patients. In [22–24,26,29,31,34,44], the virtual anatomical model is turned into a tangible physical replica by using 3D printing technologies and casting fabrication processes. For example, in [34], the authors fabricate a silicone model using a casting technique based on a 3D printed forelimb prototype of a beagle dog.

The remaining studies explored the use of 3D printing with the resin and acrylonitrile butadiene styrene (ABS). The resin is used to mimic the skull bone in [22] and to manufacture anatomical structures and surgical tools in [31]. In addition, in [22] the authors improve the model according to a handmade process with a platinum-cure silicone (Dragon Skin; Smooth-On, Inc, Macungie, PA, USA), mixed with some additives in order to mimic human tissue properties such as textures, consistencies, and mechanical resistance. Instead, ABS is employed to 3D print a hip models in [23] because it adequately approximates the mechanical behavior of the bony natural tissue. After that, the hip model is embedded in a soft synthetic foam and covered with a skin-like material which allows an accurate simulation of palpation and incision. In addition, in [24,26,44] the ABS material is used to 3D print molds for anatomical replicas. In [24], the hybrid simulator includes a physical commercial trunk phantom with replicas of the liver, gallbladder, pancreas, and stomach. The physical environment is enriched with coherent virtual models of the entire abdomen.

The replicas are obtained using casting processes of silicone materials and pigment powders. In addition, the stomach and liver are EM sensorized to quantify deformations caused by surgical action. In [26,44], the hybrid simulator developed by Viglialoro et al. includes both patient-specific models (e.g., liver, gallbladder, pancreas, abdominal aorta, esophagus–stomach–duodenum) and non-patient-specific synthetic organs designed in a CAD environment (e.g., arterial tree, biliary tree, and connective tissue). The strategy used to manufacture patient-specific replicas is the same as that used in [24]. The manufacturing process of the arterial tree and biliary tree involves the use of nitinol tubes joined together by tin wires and covered by a thin silicone layer. In addition, EM sensors are inserted inside the nitinol tubes to implement an AR solution allowing the real-time visualization of the Calot's triangle. Finally, the synthetic tissue is produced in the form of thin sheets in gelatinous material (Psyllogel Fiber powder).

The research in [28] developed a hybrid simulator that integrates a 3D virtual dentoskeletal model with the real dental cast model using the reference splint. However, the authors do not provide details on the manufactured process used to create the dental cast model.

Only five studies employ commercial phantoms. Among these, four are anthropomorphic [30,37,41,43]. In [41,43], both studies employ a plastic foam femur surrogate (Sawbones AG, Karlihof, Switzerland) to fabricate a hybrid simulator for wire navigation in orthopedic surgery. The research reported in [30] completes a commercial physical mannequin for internal jugular vein central line insertion with AR glasses. Finally, in [37] the authors customize the ProMIS simulator with a gallbladder model (Limbs & Things, Bristol, UKd) to perform a cholecystectomy procedure.

In [40], the authors report the use of commercial non-anthropomorphic phantoms. In detail, they employ two Phantom Omni (a six DOF haptic device) with one stylus that mimics the percutaneous needle during the simulation of percutaneous nephrolithotomy.

Finally, the research in [39] reports the use of toy as the main physical component of a simulator developed for training of veterinarians: two commercial Phantom Premium 1.5 haptic devices are positioned on either side of a toy cat with virtual representations of the chest and abdominal organs superimposed on the physical model.

3.5.2. Sensors Types (GQ4)

In addition to the use of position sensors for the tracking of tools and anatomical structures, in [40,42] force sensors are used to measure the puncture force during percutaneous renal access [40] and the retracting force of soft biological tissues [42].

3.6. Patient-Specific Simulation (GQ5)

As reported by Ryu et al. [49], the patient-specific simulation is very useful because it provides an accurate representation of intraoperative conditions related to the patient anatomy and the target surgical technique, and it allows trainees to try different approaches that can translate into training for complication avoidance.

Among all the studies analyzed, 13 report the use of a patient-specific simulator. In two studies [28,40], the 3D models are purely virtual, whereas in nine studies [22–24,27,29,31,34,35,38] virtual models are combined with physical replicas to create a more complex environment; finally, in only two studies [26,44] the patient-specific models are purely physical. All 3D models are obtained starting from the segmentation of the CT images of real patients.

3.7. Reusability of Simulator Components (GQ6)

Two key challenges to the reduction of the training costs are the reusability of the medical simulator components and the minimization of spare parts cost. With regard to question GQ6 ("Are the simulator components reusable?"), in the largest part of the studies analyzed [22–25,27–35,38–41,43] the entire simulator is reusable. This is due to the fact that the authors perform only non-destructive tasks such as palpation, basic laparoscopic tasks (i.e., instrument navigation, peg transfer, clipping of virtual objects, etc.), insertion of tools (i.e., wire navigation, intravenous injection, etc.), and surgical planning. In particular, the authors use materials that are extremely durable over time such as silicone rubbers, polyurethane, and plastic materials.

In studies [26,44], the authors have designed solutions to make all anatomical components reusable such as the liver, gallbladder, pancreas, abdominal aorta, esophagus–stomach–duodenum, arterial tree, and biliary tree, except the connective tissue which must be dissected during each training session. Finally, only in four studies [22,29,36,37] was the entire simulator substituted after each training session.

3.8. General Features of Simulation Systems (GQ7–9, FQ7–10)

The key feature of simulation-based medical education is the knowledge of the results of the trainee performance during a learning experience because that leads to effective learning. Other important simulation features include the possibility to create medical scenarios of progressive difficulty and the portability of the medical simulators [50]. Each feature will be explained in the next three subsections.

3.8.1. Performance Evaluation Metrics (GQ7, FQ7–8)

The assessment of clinical competence is one of the most difficult and important tasks in medical education because it provides feedback to trainees about their clinical skills, supports self-paced learning, assures the public, and provides evidence toward the certification of achievement of clinical competencies.

There are several methods of assessment, each with its own strengths and limitations. As reported by Epstein in [51], the main strategies include written examinations, direct observation or video review, assessments by supervising clinician, clinical simulation, and multisource ("360-degree") assessments and portfolios. The appropriateness of each method depends on the goal that is addressed (i.e., measuring performance or skill acquisition, etc.) and on the level of the learner's education.

Ryall et al. [52] present a systematic review of the simulation as a clinical assessment tool. They suggest that the simulation can be a valid and reliable method to assess the technical skills and to determine the skill level and the capability to practice safely. Indeed, the simulation can both differentiate performance between experts and novices on given tasks and also identify poor performers.

With regard to question GQ7 ("Is a clinical performance evaluation performed?"), a total of eight studies assess clinical performance. In answering question FQ8 ("Which metric is used for performance evaluation?"), two methods of performance evaluation are used [53]: the first technique is based on the human rater's score performance using checklists on scoring rubrics, and it is used in [30]; instead, the second method is based on the automated scoring of measurements integrated into the simulator itself, and it is used in the remaining studies [25,33,34,37,40,41,43].

The results in answering question FQ7 ("What kind of artificial intelligence technique is implemented?") are that one of six studies used an automated scoring based on artificial neural networks [40].

3.8.2. Implementation of Different Levels of Complexity (GQ8)

To design an effective learning experience in simulation-based medical education, an important factor is the possibility to offer a wide range of task difficulty levels. An appropriate level of training allows the trainee to increase the mastery of skills; the learners have opportunities to engage in the practice of medical skills, starting from basic techniques (novice levels) and proceeding to train at progressively higher difficulties (expert levels) [50]. Five of the 23 articles address question GQ8 ("Does the simulator allow selection of different scenarios based on trainee's needs?").

In [33], the authors propose an AR laparoscopic simulator including a box-trainer, a camera, and a set of laparoscopic tools equipped with custom-made sensors. Such a system allows the trainee to interact with various VR training elements. To this, the authors implement three different training tasks: instrument navigation, to improve the perception of depth of field; peg transfer, for hand-eye coordination skills; and clipping, for bimanual operation.

In [40], the authors developed an AR simulator (SimPCNL) for percutaneous nephrolithotomy and successively compared it with the commercial virtual simulator, PERC Mentor (Simbionix, Cleveland, OH). Both simulators allow the trainees to practice basic tasks for percutaneous access procedures performed under real-time fluoroscopy on a variety of virtual patients.

Two studies [25,37] concern two laparoscopic commercial simulators: the LapSim®virtual simulator (Surgical Science Inc, Minneapolis, MN, USA) and the ProMIS hybrid simulator (Haptica, Dublin, Ireland) that offer different training scenarios with different levels of complexity. No outcome has been reported on this aspect of simulation. The former simulator (the LapSim) is a high-fidelity simulator available in two versions: with and without haptic feedback. This modular system consists of laparoscopic instruments as interfaces connected to a computer. Modules include basic laparoscopic skills, ranging from navigation to more advanced skills (e.g., coordination, grasping, cutting, clip applying, suturing, etc.) and multiple surgical procedures (e.g., cholecystectomy, appendectomy, laparoscopic gynecology, etc.). The latter system (the ProMIS) combines a laparoscopic mannequin connected to a laptop with integration also into a virtual environment. It uses real surgical instruments which are tracked during the tasks to provide an accurate and objective assessment of the user's performance. The system includes both basic laparoscopic tasks and entire surgical procedures, such as appendectomy, colectomy, cholecystectomy, etc. Different physical models (such as suturing pads) can be inserted into the mannequin; for example, in [25] the authors used the MISTELS (McGill Inanimate System for Training and Evaluation of Laparoscopic Skills) task set, whereas in [37] the authors used an object-positioning module and a gallbladder model during the training sessions.

In [44], the authors developed an AR simulator for laparoscopic cholecystectomy. The key feature of this system is the capability to create physical and virtual scenarios with different degrees of complexity, allowing the trainee to acquire both the dexterity necessary for good practice and the decision-making skills. Due to the morphological and topological variations that occur naturally in human hepatobiliary anatomy, the authors predisposed physical models of different anatomical variations of the arterial and biliary trees and implemented an easy connection/disconnection coupling to facilitate any substitution on demand. This gives the tutor the possibility to choose the anatomical variations according to the trainee's level of experience.

3.8.3. Portability (GQ9)

The portability of a simulator is a major factor in spreading the use of medical simulators in educational and training settings. In answering question GQ9 ("How portable is the simulator? (very portable, portable, not portable)"), we have defined three levels of portability:

- A very-portable simulator is a commercial or custom system designed to be held in the hands and/or on the head or that can be easily carried. Seven studies [22,23,25,30,32,35,37] report the use of very portable simulators.
- A portable simulator is a system designed to have a simple assembly/disassembly of the setup and (eventually) an easy calibration procedure. Thirteen studies [24,26–28,31,33,34,36,39,41,43,44] report the use of portable simulators.
- A non-portable simulator is a system that requires a dedicated room and/or has a complex assembly/disassembly of the setup and (eventually) a difficult calibration procedure. Two studies [29,42] report the use of non-portable simulators.

In [40], the authors use two simulators: one commercial, identified as very portable; and one custom, identified as portable.

3.9. Evaluation of Simulators (FQ9–10)

To guarantee proper simulator-based training it is important to verify whether improvements in performance on medical simulators translate into improved performance on real patients. In [53], the authors affirm that the evaluation of medical simulators has to satisfy two main criteria that are "validity" and "reliability".

Overall, the "validity" is the degree to which a method measures something. The main types of validity are face, content, construct, concurrent, and predictive validity. In the medical simulation context:

- Face validity refers to simulator realism, and it is assessed by experts by means of questionnaires or surveys;
- Content validity measures the appropriateness and usefulness of the simulator as a training tool, and it is typically assessed by experts with checklists;
- Construct validity determines the ability of simulator to differentiate between expert and novices;
- Concurrent validity indicates the correspondence between trainees' performance tested on a simulator and on a gold standard method or against another, previously validated, simulator;
- Predicitive validity denotes the ability of the simulator to predict future performance in real scenarios [53,54].

"Reliability" refers to the consistency of measurements. However, there are two other less important criteria that are "fairness" and "usability": the first is an aspect of validity, and it is refers to absence of any bias (test free of bias, lack of favoritism toward test takers, accessibility, and validity of score interpretations), while the second concerns implementation costs, time required, ease of administration, and comprehensibility of the results for the users [53,54].

To answer question FQ9 ("Which evaluation method is performed to validate the simulator? (technical, validity, technical + validity)"), we have defined three evaluation stages: only technical evaluation, only validity evaluation, both validity and technical evaluations.

The technical evaluation concerns accuracy, reliability, and efficiency, and only nine studies out of 23 report a technical evaluation [22,27,28,31,35,36,38,42,43]. In [35,38], the authors evaluate the displays in terms of registration accuracy [35,38] and frames-per-second (FPS) during the visualization of surface and volume data [35].

Measurements of force are performed in [27,42]. Fuerst et al. [27] evaluate the physical components of the simulator measuring the average force during transpedicular insertions performed on six vertebral models to perform a comparison with human specimens. Tsujita et al. [42] instead evaluate whether the developed haptic interface and the mechanical components satisfy the specifications in terms of force requirements.

In [23,28,36,43], the authors evaluate the accuracy of simulators that include an AR component. Among them, Condino et al. in [23] evaluate the accuracy of a simulator developed for Microsoft HoloLens. The accuracy was evaluated in terms of the perceived position of AR targets; moreover, the authors evaluate the workload and usability of the HoloLens for their application considering visual and audio perception, interaction, and ergonomics issues.

In [31], the authors evaluate the reliability and efficiency of the simulator. The authors evaluate the accuracy of the registration between real and virtual scenarios using the Euclidean distance between the 3D point where the resident hit the equipment in the simulation model and the actual 3D point in the real world, and the robustness, checking if the registration error depended on landmark points. Additionally, the authors demonstrated the efficiency of the system.

Validity evaluation: Eleven studies out of 23 report face/content/construct/concurrent/predictive validity tests [22,25,29,30,32–34,37,39,40]. Among them, three studies [29,32,39] perform a non-detailed preliminary evaluation of simulators, and the results obtained should be confirmed in larger studies. The sample sizes are five (expert physicians), five (undergraduate students), and seven (veterinary students), respectively. In [29], the authors evaluate the effectiveness of the system to teach anatomy and to grasp the basics of a specific orthopedic surgery. In [32], both content validity and usability evaluation are performed in terms of how easy to use the simulator is. In [39], the authors perform only face validity.

In [40], the authors report face, content, construct, skills improvement validity, and criterion validity (often divided into concurrent and predictive validity). They compare the developed simulator and the PERC Mentor.

Simulator's face and content validity are evaluated by 38 expert surgeons in [22] and by 40 subjects in [34]. In both of these studies, a questionnaire on the realism and the usefulness of simulators is used, and in [22] the authors also address questions on the value of AR for medical training. Overall, the opinions of the users are very positive in all studies. Finally, in [34], proficiency level is also assessed.

Concurrent validity is reported in four studies [25,30,37,40]. In [25], the authors evaluate the performance of 20 medical students in robotic surgery sessions before and after training using ProMIS and the LapSim. The results show that the use of ProMIS and LapSim simulators in conjunction with each other can improve robotic console performance. In [37], laparoscopic skills are assessed in ProMIS tasks before and after LapSim training to clarify whether this training improves operation skills: the results confirm an improvement. In [30], the authors compare physical simulation and AR simulation of central venous catheters mannequin. The results show a significant difference in the adherence level between the AR group and the non-AR group, owing to the real-time feedback the AR group received as they performed the procedure. Additionally, tests of usability, workload, and ergonomics of AR glasses are performed.

Lahanas et al. [33] report both face and construct validity of their simulator. Face validity is evaluated by 20 users (10 novices and 10 expert surgeons) using a questionnaire about the realism of the VR objects and the interaction between the instruments and the VR objects, and the difficulty of the task and the lack of force feedback during tool-object interaction. Construct validity is evaluated in three tasks between two experience groups. The results demonstrate highly significant differences in all performance metrics.

Validity and technical evaluation: Four studies out of 23 report face and content validity and technical evaluation [24,26,41,44].

With regard to face and content validity, all studies use a questionnaire on the realism and the usefulness of the simulators; in [26,44], the questions also address the value of AR for medical training. Overall, the opinions of the users are very positive. Additionally, in [26,44] the authors evaluate the robustness of the simulator hardware. The users enrolled in all studies are five expert surgeons in [26], 13 clinicians in [24], 10 expert surgeons in [44], six novices, and four expert surgeons in [41].

With regard to the technical evaluation, in [26,44] the accuracy of AR visualization is evaluated as adequate for training purposes. In [24], the authors perform three tests to measure eventual damage of EM sensors during embedding steps, the correspondence between planned and actual sensor positions, and the correspondence between real and virtual scenarios; all the results were coherent.

In [41], the authors assess both the simulator reliability measuring the precision of the tracking and the simulator face, content, and construct validity. All users agree on the realism of the simulator and on the fact that practice on the simulator would improve their intraoperative wire navigation performance. About the content validity assessment, the authors compare the desired task characteristics from the design specification checklist with the features of the assembled simulator. Additionally, construct validity results confirm the ability of a simulator to differentiate performance between experts and novices.

With regard to question FQ10 ("Is a statistical analysis performed?"), 16 studies out of 23 conducted a statistical analysis [22–28,30,31,33,34,37,40,41,43,44]. One criticism of these studies is that often the number of participants was small: only five studies involved more than 20 subjects [22,30,34,40,43], so further studies are needed to generalize the findings obtained.

3.10. Trends of Simulation Techniques in Healthcare (SQ1–4)

This review also reports the trends of simulation techniques in healthcare and the types (commercial or custom-made) of simulators used to integrate the chosen approach or to compare two or more different approaches.

The statistical data collected in this section are obtained by the answering the statistical questions SQ1 ("How many commercial simulators are used?"), SQ2 ("How many MR simulators?"), SQ3 ("How many AR simulators?"), and SQ4 ("How many hybrid simulators?"). Figure 2 shows the percentage of studies using commercial and custom-made simulators: it can be seen that 22% used commercial simulators, and 78% custom-made simulators.

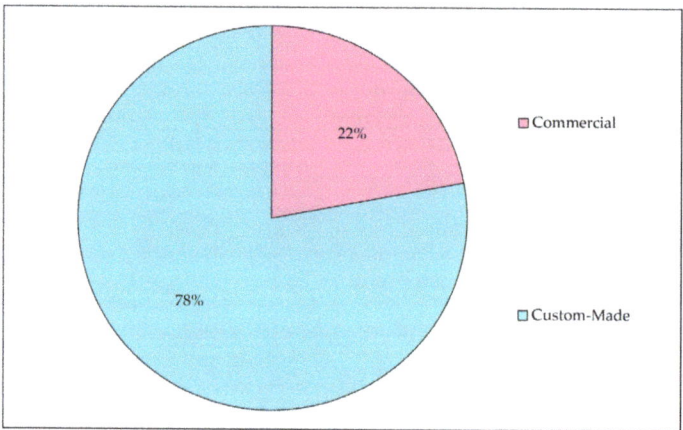

Figure 2. The pie chart shows the percentages of studies using commercial (22%) and custum-made (78%) simulators.

Figure 3 shows the distribution of the approaches used in the implementation of medical simulators: 43% of selected studies combine two approaches (MR and hybrid), 22% combine all three approaches, 26% employed only the hybrid approach, and 9% applied only the MR approach.

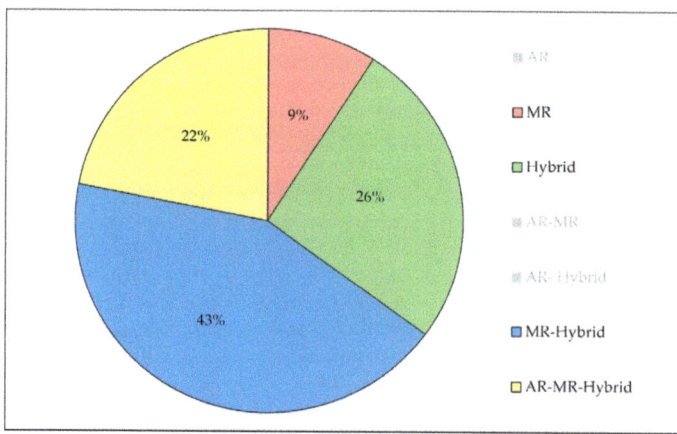

Figure 3. The pie chart shows the distribution of analyzed papers in terms of the approaches used in the implementation of medical simulators. The categories grayed out (augmented reality (AR), AR-mixed reality (MR), and AR-Hybrid) are associated with a percentage of 0%.

4. Discussion

This systematic review investigates the impact of AR, MR, and hybrid approaches on medical simulation and reveals that most of the selected studies (43%) combine MR and hybrid approaches.

Most studies use simulation predominantly as a medical/surgical training tool addressing both technical and non-technical skills. Eight of them use the simulator also as an automatic assessment tool for the evaluation of the user performance. However, given the promising role of simulation in objective skill assessment, we believe that more research is needed to integrate such functionalities in AR, MR, and hybrid simulators.

Furthermore, the review examines how the virtual and physical components are implemented. As for the virtual component, we analyzed the following core elements: the tracking approach for deriving the spatiotemporal relationship between the real and virtual worlds, the display technologies, and the implementation of software haptic feedback and AI techniques.

Tracking methods commonly employed for simulators include the use of EM sensors, vision-based approaches (mainly with planar printable markers), and hybrid methods. The latter use marker-based procedures combined with marker-less or sensor-based methods.

Concerning the visualization modality, most of the revised simulators use a traditional 2D display; six studies report the use of HMDs, and only two a hand-held display.

As for haptic feedback, it is mostly obtained through actual interaction with a physical replica of the anatomy. However, two simulators integrate a commercial haptic interface. More specifically, in one study, interaction with the physical environment is enriched by virtual haptic feedback generated by means of commercial haptic interfaces used to interact with internal organs not reproduced in the mannequin.

Actually, in the literature, AI algorithms are studied but not yet robustly integrated. Indeed, among all the studies analyzed, only four report the use of AI methods. The use of AI techniques is increasing in the development of surgical simulators, as the AI potential is huge for automatic performance evaluation, metrics extraction, simulation level adaptation to the trainee performance, and realistic force feedback implementation. Thus, we believe that this issue deserves future attention for the development of high performance AR, MR, and hybrid simulators.

Among all the studies analyzed, 78% use custom-made simulators. The manufacturing process for most custom-made phantoms starts with extracting 3D models from CT images of real patients. The 3D model is turned into a tangible physical replica using 3D printing technologies and casting fabrication processes. Printing materials such as resin and ABS are used to reproduce rigid parts (i.e., bones), and they adequately approximate the mechanical behavior of the natural tissue. Silicone mixtures and polyurethane materials are used for the manufacturing of soft parts to mimic human tissue properties. Among the revised custom-made phantoms, two include both patient-specific and non-patient specific synthetic organs. In addition, some authors equip the phantoms with EM sensors to implement AR applications. Overall, the manufacturing materials used are extremely durable over time allowing the reusability of the phantom (where is it possible) and thus a reduction in training costs. Given the importance of physical interaction in the skill acquisition for surgery, it is essential in the future both to study deeply the most suitable materials to mimic soft tissues and bones and to validate the realism of the interaction between physical models and surgical instrumentation.

Other aspects investigated by this review include the complexity of the medical scenario, the integration of methods for evaluating clinical performance, and the level of portability of the simulator. Despite the importance of the first two aspects on learning effectiveness, only a few studies have addressed these issues. Regarding portability (a significant factor in the widespread use of medical simulators in educational and training settings), the review shows that most simulators are simple to assemble/disassemble, and some can be easily transported.

Finally, concerning the evaluation of simulators, most articles conduct either a technical or a validity evaluation or, more rarely, both. However, a common limitation of the reviewed studies is the small number of participants (only five studies involved more than 20 subjects [22,30,34,40,43]) recruited to test simulator. More specifically, with regard to the validity assessment, the number of experts enrolled to validate simulators is often small (only two studies involved more than 10 experts [22,30]). Thus, although preliminary results are encouraging, further research is needed to validate existing AR, MR, and hybrid simulators for surgical training and to test whether improvements in performance on a simulated scenario translate into better performance on real patients.

At the time of the literature search, there was no systematic review covering the topic of simulation techniques based on AR, MR, and hybrid approaches in healthcare. Only one review in English [55] was found on augmented reality-based simulators in laparoscopic surgery. More specifically, the authors described five commercial AR simulators in terms of the features of simulators (modules and tested skills, recorded parameters, and feedback), an overview of measurements (need for observer and instructions), the assessment methods of performance, the most important aspects, shortcomings, validity, and costs of the simulators. However, our review provides a wider range of studies on medical simulation techniques not limited to AR but including also MR and hybrid approaches, providing a complete analysis of virtual and physical components of commercial and custom-made simulators and identifying current trends in the choice of simulation approaches.

Author Contributions: Conceptualization, M.G. and V.F.; methodology, R.M.V., S.C., G.T. and M.C.; investigation, R.M.V., S.C., G.T. and M.C.; data curation, R.M.V., S.C., G.T. and M.C.; writing—original draft preparation, R.M.V., S.C., G.T. and M.C.; writing—review and editing, G.T. and S.C.; supervision M.G. All authors have read and agreed to the published version of the manuscript.

Funding: This work was supported by the Italian Ministry of Education and Research (MIUR) in the framework of the CrossLab project (Departments of Excellence) of the University of Pisa, Laboratory of Augmented Reality.

Institutional Review Board Statement: Not applicable.

Informed Consent Statement: Not applicable.

Data Availability Statement: Not applicable.

Conflicts of Interest: The authors declare no conflict of interest.

References

1. Kerr, B.; O'Leary, J. The training of the surgeon: Dr. Halsted's greatest legacy. *Am. Surg.* **1999**, *65*, 1101–1102. [PubMed]
2. Scott, D.J.; Cendan, J.C.; Pugh, C.M.; Minter, R.M.; Dunnington, G.L.; Kozar, R.A. The changing face of surgical education: Simulation as the new paradigm. *J. Surg. Res.* **2008**, *147*, 189–193. [CrossRef]
3. Tan, S.S.Y.; Sarker, S.K. Simulation in surgery: A review. *Scott. Med. J.* **2011**, *56*, 104–109. [CrossRef]
4. Meier, A.H.; Rawn, C.L.; Krummel, T.M. Virtual reality: Surgical application–challenge for the new millennium. *J. Am. Coll. Surg.* **2001**, *192*, 372–384. [CrossRef]
5. Hutter, M.M.; Kellogg, K.C.; Ferguson, C.M.; Abbott, W.M.; Warshaw, A.L. The impact of the 80-hour resident workweek on surgical residents and attending surgeons. *Ann. Surg.* **2006**, *243*, 864–875. [CrossRef] [PubMed]
6. Sutherland, L.M.; Middleton, P.F.; Anthony, A.; Hamdorf, J.; Cregan, P.; Scott, D.; Maddern, G.J. Surgical simulation: A systematic review. *Ann. Surg.* **2006**, *243*, 291–300. [CrossRef]
7. The Southern Surgeons Club; Moore, M.J.; Bennett, C.L. The learning curve for laparoscopic cholecystectomy. *Am. J. Surg.* **1995**, *170*, 55–59. [CrossRef]
8. Scott, D.J. Patient Safety, Competency, and the Future of Surgical Simulation. *Simul. Healthc.* **2006**, *1*, 164–170. [CrossRef]
9. Stefanidis, D.; Sevdalis, N.; Paige, J.; Zevin, B.; Aggarwal, R.; Grantcharov, T.; Jones, D.B. Simulation in surgery: What's needed next? *Ann. Surg.* **2015**, *261*, 846–853. [CrossRef]
10. Vozenilek, J.; Huff, J.S.; Reznek, M.; Gordon, J.A. See One, Do One, Teach One: Advanced Technology in Medical Education. *Acad. Emerg. Med.* **2004**, *11*, 1149–1154. [CrossRef]
11. Bradley, P. The history of simulation in medical education and possible future directions. *Med. Educ.* **2006**, *40*, 254–262. [CrossRef] [PubMed]
12. Gaba, D.M. The future vision of simulation in healthcare. *Simul. Healthc.* **2007**, *2*, 126–135. [CrossRef] [PubMed]
13. Lateef, F. Simulation-based learning: Just like the real thing. *J. Emerg. Trauma. Shock.* **2010**, *3*, 348–352. [CrossRef]

14. Ziv, A.; Wolpe, P.R.; Small, S.D.; Glick, S. Simulation-based medical education: An ethical imperative. *Acad. Med.* **2003**, *78*, 783–788. [CrossRef] [PubMed]
15. Ziv, A.; Small, S.D.; Wolpe, P.R. Patient safety and simulation-based medical education. *Med. Teach.* **2000**, *22*, 489–495. [CrossRef] [PubMed]
16. de Visser, H.; Watson, M.O.; Salvado, O.; Passenger, J.D. Progress in virtual reality simulators for surgical training and certification. *Med. J. Aust.* **2011**, *194*, S38–S40. [CrossRef] [PubMed]
17. Gurusamy, K.; Aggarwal, R.; Palanivelu, L.; Davidson, B. Systematic review of randomized controlled trials on the effectiveness of virtual reality training for laparoscopic surgery. *Br. J. Surg.* **2008**, *95*, 1088–1097. [CrossRef]
18. Loukas, C. Surgical Simulation Training Systems: Box Trainers, Virtual Reality and Augmented Reality Simulators. *Int. J. Robot. Autom.* **2016**, *1*, 1–9. [CrossRef]
19. Badash, I.; Burtt, K.; Solorzano, C.A.; Carey, J.N. Innovations in surgery simulation: A review of past, current and future techniques. *Ann. Transl. Med.* **2016**, *4*, 453. [CrossRef]
20. Dunkin, B.; Adrales, G.L.; Apelgren, K.; Mellinger, J.D. Surgical simulation: A current review. *Surg. Endosc.* **2007**, *21*, 357–366. [CrossRef] [PubMed]
21. Moher, D.; Liberati, A.; Tetzlaff, J.; Altman, D.G.; The, P.G. Preferred Reporting Items for Systematic Reviews and Meta-Analyses: The PRISMA Statement. *PLoS Med.* **2009**, *6*, e1000097. [CrossRef] [PubMed]
22. Coelho, G.; Rabelo, N.N.; Vieira, E.; Mendes, K.; Zagatto, G.; Santos de Oliveira, R.; Raposo-Amaral, C.E.; Yoshida, M.; de Souza, M.R.; Fagundes, C.F.; et al. Augmented reality and physical hybrid model simulation for preoperative planning of metopic craniosynostosis surgery. *Neurosurg. Focus* **2020**, *48*, E19. [CrossRef]
23. Condino, S.; Turini, G.; Parchi, P.D.; Viglialoro, R.M.; Piolanti, N.; Gesi, M.; Ferrari, M.; Ferrari, V. How to Build a Patient-Specific Hybrid Simulator for Orthopaedic Open Surgery: Benefits and Limits of Mixed-Reality Using the Microsoft HoloLens. *J. Healthc. Eng.* **2018**, *2018*, 5435097. [CrossRef] [PubMed]
24. Condino, S.; Carbone, M.; Ferrari, V.; Faggioni, L.; Peri, A.; Ferrari, M.; Mosca, F. How to build patient-specific synthetic abdominal anatomies. An innovative approach from physical toward hybrid surgical simulators. *Int. J. Med. Robot. Comput. Assist. Surg.* **2011**, *7*, 202–213. [CrossRef]
25. Feifer, A.; Al-Ammari, A.; Kovac, E.; Delisle, J.; Carrier, S.; Anidjar, M. Randomized controlled trial of virtual reality and hybrid simulation for robotic surgical training. *BJU Int.* **2011**, *108*, 1652–1656, discussion 1657. [CrossRef] [PubMed]
26. Ferrari, V.; Viglialoro, R.M.; Nicoli, P.; Cutolo, F.; Condino, S.; Carbone, M.; Siesto, M.; Ferrari, M. Augmented reality visualization of deformable tubular structures for surgical simulation. *Int. J. Med. Robot.* **2016**, *12*, 231–240. [CrossRef]
27. Fuerst, D.; Hollensteiner, M.; Schrempf, A. A novel augmented reality simulator for minimally invasive spine surgery. In Proceedings of the 2014 Summer Simulation Multiconference, Monterey, CA, USA, 6–10 July 2014; p. 28.
28. Fushima, K.; Kobayashi, M. Mixed-reality simulation for orthognathic surgery. *Maxillofac. Plast Reconstr. Surg.* **2016**, *38*, 13. [CrossRef] [PubMed]
29. Halic, T.; Kockara, S.; Bayrak, C.; Rowe, R. Mixed reality simulation of rasping procedure in artificial cervical disc replacement (ACDR) surgery. *BMC Bioinform.* **2010**, *11* (Suppl. 6), S11. [CrossRef]
30. Huang, C.Y.; Thomas, J.B.; Alismail, A.; Cohen, A.; Almutairi, W.; Daher, N.S.; Terry, M.H.; Tan, L.D. The use of augmented reality glasses in central line simulation: "see one, simulate many, do one competently, and teach everyone". *Adv. Med. Educ. Pract.* **2018**, *9*, 357–363. [CrossRef]
31. Jain, S.; Lee, S.; Barber, S.R.; Chang, E.H.; Son, Y.-J. Virtual reality based hybrid simulation for functional endoscopic sinus surgery. *IISE Trans. Healthc. Syst. Eng.* **2020**, *10*, 127–141. [CrossRef]
32. Keebler, J.R.; Lazzara, E.H.; Patzer, B. Building a Simulated Medical Augmented Reality Training System. *Proc. Hum. Factors Ergon. Soc. Annu. Meet.* **2014**, *58*, 1169–1173. [CrossRef]
33. Lahanas, V.; Loukas, C.; Smailis, N.; Georgiou, E. A novel augmented reality simulator for skills assessment in minimal invasive surgery. *Surg. Endosc.* **2015**, *29*, 2224–2234. [CrossRef] [PubMed]
34. Lee, S.; Lee, J.; Lee, A.; Park, N.; Lee, S.; Song, S.; Seo, A.; Lee, H.; Kim, J.I.; Eom, K. Augmented reality intravenous injection simulator based 3D medical imaging for veterinary medicine. *Vet. J.* **2013**, *196*, 197–202. [CrossRef]
35. Lin, Y.-K.; Tsai, K.-L.; Yau, H.-T. The Development of Optical See-through Display Based on Augmented Reality for Oral Implant Surgery Simulation. *Comput. Aided Des. Appl.* **2012**, *9*, 111–120. [CrossRef]
36. Loukas, C.; Lahanas, V.; Georgiou, E. An integrated approach to endoscopic instrument tracking for augmented reality applications in surgical simulation training. *Int. J. Med. Robot.* **2013**, *9*, e34–e51. [CrossRef]
37. Nomura, T.; Mamada, Y.; Nakamura, Y.; Matsutani, T.; Hagiwara, N.; Fujita, I.; Mizuguchi, Y.; Fujikura, T.; Miyashita, M.; Uchida, E. Laparoscopic skill improvement after virtual reality simulator training in medical students as assessed by augmented reality simulator. *Asian J. Endosc. Surg.* **2015**, *8*, 408–412. [CrossRef]
38. Onishi, K.; Mizushino, K.; Ikemoto, H.; Noborio, H. AR Dental Surgical Simulator Using Haptic Feedback. In Proceedings of the International Conference on Human-Computer Interaction HCI 2013, Las Vegas, NV, USA, 21–26 July 2013; Springer: Berlin/Heidelberg, Germany, 2013; pp. 202–205.
39. Parkes, R.; Forrest, N.; Baillie, S. A mixed reality simulator for feline abdominal palpation training in veterinary medicine. *Stud. Health Technol. Inform.* **2009**, *142*, 244–246. [PubMed]

40. Yonghang, T.; Wei, L.; Zhou, H.; Peng, J.; Li, Q.; Li, F.; Zhang, J.; Shi, J. Augmented-reality-driven medical simulation platform for percutaneous nephrolithotomy with cybersecurity awareness. *Int. J. Distrib. Sens. Netw.* **2019**, *15*. [CrossRef]
41. Thomas, G.W.; Johns, B.D.; Kho, J.Y.; Anderson, D.D. The Validity and Reliability of a Hybrid Reality Simulator for Wire Navigation in Orthopedic Surgery. *IEEE Trans. Hum. Mach. Syst.* **2015**, *45*, 119–125. [CrossRef]
42. Tsujita, T.; Sase, K.; Chen, X.; Tomita, M.; Konno, A.; Nakayama, M.; Nakagawa, A.; Abe, K.; Uchiyama, M. Development of a Surgical Simulator for Training Retraction of Tissue with an Encountered-Type Haptic Interface Using MR Fluid. In Proceedings of the 2018 IEEE International Conference on Robotics and Biomimetics (ROBIO 2018), Kuala Lumpur, Malaysia, 12–15 December 2018; pp. 898–903.
43. van Duren, B.H.; Sugand, K.; Wescott, R.; Carrington, R.; Hart, A. Augmented reality fluoroscopy simulation of the guide-wire insertion in DHS surgery: A proof of concept study. *Med. Eng. Phys.* **2018**, *55*, 52–59. [CrossRef]
44. Viglialoro, R.M.; Esposito, N.; Condino, S.; Cutolo, F.; Guadagni, S.; Gesi, M.; Ferrari, M.; Ferrari, V. Augmented Reality to Improve Surgical Simulation: Lessons Learned Towards the Design of a Hybrid Laparoscopic Simulator for Cholecystectomy. *IEEE Trans. Biomed. Eng.* **2019**, *66*, 2091–2104. [CrossRef]
45. Lynch, A. Simulation-based acquisition of non-technical skills to improve patient safety. *Semin. Pediatric Surg.* **2020**, *29*, 150906. [CrossRef]
46. Agha, R.A.; Fowler, A.J.; Sevdalis, N. The role of non-technical skills in surgery. *Ann. Med. Surg.* **2015**, *4*, 422–427. [CrossRef]
47. Escobar-Castillejos, D.; Noguez, J.; Neri, L.; Magana, A.; Benes, B. A Review of Simulators with Haptic Devices for Medical Training. *J. Med. Syst.* **2016**, *40*, 104. [CrossRef] [PubMed]
48. Turini, G.; Condino, S.; Parchi, P.D.; Viglialoro, R.M.; Piolanti, N.; Gesi, M.; Ferrari, M.; Ferrari, V. A Microsoft HoloLens Mixed Reality Surgical Simulator for Patient-Specific Hip Arthroplasty Training. In Proceedings of the International Conference on Augmented Reality, Virtual Reality and Computer Graphics (AVR 2018), Otranto, Italy, 24–27 June 2018; Springer: Cham, Switzerland, 2018; pp. 201–210.
49. Ryu, W.H.A.; Dharampal, N.; Mostafa, A.E.; Sharlin, E.; Kopp, G.; Jacobs, W.B.; Hurlbert, R.J.; Chan, S.; Sutherland, G.R. Systematic Review of Patient-Specific Surgical Simulation: Toward Advancing Medical Education. *J. Surg. Educ.* **2017**, *74*, 1028–1038. [CrossRef]
50. Issenberg, B.; McGaghie, W.; Petrusa, E.; Gordon, D.; Scalese, R. Features and uses of high-fidelity medical simulations that lead to effective learning: A BEME systematic review. *Med. Teach.* **2005**, *27*, 10–28. [CrossRef] [PubMed]
51. Cox, M.; Irby, D.; Epstein, R. Assessment in Medical Education. *N. Engl. J. Med.* **2007**, *22*, 13–16.
52. Ryall, T.; Judd, B.K.; Gordon, C.J. Simulation-based assessments in health professional education: A systematic review. *J. Multidiscip. Healthc.* **2016**, *9*, 69–82. [PubMed]
53. Bewley, W.; Oneil, H. Evaluation of Medical Simulations. *Mil. Med.* **2013**, *178*, 64–75. [CrossRef]
54. Moglia, A.; Ferrari, V.; Morelli, L.; Ferrari, M.; Mosca, F.; Cuschieri, A. A Systematic Review of Virtual Reality Simulators for Robot-assisted Surgery. *Eur. Urol.* **2016**, *69*, 1065–1080. [CrossRef]
55. Botden, S.M.; Jakimowicz, J.J. What is going on in augmented reality simulation in laparoscopic surgery? *Surg. Endosc.* **2009**, *23*, 1693–1700. [CrossRef] [PubMed]

MDPI
St. Alban-Anlage 66
4052 Basel
Switzerland
Tel. +41 61 683 77 34
Fax +41 61 302 89 18
www.mdpi.com

Applied Sciences Editorial Office
E-mail: applsci@mdpi.com
www.mdpi.com/journal/applsci

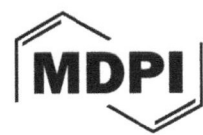

www.ingramcontent.com/pod-product-compliance
Lightning Source LLC
LaVergne TN
LVHW070657100526
838202LV00013B/983